D0753479

San Diego Christian College
2100 Greenfield Drive
El Cajon, CA 92019

Medical Adherence and Aging

Medical Adherence and Aging

SOCIAL AND COGNITIVE PERSPECTIVES

EDITED BY

Denise C. Park
Linda L. Liu

AMERICAN PSYCHOLOGICAL ASSOCIATION
WASHINGTON, DC

Published by
American Psychological Association
750 First Street, NE
Washington, DC 20002
www.apa.org

To order
APA Order Department
P.O. Box 92984
Washington, DC 20090-2984
Tel: (800) 374-2721
Direct: (202) 336-5510
Fax: (202) 336-5502
TDD/TTY: (202) 336-6123
Online: www.apa.org/books/
E-mail: order@apa.org

In the U.K., Europe, Africa, and the Middle East, copies may be ordered from
American Psychological Association
3 Henrietta Street
Covent Garden, London
WC2E 8LU England

Typeset in Goudy by World Composition Services, Inc., Sterling, VA

Printer: Maple–Vail Press, Binghamton, NY
Cover Designer: Berg Design, Albany, NY
Technical/Production Editor: Devon Bourexis

The opinions and statements published are the responsibility of the authors, and such opinions and statements do not necessarily represent the policies of the American Psychological Association.

Library of Congress Cataloging-in-Publication Data

Medical adherence and aging : social and cognitive perspectives / edited by Denise C. Park and Linda L. Liu.
    p. ; cm.
  Includes bibliographical references and index.
  ISBN-13: 978-1-59147-731-0
  ISBN-10: 1-59147-731-X
  1. Older people—Health and hygiene. 2. Patient compliance. 3. Medicine and psychology. I. Park, Denise C. II. Liu, Linda L. III. American Psychological Association.
  [DNLM: 1. Patient Compliance. 2. Aged. 3. Cognition. 4. Patient Compliance—psychology. W 85 M489 2007]

R727.43.M4322 2007
616—dc22

2006024262

British Library Cataloguing-in-Publication Data
A CIP record is available from the British Library.

Printed in the United States of America
First Edition

CONTENTS

CONTRIBUTORS

Scott C. Brown, University of Miami Miller School of Medicine, Miami, FL

Charlene Caburnay, St. Louis University, St. Louis, MO

Emily Chan, The Colorado College, Colorado Springs

Manfred Diehl, Colorado State University, Fort Collins

Gilles O. Einstein, Furman University, Greenville, SC

Arthur D. Fisk, Georgia Institute of Technology, Atlanta

Julie A. Garcia, University of Michigan, Ann Arbor

Peter M. Gollwitzer, New York University, New York, NY

Richard Gonzalez, University of Michigan, Ann Arbor

Matthew W. Kreuter, St. Louis University, St. Louis, MO

Elaine A. Leventhal, Robert Wood Johnson Medical School, New Brunswick, NJ

Howard Leventhal, Rutgers, The State University of New Jersey, New Brunswick

Linda L. Liu, University of Michigan, Ann Arbor

Mark A. McDaniel, Washington University, St Louis, MO

Anne Collins McLaughlin, Georgia Institute of Technology, Atlanta

Michelle L. Meade, University of Illinois at Urbana–Champaign

Gabriele Oettingen, New York University, New York, NY

Sheina Orbell, University of Essex, Colchester, England

Denise C. Park, University of Illinois at Urbana–Champaign

Joel Rodriguez, University of Michigan, Ann Arbor

Wendy A. Rogers, Georgia Institute of Technology, Atlanta

Angelenia Semegon, University of Florida, Gainesville

Pamela Whitten, Michigan State University, East Lansing

Ricardo Wray, St. Louis University, St. Louis, MO

Oscar Ybarra, University of Michigan, Ann Arbor

Lise M. Youngblade, Colorado State University, Fort Collins

PREFACE

As the projected life span of individuals increases, issues surrounding the health care of older adults have shifted from focusing on recuperation and rehabilitation toward goals of disease prevention and self-management of health concerns. In particular, older adults are expected to play a more active role in managing their own care and treatment, including setting and striving to achieve health improvement goals, coordinating their medical regimens, researching and making decisions about their treatment options, and integrating new technologies into their daily lives. All of these medical behaviors must be performed against a backdrop of age-related cognitive changes that may affect older patients' ability to comprehend and remember medical instructions.

This volume adopts a multidisciplinary approach toward issues that influence medical adherence and how patients follow medical instructions, with a focus on older adults. The goal is to provide a means for theoretical issues in cognitive and social psychology to inform and improve how medical instructions and treatment plans are presented to and understood by elderly patients. To this end, this book brings together behavioral scientists, some of whom are specialists in aging and others who are not, to discuss important issues at the intersection of social psychology, cognition, and medicine. It focuses on the theoretical frameworks proposed by leading cognitive and social psychologists as the basis for understanding how patients process medical and health information, adhere to their doctors' medical instructions, and use medical information technology.

The book is unique because it provides an opportunity for cognitive and social psychological perspectives to inform key issues in health care such as patient comprehension of and compliance with medical instruction. The chapters are presented by experts in the field of cognitive or social psychology, by researchers in aging, and by specialists in medicine and health care (many of the authors are experts in more than one of these areas).

The unifying theme of the book is the relevance and potential contributions of theories of cognitive and social psychology to facilitating older adults' ability to translate their doctors' instructions into appropriate behaviors in their daily lives. Part I, Theoretical Framework, lays the theoretical groundwork and provides an overview of basic cognitive psychological processes that are relevant to how patients understand and comply with their medical care instructions. These four chapters survey the work on cognitive processing, motivation, and prospective memory and serve as a backdrop for the remaining chapters. Part II, Understanding Doctors' Instructions, focuses on factors that influence the comprehension of medical information, such as patients' existing beliefs about their illnesses, the familiarity of the information presented, and the changes in susceptibility to deception that occur with age. Part III, Adherence to Treatment, addresses the issue of medical compliance and illustrates how cognitive and social psychological theories on motivation and decision making can inform the development of simple and practical strategies to improve patient compliance with medical directives. Part IV, Technology and Treatment, explores the role of technology in health care and discusses ways in which access to this technology can be improved for senior adults.

This book is the result of a conference sponsored by the Roybal Center for Aging and Cognition: Health, Education, and Training (sponsored by the National Institute on Aging [NIA]). We are grateful for the support of the NIA.

I
THEORETICAL
FRAMEWORKS

1

A BROAD VIEW OF MEDICAL ADHERENCE: INTEGRATING COGNITIVE, SOCIAL, AND CONTEXTUAL FACTORS

DENISE C. PARK AND MICHELLE L. MEADE

Put very simply, *medical adherence* refers to the probability that a patient will follow a doctor's health instructions. Most conceptual models as well as research on the topic of medical adherence have focused primarily on medication adherence, that is, the probability that a patient will take pills or other medications prescribed by a physician in the appropriate amounts and at the appropriate times. The topic of medical adherence is much broader and encompasses a range of medical behaviors, for example, (a) adhering to lifestyle recommendations made by a physician or other health care provider, such as dietary or activity changes; (b) using medical equipment, such as an oxygen tank, properly; (c) implementing recommended medical procedures, such as regularly changing a dressing or monitoring blood glucose; and (d) taking prescribed medications accurately. Virtually all successful health care outcomes require that the recipient of the services follow a set of instructions to ensure recovery from a surgery or management of a chronic illness. In many cases, services are provided to the patient by family members or friends, so there are many cases in which it is appropriate to think of adherence from a systems perspective and consider the psychosocial, cognitive, and contextual variables associated with caregiving to determine whether instructions will be followed. Despite the centrality of the medical adherence issue to successful outcomes, the focus of most health care research dollars is directed toward improving medical procedures, technologies, and drugs, with relatively little concern directed toward the variables that influence whether patients can or will successively complete treatment requirements. In this chapter (and indeed in the entire volume), variables that affect patients' adherence to medical instructions are examined in an effort to better understand how to positively impact adherence to treatment regimens.

It is useful to think of three important components that contribute to medical adherence behaviors, some of which have received relatively little attention. The first component involves psychosocial influences on adherence. Variables such as belief systems, motivational states, social networks, and relationship to physician or health care provider are explored under this rubric. Although much work remains to be done, this area has received more rather than less attention, particularly in the area of belief systems and cognitive models of adherence, exemplified by the large body of literature related to the self-regulatory model proposed by Leventhal and Cameron (1987; Cameron & Leventhal, 2003; see also chap. 4, this volume) as well as the health beliefs model (Becker, 1989; Rosenstock, 1990).

A second domain that has recently received more attention is the role of cognitive function in medication adherence, particularly as it relates to an aging population. Our lab has taken an active role in understanding this topic (e.g., Brown & Park, 2002; Morrell, Park, Kidder, & Martin, 1997; Park et al., 1999; Park, Willis, Morrow, Diehl, & Gaines, 1994; Shifren, Park, Bennett, & Morrell, 1999; Skurnik, Yoon, Park, & Schwarz, 2005), with some significant findings from our work being counterintuitive. For example, we have frequently reported that older adults are more adherent to pill regimens than are young adults, despite diminished cognitive capacity (Brown & Park, 2003; Morrell et al., 1997; Park et al., 1999). In this chapter, we discriminate between situations in which decreased cognition does affect adherence negatively and those in which declining cognition is relatively unimportant or is compensated for by more powerful variables.

This leads to the third domain—which remains relatively unexplored in the study of medical adherence—and that is the role that contextual variables play in whether patients adhere to treatment regimens. The environment in which an individual functions, the magnitude of the routines that govern individual behaviors, and the level of busyness or engagement that characterizes a person are all important predictors of adherence (Martin & Park, 2003; Park, 1996; Park et al., 1999). Moreover, as we describe in this chapter, one can capitalize on the predictability of an environment to enhance the prospect of medical adherence (Liu & Park, 2004).

In this chapter, we focus primarily on the role of cognitive and contextual factors in medical adherence, while integrating psychosocial variables and belief systems into our discussion whenever appropriate. We discuss initially the role that limited cognitive capacity may play in affecting medical adherence, and we distinguish between effortful and automatic processes as they relate to cognitive capacity and adherence. Then we make an important distinction between the early stages of adherence (comprehending and remembering medical instructions, protocols, or regimens) and later stages (actual implementation of medical instructions), as well as what variables influence these different stages of adherence. We conclude with promising future directions for research development to facilitate adherence to medical instructions.

DIMINISHED COGNITION AND MEDICAL ADHERENCE

It is important to recognize that the population of individuals who must follow medical instructions comprises many individuals with diminished cognition. Older adults consume a disproportionate amount of health care, and there is clear evidence that with age many cognitive functions, including speed of information processing, working memory capacity, and long-term memory, decline (Park et al., 2002). Additionally, many patients with psychiatric or neurologic disorders, as well as some HIV patients, show evidence of cognitive compromise, and patients in these diagnostic categories have high adherence requirements. Finally, patients who are ill (e.g., feverish) or in pain may also temporarily have less cognitive capacity available to them. Thus, the group of individuals who are cognitively compromised in some way and must follow medical instructions is a large one. For this reason, it makes sense to consider the implications of declining cognition for medical adherence. Although the implications would appear to be obvious— that with less cognitive capacity, individuals will have more trouble adhering—there is considerable research that suggests this is not always the case. It is important to recognize that both effortful and automatic processes are important in medication adherence and that decreases in cognition that occur with age or in other compromising conditions occur primarily in effortful but not automatic processes (Brown & Park, 2003). To the extent that adherence involves automatic processes, diminished cognition will not play an important role.

The term *effortful process* refers to cognition that involves activation of executive processes and deliberate efforts to encode, retrieve, inhibit, or manipulate information. Effortful processes have often been described as conceptually driven or top-down processes (e.g., Jacoby, 1983). Examples of effortful cognitive processes include learning a list of words and then later trying to recall it, or studying a set of medical instructions and consciously attempting to translate the instructions into a personal plan of action. There are marked, easily documented changes in cognitive function that occur in effortful processes with age (Park et al., 2002).

In contrast, *automatic processes* operate often without the individual's conscious awareness and require little engagement of executive function and deliberate processing of information. Automatic cognition is often described as data driven or bottom-up, reflecting the important role that external environmental cues play in determining information that automatically comes to consciousness without active encoding or retrieval effort. Examples of automatic processes include completing a three-letter word stem with a word that you just heard earlier, or after brushing your teeth in the morning, reaching for the bottle of pills on the bathroom counter that you take every morning as soon as you put down your toothbrush. There is some debate as to whether automatic processes may operate slightly less efficiently with age (La Voie & Light, 1994; Park & Shaw, 1992), but there is strong agreement that the deficits (if any) in automatic processes with age are much less pronounced than in effortful processes. Thus, when thinking about medical adherence processes, it is important to recognize that cognitively compromised populations will likely only show deficits in the facets of medical adherence that involve effortful processes, unless they are severely compromised, as might be the case in some very advanced stages of HIV and would always be the case for advanced cases of Alzheimer's disease.

THE EARLY STAGES OF MEDICAL ADHERENCE: COMPREHENDING AND REMEMBERING MEDICAL INSTRUCTIONS

Medical adherence is not a global behavior and has a number of component processes (Park, 1992). To take medication successfully or follow medical instructions appropriately, an individual must first be able to comprehend the instructions, then later remember the instructions or, at least, have the written instructions directly available at the time of implementation. Given that an individual successfully comprehends and remembers the instructions, he or she must then prospectively remember to perform or implement the instructed action. Much of the adherence literature focuses on remembering to take medications and relatively little addresses the issue of accurate comprehension and memory for what is to be done. We argue that it is this early phase—particularly comprehension of a regimen or instruction—that is most compromised by cognitive frailty and a domain to which much more attention needs to be directed, particularly in the area of medical equipment (see chap. 11, this volume).

We initially investigated the problem of comprehension by orally presenting young and old adults with a series of fictitious prescriptions, as if they were receiving instructions from a physician (Morrell, Park, & Poon, 1989). We found consistent evidence that older adults showed not only poorer memory for the instructions but also poorer comprehension than young adults of the materials. When young and older adults had the medication available to them in writing and could consult the information when developing a plan for when to take the medications, older adults consistently made more errors. Morrell et al. (1989) also reported that when given as much time as desired to study the medical information prior to a memory test, older adults still made more mistakes on a memory test compared with young adults. Of particular concern was that when participants had unlimited study time, younger adults chose to study the medication information significantly longer than did older adults before indicating they were ready to take the memory test. This finding illustrates that older adults may have metacognitive failures (not knowing that they do not know the medical regimen or procedure) that contribute to nonadherence.

In basic laboratory research, we have consistently reported that older adults have intact picture recognition memory (Park, Puglisi, & Smith, 1986; Park, Royal, Dudley, & Morrell, 1988), so in a later study, we redesigned medication labels to have a pictorial format (Morrell, Park, & Poon, 1990) and compared younger and older adults' memory for pictorial labels with their memory for well-organized verbal labels. An example of the pictorial labels appears in Figure 1.1. Morrell et al. (1990) found somewhat surprisingly that the pictorial labels did not facilitate memory in the older adults relative to the verbal labels, but they did facilitate memory in the young adults. It seemed that the novel format for the pictorial labels required more cognitive effort to use for the older adults than the more familiar verbal labels. Similar findings were reported by Morrow, Leirer, and Andrassy (1996), who showed older adults were better able to paraphrase medication schedules when the information was presented in text format than when presented with icons of clocks pictorially depicting the schedule. These findings highlight the importance of relying on familiar formats and procedures in interventions to improve adherence. Although it would be an oversimplification to suggest that new formats will not be successful, it is important to recognize that novelty likely introduces cognitive load for older adults, at least until a high degree of familiarity is achieved with the intervention.

One commonly available and frequently used intervention to assist in medication adherence is various medication organizers or medication containers that are sold over the counter. These devices typically have bins

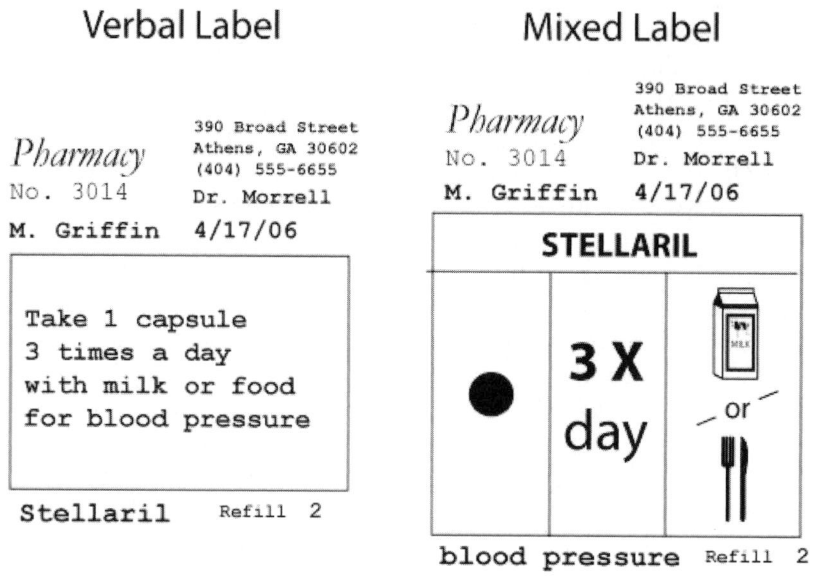

Verbal Label

Pharmacy
No. 3014

390 Broad Street
Athens, GA 30602
(404) 555-6655

Dr. Morrell

M. Griffin   4/17/06

Take 1 capsule
3 times a day
with milk or food
for blood pressure

Stellaril   Refill 2

Mixed Label

Pharmacy
No. 3014

390 Broad Street
Athens, GA 30602
(404) 555-6655

Dr. Morrell

M. Griffin   4/17/06

STELLARIL

● | **3 X day** | _or_

blood pressure   Refill 2

Figure 1.1. Examples of labels used in experiment. From "Effects of Labeling Techniques on Memory and Comprehension of Prescription Information in Young and Old Adults," by R. W. Morrell, D. C. Park, and L. W. Poon, 1990, *Journals of Gerontology: Psychological Sciences, 45*, p. P168. Copyright © The Gerontological Society of America. Reproduced by permission of the publisher.

or wells marked with days or times, or both. Consumers are to load the organizers with their medications, typically for a week, and then carry the organizer around with them. The organizers solve the problem of remembering whether a medication has been taken, because if it has not been, it will be obvious by looking at the date–time slot. At the same time, once the consumer takes medications out of the original prescriptions vials, all information about the medication, including name, quantity, and time to be taken, is lost. Hence, if the consumer loads the medication organizers incorrectly, this has the potential to be quite dangerous. To investigate the safety of these devices, we tested the ability of a group of patients with arthritis taking multiple medications to correctly load different types of organizers with their own medications (Park, Morrell, Frieske, Blackburn, & Birchmore, 1991). There are many different types of devices, but two of the most common are shown in Figure 1.2. The top organizer, referred to as a *7-day with times organizer* had a much lower rate of loading errors than the bottom one, referred to as a *7-day without times organizer*. The failure to load correctly the 7-day without times organizer is particularly disturbing because consumers lose all identity information about the medication—even what time of day it is to be taken, which likely further compounds the errors that occur after it is initially incorrectly loaded. In contrast, the 7-day with times

7-Day With Times Organizer

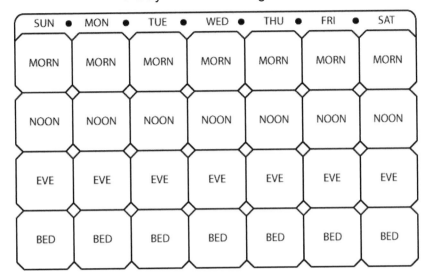

7-Day Without Times Organizer

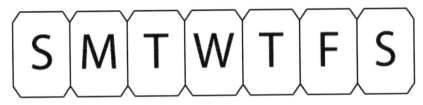

Figure 1.2. Schematic representation of the three types of organizers used in the study. From "Cognitive Factors and the Use of Over-the-Counter Medication Organizers by Arthritis Patients," by D. C. Park, R. W. Morrell, D. Frieske, B. Blackburn, and D. Birchmore, 1991, *Human Factors, 33,* p. 60. Copyright 1991 by the Human Factors and Ergonomics Society. Reprinted with permission.

organizer had quite a low error rate (about 5%); we believe that the organizer actually serves to structure consumers' cognition, and the act of loading it may actually enhance comprehension of a medication regimen. Nevertheless, these findings illustrate the potential risks associated with over-the-counter medication organizers, as well as the fact that generally they are designed to facilitate the act of implementation of a prescription regimen and that good comprehension of the regimen is essential if these organizers are to be loaded correctly.

In a subsequent effort to understand the role of enhancing comprehension of medical information on adherence, Park, Morrell, Frieske, and Kincaid (1992) studied adults ages 60 and over taking four or more medications and provided them with materials designed to enhance comprehension.

One group received a poster for their refrigerator developed by the experimenters that provided detailed information, day by day, hour by hour, on exactly which medications were to be taken at a given time. There was a check-off area on the poster, so that participants could mark when they took the medication. The poster relieved participants of any need to comprehend their regimen—they merely picked up the appropriately marked vial at the stated time. In short, participants continued to have a prospective memory task to adhere—remembering to take the medication—but the comprehension burden was considerably diminished. Another group received a 7-day with times organizer that the experimenter loaded with each participant's medications. This also relieved the comprehension burden of a regimen but still required prospective memory to take the medications. A third group received both types of cognitive supports, and the fourth group was a no-treatment control group that took their medications without any of the cognitive aids. Medication adherence was monitored for 1 month with sensitive barcode scanners, providing relatively accurate measures of adherence.

The results were initially surprising. A median split of participants into a young-old (ages 70 and younger) and old-old (ages 71 and greater) showed that adults in the young-old control group had a 94% adherence rate, and because adherence was already so high, the interventions did not improve adherence rates in this group. In contrast, the adults in the old-old group had a lower adherence rate (82%) and showed significantly greater levels of adherence when they received the two comprehension aids—a medication organizer and a medication refrigerator poster. This is an important set of findings, first, because it indicates that adherence rates in young-old adults are actually quite high and that this group is not at particularly high risk of nonadherence. Second, the findings suggest that very old adults are at risk of nonadherence and that the nonadherence is primarily due to comprehension difficulties in them, because providing older adults with the dual cognitive aids increased their adherence to 98%. It is important to recognize that this magnitude of adherence was obtained without any prospective reminders, suggesting that comprehension, not prospective remembering, is the biggest barrier to adherence in this population.

The work just described, because it focused on the role of medication organizers and specific medication instructions, provides relatively little insight into issues associated with following instructions about medical conditions and medical procedures. Individuals who are experiencing memory decline as a result of either age or medical condition will, of course, be at risk of having some difficulty remembering medical information or following medical instructions. Brown and Park (2002) reported that older adults had more difficulty than young adults in acquiring information presented to them about a disease. It is surprising that they were particularly resistant to acquiring new information about a familiar disease (e.g., breast cancer) compared with an unfamiliar one (e.g., acromegaly). It appears that patients may resist changing existing schemas about familiar diseases and are more open to learning novel information about a disorder for which they have no preconceived notions.

Individuals who are cognitively frail may also be prone to distortions of presented instructions. For example, Skurnik et al. (2005) demonstrated how the illusion of truth associated with familiar information can make false information seem true to older adults. There is a well-documented finding (called the *illusion of truth effect*) that demonstrates that familiar information, even if the individual understood it to be false at the time of acquisition, feels true later on because of its familiarity and the loss of context about a statement's truth value (Hasher, Goldstein, & Toppino, 1977). Because older adults rely more on familiarity to remember things than do young adults (Jacoby, 1999), they should be unusually susceptible to the illusion of truth. Skurnik et al. (2005) presented young and old adults with medical statements during acquisition, along with the truth value of each statement (e.g., true or false). Some statements were presented once and others three times. After 3 days, participants were presented with the old statements as well as some new statements, and they had to indicate whether the medical statements were new or were statements they had been told were true or false. Older adults were more certain that statements they had studied as false three times were true than statements they had studied as false only once! In contrast to older adults, younger adults did remember statements they were told were false three times were false but had a bias to remember items presented only once as true, as shown in Figure 1.3. In short, the more frequent statements felt familiar to the older adults, and familiar information feels true, so they were more likely to misremember medical information repeatedly presented to them as false. The younger adults, however, did remember the context and so had explicit memory for the false items as false when they were presented three times.

The basic message from Skurnik et al.'s (2005) study is that older adults will often remember medical instructions that they hear but forget the context in which they learned it. Thus, telling older adults, for example, "Some people think this medication is safe to take with food. That's not true." might be less effective than instructing them, "Never eat at the time you take this medication." They might forget the truth value of the former statement and remember only "medication is safe to take with food" and make a serious mistake. Presenting medical instructions and then negating them (as in "It's safe to smoke around your oxygen tank, right? Don't do it!") is a dangerous practice with older adults, as they may remember the initial false statement and not the disconfirming sentence that follows it.

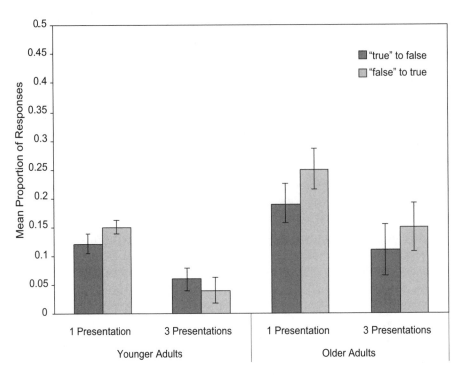

Figure 1.3. Memory for truth and falsity when truth value is disclosed on each presentation, by age and repetition. From "How Warnings About False Claims Become Recommendations," by I. Skurnik, C. Yoon, D. C. Park, and N. Schwarz, 2005, *Journal of Consumer Research, 31,* p. 717. Copyright 2005 by the University of Chicago Press. Reprinted with permission.

Once older adults come to believe an inaccurate health statement as true, it may be difficult for them to remember contradictory (yet accurate) information. Rice and Okun (1994) tested participants' memory for accurate statements about osteoarthritis. Participants were less likely to remember the accurate statements that contradicted their previous misconceptions than they were to remember accurate statements that were consistent with their previous beliefs. Follow-up research indicated that older adults were even less likely to remember disconfirming, accurate statements when the information was personally relevant to them because they had the disease (Okun & Rice, 2001). These findings suggest that once participants believe inaccurate information, they are resistant to changing it.

Another aspect that may play into tendencies to adhere is the wealth of information about medical conditions and treatments available through the media, particularly the ability to find detailed information about a particular illness or treatment on the Internet within a matter of seconds by initiating a simple search. Increasingly, the Internet is finding its way into the everyday lives of older adults, and the magnitude of this will only increase as the baby boomers age. There is even direct marketing of medical information to consumers, as well as tailoring of individual messages that are designed to be particularly motivating to individuals with a particular configuration of characteristics (see chap. 10, this volume). The potential for environmental influences via the Internet and media outlets affecting or biasing memory and comprehension of medical instructions is something that will play an ever greater role in following medical instructions and will be difficult to comprehend or control in understanding medical adherence, as environmental factors will vary considerably across individuals.

Another domain that will be important in affecting the comprehension–memory component of medication adherence is that of collaborative cognition. It is often the case that patients operate as dyads with another family member (e.g., spouses, elder parent with child, or caregiver with patient) when developing treatment adherence plans. In understanding the dynamics associated with comprehending a medical regimen or instructions, it may be important to treat patients as a dyadic unit and assess whether members of the dyad have sufficient information to adhere to a plan. Alternatively, it may be more important that a caregiver understand adherence plans than the patient, although sometimes the instructions may be delivered by the patient. It is important to recognize that the caregiver may be the same age, or even older, than the patient and that the existence of a caregiver does not necessarily mitigate problems with instructions. Understanding how to use dyads effectively to improve comprehension and memory of a medical regimen is an important direction for future research of medical adherence.

Another important issue with respect to comprehension of medical instructions is the clarity of the material actually presented to patients. In 1991, the Patient Self-Determination Act (1990; Omnibus Budget Reconciliation Act, 1990) became effective and required that hospital and nursing home patients be given information about legal rights regarding living wills and durable powers of attorney for health care. Park, Eaton, Larson, and Palmer (1994) surveyed hospital administrators regarding problems with implementing the law. The second most common problem cited was the inability of patients to comprehend the information that was presented, confirming the difficulty medical institutions have in presenting complex information in a format readily comprehended by patients. In a later study comparing nursing homes with hospitals, 74% of both nursing homes and hospitals cited "difficulty in conveying information to residents/patients" as a significant problem encountered in implementing the Patient Self-Determination Act, again suggesting that patients often receive information and materials that even those delivering the information suspect cannot be understood.

There is a substantial body of research on how to make both written text and spoken language more comprehensible to older adults. If fact, some researchers have focused specifically on the topic of increasing comprehensibility of medical instructions for older adults. Rice, Meyer, and Miller (1989) demonstrated that organization plays an important role in older adults' memory for medical information. Older adults remembered significantly more information from medical passages organized so that the most important information was presented at the highest level of content structure. Presentation format can also influence older adults' processing of medical information. Morrow, Leirer, and Altieri (1995) found that older adults' comprehension and subsequent memory for medical information are improved when the information is presented in a list format (rather than a paragraph format). Further, presenting medical information in a list format reduced age differences in comprehension, memory, and making inferences (Morrow, Leirer, Andrassy, Hier, & Menard, 1998). Repeating medical information also helps older adults better remember it (Morrow, Leirer, Carver, Tanke, & McNally, 1999b), and it is interesting to note that when given the option to repeat a medical message, both young and older adults often choose repetition, thereby improving their memory (Morrow, Leirer, Carver, Tanke, & McNally, 1999a). In her testimony to the U.S. Senate Special Committee on Aging given on June 2005, Denise Park reviewed an array of brochures designed to present information to older adults that were of limited clarity and proposed that congressional standards requiring design and review of government-produced materials for comprehensibility be implemented (*Consumer Fraud and the Aging Mind*, 2005).

LATER STAGES OF MEDICAL ADHERENCE: IMPLEMENTING MEDICAL INSTRUCTIONS

We now turn to a discussion of the act of implementing medical instructions, once comprehended. The act of remembering to perform a medical instruction is often called a *prospective memory task* (see chap. 3, this volume), that is, remembering to perform a planned action. The data presented earlier in this chapter suggested that when electronic monitors were used, older adults had a relatively high rate of adherence (Morrell et al., 1997; Park et al., 1992). However, in these studies, participants were required to carry a wallet with a small bar-code scanner in it and to scan the appropriate code each time they took a medication, thus recording the date and time. Carrying around the bar-code scanner and wallet made the act of remembering to take medications relatively salient, and the wallet could have served as a memory cue.

In a later study, Park et al. (1999) attempted to get a more naturalistic measure of medication adherence by using the Medication Event Monitoring System (MEMS). With this system, participants received new lids for their medication bottles that had a microchip embedded in them. Each time they opened the bottle to take a medication, the date and time were recorded. The use of the MEMS system provided a relatively unobtrusive way to monitor medication adherence. Park et al. recruited 122 patients with rheumatoid arthritis ranging in age from 34 to 84 and collected detailed psychosocial, cognitive, and health status information from the patients, and even collected measures of disease severity from patients' physicians. Patients were all taking a large number of medications, and all of their medications were outfitted with the MEMS system. Patients left the laboratory and medication events were monitored for 4 weeks, providing detailed information about medication behaviors. The extensive battery collected provided a plethora of individual differences measures. Structural equation modeling was used on these individual differences measures to determine the causal factors associated with nonadherence.

The results were somewhat surprising. As in the earlier studies (Morrell et al., 1997; Park et al., 1992), younger adults were less adherent than older adults (see Hinkin et al., 2004, for similar conclusions regarding young and older adults' adherence to AIDS medications). Given this finding, it is not surprising that higher cognitive function was not the best predictor of adherence. Nor did beliefs about illness, depression, anxiety, or disease severity prove to be strong predictors of adherence. Rather, the best predictor of adherence was how busy and routine patients reported their lives to be using the Martin and Park (2003) Busyness Questionnaire. The busier and less routine patients' lives were, the more likely they were to be nonadherent. Because middle-aged adults reported leading the busiest lives, they also tended to be the most nonadherent. Thus, not only did the finding from earlier studies replicate, but the mechanism underlying the apparent superiority of older adults for this phase of adherence was isolated.

Both the constructs of busyness and routinization are important in understanding why older adults have such high adherence rates. A low level of busyness provides older adults with sufficient unstructured time to monitor the activities they need to perform for the day. Busy middle-aged individuals who are multitasking are less likely to have the time available to monitor future obligations, and thus are more likely to miss the appropriate time window when they must perform a prospective task. Additionally, however, we believe that a high level of routinization in one's life (which also was more characteristic of older adults) operates to automatize prospective behaviors that must be performed on a regular basis (Brown & Park, 2003). If an individual is required to take their medication every morning with food and he or she leads a routine life, it is likely that the individual will eat breakfast at a regular time (and often even eat the same thing for breakfast). As an example, perhaps one might place one's medication on the kitchen table and take it each morning after drinking orange juice. After a few days of remembering to take one's medications after the orange juice, there will be a tendency to spontaneously or automatically reach for the medication after taking the orange juice without conscious thought that it is time for medication, much as one might spontaneously reach for a toothbrush upon entering the bathroom in the morning. After a few days of remembering, the orange juice automatically cues reaching for the medication bottle. This seems like a particularly plausible basis for the good adherence behavior of older adults given the high scores they achieve on levels of routinization (Martin & Park, 2003) combined with the high levels of adherence they evidence.

Brown and Park (2003) argued that adherence to medications and medical procedures might be improved by exploiting the component of memory and cognition that remains relatively unchanged with age—automatic processes. Thus, Liu and Park (2004) attempted to engage automatic processes to enhance medical adherence in a sample of older adults, relying on a technique used by Brandstätter, Lengfelder, and Gollwitzer (2001; see also chap. 2, this volume). Brandstätter et al. reported that young adults who were required to imagine the specific steps involved in implementing a desired behavior were more likely to complete the imagined behavior in the future than a control group. They suggested that forming detailed implementation plans enhanced goal achievement through the engagement of automatic processes and a tendency to act when they later encountered some of the cues they imagined. Chasteen, Park, and Schwarz (2001) demonstrated that the development of such implementation intentions was effective for improving older adults' performance of a simple prospective memory task in the laboratory. On the basis of these findings, Liu and Park (2004) hypothesized that implementation intentions would facilitate the performance of a more complex health adherence behavior by older adults outside of the laboratory. They trained older adults who had never used a glucose monitor and had no history of diabetes to use a glucose monitor to record the date and time the glucose was measured. Then, the adults were divided into one of three groups. The implementation group imagined exactly what they would be doing the next day at four different times when they were to draw blood from their finger with a lance and test it with the glucose monitor. A rehearsal group repeated the instructions multiple times across a rehearsal interval, and a third group wrote the pros and cons of testing their blood glucose. Then, participants left the laboratory and were instructed to use the blood glucose monitor at the same appointed times everyday for 3 weeks.

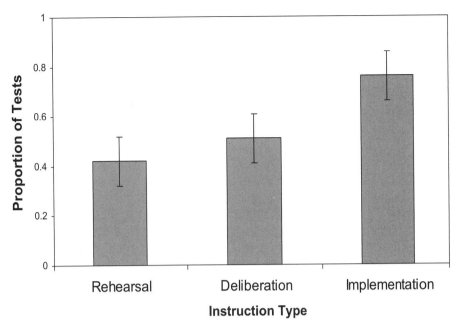

Figure 1.4. Average proportion of blood glucose tests performed correctly as a function of instruction type received. Error bars represent ±1 *SE* of the mean. Prop. = proportion. From "Aging and Medical Adherence: The Use of Automatic Processes to Achieve Effortful Things," by L. L. Liu and D. C. Park, 2004, *Psychology and Aging, 19,* p. 321. Copyright 2004 by the American Psychological Association.

Results are shown in Figure 1.4 and indicate that the implementation instructions were superior in maintaining adherence to the glucose monitoring regimen over the other two rehearsal conditions. Of particular interest is the finding that the behavior continued to increase over the 3-week period—a truly remarkable finding given that participants engaged in only one 5-minute session before the 1st day. The improvement in the latter part of the time period speaks to the automatization of the behavior through routine. Once participants began performing the behavior (as a result of the implementation instructions), they began to integrate it into their daily routine such that the performance of the behavior each day served to increase the probability that it would be performed on subsequent days as a result of the increased likelihood that more environmental cues would be encountered that were associated with the behavior and enhance adherence. The finding that a simple 5-minute practice session enhanced and maintained adherence over a 3-week period speaks to the importance of automatic processes in controlling adherence behavior as well as the ability to harness such processes in older adults to maintain adherence behaviors.

DIRECTIONS FOR THE FUTURE

There is much innovative research that remains to be done on the topic of medical adherence, particularly in the interaction of cognitive processes with environmental cues and demands. The data we have presented suggest that the most problematic aspect of following medical directions in cognitively frail populations has to do with comprehension and memory of instructions rather than in actually remembering to perform the adherence task. Moreover, the data suggest that it is likely easier to improve the implementation component of medical adherence even further in older adults by exploiting the component of memory that remains intact with advanced age or decreasing cognitive function—automatic processes. The challenge to researchers is to understand how to structure information and instructions so that they will be effective. Although much is known about typeface, luminance, and other variables affecting visual perception and aging, considerably less is known about the most effective medium for presenting medical instructions, how effective video training tapes might be for the use of complex equipment, and what role the Internet and other media might play in affecting interpretation and retention of medical information and instructions. It is likely that the move to decreased hospitalization will continue over time, with increased caregiving by relatives or unskilled adults. It is critically important that a better understanding be achieved of how to present medical information so that it can be comprehended and remembered, and also what social contexts and motivational states maximally facilitate adherence in cognitively frail adults. It is not always the case that cognition is the limiting factor in adherence, even in cognitively compromised adults. As this chapter illustrates, sometimes context plays a more important role than cognition. Understanding the role of these variables individually is important, but a full understanding of adherence will be achieved only when naturalistic studies are done that examine the behavior and variables that affect it in complex settings and integrate social, contextual, and cognitive perspectives.

REFERENCES

Becker, L. A. (1989). Family systems and compliance with medical regiments. In C. N. Ramsey Jr. (Ed.), *Family systems in medicine* (pp. 416–431). New York: Guilford Press.

Brandstätter, V., Lengfelder, A., & Gollwitzer, P. M. (2001). Implementation intentions and efficient action initiation. *Journal of Personality and Social Psychology, 81,* 946–960.

Brown, S. C., & Park, D. C. (2002). Roles of age and familiarity in learning of health information. *Educational Gerontology, 28,* 695–710.

Brown, S. C., & Park, D. C. (2003). Theoretical models of cognitive aging and implications for translational research in medicine. *The Gerontologist, 43,* 57–67.

Cameron, L. D., & Leventhal, H. (2003). Self-regulation, health, and illness: An overview. In L. D. Cameron & H. Leventhal (Eds.), *The self-regulation of health and illness behavior* (pp. 1–13). New York: Routledge.

Chasteen, A. L., Park, D. C., & Schwarz, N. (2001). Implementation intentions and facilitation of prospective memory. *Psychological Sciences, 6,* 457–461.

Consumer Fraud and the Aging Mind, 109th Cong., 59 (2005) (testimony of Denise C. Park).

Hasher, L., Goldstein, D., & Toppino, T. (1977). Frequency and the conference of referential validity. *Journal of Verbal Learning and Verbal Behavior, 16,* 107–112.

Hinkin, C. H., Hardy, D. J., Mason, K. I., Castellon, S. A., Durvasula, R. S., Lam, M. N., & Stefaniak, M. (2004). Medication adherence in HIV-infected adults: Effect of patient age, cognitive status, and substance abuse. *AIDS, 18,* 19–25.

Jacoby, L. L. (1983). Remembering the data: Analyzing interactive processes in reading. *Journal of Verbal Learning and Verbal Behavior, 22,* 485–508.

Jacoby, L. L. (1999). Ironic effects of repetition: Measuring age-related differences in memory. *Journal of Experimental Psychology: Learning, Memory, and Cognition, 25,* 3–22.

La Voie, D., & Light, L. L. (1994). Adult age differences in repetition priming: A meta-analysis. *Psychology and Aging, 9,* 539–553.

Leventhal, H., & Cameron, L. (1987). Behavioral theories and the problem of compliance. *Patient Education and Counseling, 10,* 117–138.

Liu, L. L., & Park, D. C. (2004). Aging and medical adherence: The use of automatic processes to achieve effortful things. *Psychology and Aging, 19,* 318–325.

Martin, M., & Park, D. C. (2003). The Martin and Park Environmental Demands (MPED) Questionnaire: Psychometric properties of a brief instrument. *Aging: Clinical and Experimental Research, 15,* 77–82.

Morrell, R. W., Park, D. C., Kidder, D. P., & Martin, M. (1997). Adherence to anti-hypertensive medications across the life span. *The Gerontologist, 37,* 609–619.

Morrell, R. W., Park, D. C., & Poon, L. W. (1989). Quality of instructions on prescription drug labels: Effects on memory and comprehension in young and old adults. *The Gerontologist, 29,* 345–353.

Morrell, R. W., Park, D. C., & Poon, L. W. (1990). Effects of labeling techniques on memory and comprehension of prescription information in young and old adults. *Journal of Gerontology, 45,* P166–P172.

Morrow, D. G., Leirer, V. O., & Altieri, P. (1995). List formats improve medication instructions for older adults. *Educational Gerontology, 21,* 151–166.

Morrow, D. G., Leirer, V. O., & Andrassy, J. M. (1996). Using icons to convey medication schedule information. *Applied Ergonomics, 27,* 267–275.

Morrow, D. G., Leirer, V. O., Andrassy, J. M., Hier, C. M., & Menard, W. E. (1998). The influence of list format and category headers on age differences in understanding medication instructions. *Experimental Aging Research, 24,* 231–256.

Morrow, D. G., Leirer, V. O., Carver, L. M., Tanke, E. D., & McNally, A. D. (1999a). Effects of aging, message repetition, and note-taking on memory for health information. *Journals of Gerontology Series B: Psychological Sciences and Social Sciences, 54B,* P369–P379.

Morrow, D. G., Leirer, V. O., Carver, L. M., Tanke, E. D., & McNally, A. D. (1999b). Repetition improves older and younger adult memory for automated appointment messages. *Human Factors, 41,* 194–206.

Okun, M. A., & Rice, G. E. (2001). The effects of personal relevance of topic and information type on older adults' accurate recall of written medical passages about osteoarthritis. *Journal of Aging and Health, 13,* 410–429.

Ominibus Budget Reconciliation Act of 1990, Pub. L. No. 101-508, 4206 and 4751, codified at 42 U.S.C. 1395cc(a) (1) (Q), 1395 mm (c) (8), 1395cc (f), 1396(a) (57), (58), 1396a (w) (1990).

Park, D. C. (1992). Applied cognitive aging research. In F. I. M. Craik & T. A. Salthouse (Eds.), *Handbook of cognition and aging* (pp. 449–493). Mahwah, NJ: Erlbaum.

Park, D. C. (1996). Aging, health, and behavior: The interplay between basic and applied science. In R. J. Resnick & R. H. Rozensky (Eds.), *Health psychology through the lifespan: Practice and research opportunities* (pp. 59–75). Washington, DC: American Psychological Association.

Park, D. C., Eaton, T. A., Larson, E. J., & Palmer, H. T. (1994). Implementation and impact of the Patient Self-Determination Act. *Southern Medical Journal, 87,* 971–977.

Park, D. C., Hertzog, C., Leventhal, H., Morrell, R. W., Leventhal, E., Birchmore, D., et al. (1999). Medication adherence in rheumatoid arthritis patients: Older is wiser. *Journal of American Geriatrics Society, 47,* 172–183.

Park, D. C., Lautenschlager, G., Hedden, T., Davidson, N., Smith, A. D., & Smith, P. (2002). Models of visuospatial and verbal memory across the adult life span. *Psychology and Aging, 17,* 299–320.

Park, D. C., Morrell, R. W., Frieske, D., Blackburn, B., & Birchmore, D. (1991). Cognitive factors and the use of over-the-counter medication organizers by arthritis patients. *Human Factors, 33,* 57–67.

Park, D. C., Morrell, R. W., Frieske, D., & Kincaid, D. (1992). Medication adherence behaviors in older adults: Effects of external cognitive supports. *Psychology and Aging, 7,* 252–256.

Park, D. C., Puglisi, J. T., & Smith, A. D. (1986). Memory for pictures: Does an age-related decline exist? *Psychology and Aging, 1,* 11–17.

Park, D. C., Royal, D., Dudley, W., & Morrell, R. (1988). Forgetting of pictures over a long retention interval in old and young adults. *Psychology and Aging, 3,* 94–95.

Park, D. C., & Shaw, R. (1992). Effect of environmental support on implicit and explicit memory in young and old adults. *Psychology and Aging, 7,* 632–642.

Park, D. C., Willis, S. L., Morrow, D., Diehl, M., & Gaines, C. L. (1994). Cognitive function and medication usage in older adults. *Journal of Applied Gerontology, 13,* 39–57.

Patient Self-Determination Act, Pub. L. No. 101-508, 104 Stat. 1388 (1990) (codified as amended at 42 U.S.C. §§ 1395cc(a) (1) (Q), 1395cc(f) (2000)).

Rice, G. E., Meyer, B. J., & Miller, D. C. (1989). Using text structure to improve older adults' recall of important medical information. *Educational Gerontology, 15,* 527–542.

Rice, G. E., & Okun, M. A. (1994). Older readers' processing of information that contradicts their beliefs. *Journal of Gerontology, 49,* 119–128.

Rosenstock, I. M. (1990). The health belief model: Explaining health behavior through expectancies. In K. Glanz, F. M. Lewis, & B. K. Reiner (Eds.), *Health behavior and health education* (pp. 39–62). San Francisco: Jossey-Bass.

Shifren, K., Park, D. C., Bennett, J. M., & Morrell, R. W. (1999). Do cognitive processes predict mental health in individuals with rheumatoid arthritis? *Journal of Behavioral Medicine, 22,* 529–547.

Skurnik, I., Yoon, C., Park, D. C., & Schwarz, N. (2005). How warnings about false claims become recommendations. *Journal of Consumer Research, 31,* 713–724.

2

THE ROLE OF GOAL SETTING AND GOAL STRIVING IN MEDICAL ADHERENCE

PETER M. GOLLWITZER AND GABRIELE OETTINGEN

From a motivational–volitional perspective, a first prerequisite for medical adherence is that people walk away from a health care provider (or from medical instructions obtained elsewhere) with a strong intention (goal) to act on the advice or instructions given. Second, and equally important, people need to effectively translate their goals into action, not only right after the advice has been given but also weeks and months thereafter. What facilitates the setting of adherence goals, and what guarantees acting on them? In this chapter we try to answer both of these questions, starting with the issue of goal setting and continuing with the problem of goal implementation. More specifically, we outline self-regulatory strategies that help people set adherence goals and attain them.

Determinants of Goal Setting

Goal pursuit starts with setting goals for oneself or adopting goals assigned by others. Most theories of motivation (Ajzen, 1991; Atkinson, 1957; Bandura, 1997; Brehm & Self, 1989; Carver & Scheier, 1998; Gollwitzer, 1990; Locke & Latham, 1990; Vroom, 1964) suggest that people prefer to choose and adopt goals that are desirable and feasible. Desirability is determined by the estimated attractiveness of likely short-term and long-term consequences of goal attainment. Such consequences may pertain to anticipated self-evaluations, evaluations of significant others, progress toward some higher order goal, external rewards of having attained the goal, and the joy–pain associated with moving toward the goal (Heckhausen, 1977).

In the medical setting, perceived desirability of following doctors' or other health care providers' instructions has been discussed as pertaining to the personal value of health, the perceived personal vulnerability, the perceived severity of the experienced illness, the perceived benefits of the regimen, the costs of following the regimen, and so forth (Hochbaum, 1958; Rosenstock, 1974). Perceived desirability may also relate to people's beliefs about whether they should adhere to the suggested medical instructions (Ajzen & Fishbein, 1980). Finally, as Brownlee, Leventhal, and Leventhal (2000) pointed out, the weight of the various health-related beliefs in determining the desirability of following a given medical instruction is influenced by how a person mentally represents the illness, how the suggested regimen fits a person's self-concept, and how the physician or health care provider manages to communicate the information relevant to the various desirability-related beliefs. The effectiveness of communication in turn depends not only on how patients and providers relate to each other (e.g., trust) but also on features of the provided message (e.g., verbal instructions only vs. verbal instructions mixed with pictorial representations; Morrell, Park, & Poon, 1990).

Feasibility of a goal depends on people's judgments of their capabilities to perform relevant goal-directed behaviors (i.e., self-efficacy expectations; Bandura, 1997), their beliefs that these goal-directed behaviors will lead to the desired outcome (i.e., outcome expectations, Bandura, 1997; instrumentality beliefs, Vroom, 1964), the judged likelihood of attaining the desired outcome (i.e., general expectations; Oettingen, 1996), or desired outcomes in general (i.e., optimism; Scheier & Carver, 1987). These various feasibility-related beliefs are informed by a person's experiences in the past (e.g., by one's own performance, by observing performances of similar others, or by persuasion of respected others; Bandura, 1997).

Thus, in the medical setting perceived feasibility of a medical instruction should be codetermined by the perceived usefulness of the behavior and the experienced confidence in one's ability to perform the required behavior (Rogers, 1983), which in turn are based on one's past experiences. Again, the strength of these beliefs should be moderated by the person's illness representations, his or her self-concept, and the quality of patient–provider communication.

Goal theories (summaries by Gollwitzer & Moskowitz, 1996; Oettingen & Gollwitzer, 2001) implicitly assume that high perceived feasibility and desirability will assure that people set strong goals (i.e., form strong goal commitments). However, research exploring the psychological processes on which goal setting is based indicated that the way people approach the task of setting a goal makes a difference. For example, whether the goal-setting determinant of feasibility will take effect depends on the mode of self-regulatory thought with which the task of setting a goal is approached (Oettingen, 1996, 1999).

Self-Regulation of Goal Setting

Oettingen (1999) suggested that feasibility beliefs are considered in goal setting only when people experience a necessity to act. In other words, high expectations lead to setting binding goals when people face the question of whether they should try to reach a desired outcome. In a series of experiments (Oettingen, Pak, & Schnetter, 2001), it has been demonstrated that a necessity to act readily emerges when people first mentally elaborate the desired future but then switch to mentally elaborating the negative reality that stands in the way of realizing the desired future. Such mental contrasting of the desired future with impeding reality makes people think of whether they have a chance to close the gap between future and reality by overcoming present obstacles. If feasibility-related beliefs are high, such mental contrasting leads to strong goal commitments; if they are low, no respective goals are formed.

In a typical study (Oettingen et al., 2001, Study 4), male freshmen enrolled in vocational schools first judged the probability of improving in mathematics, the most important subject in their 1st year of study. Participants then generated positive aspects of improving in mathematics (e.g., pride, career prospects) and negative aspects of impeding reality (e.g., being distracted, being disinterested). They then were divided into three groups to form mental elaborations of these aspects. In the positive fantasy/negative reality contrast group, participants mentally elaborated positive aspects of improving in math and negative aspects of reality standing in its way, in alternating order, beginning with a positive aspect. In the positive fantasy or indulging group, participants mentally elaborated only the positive aspects of improving in math; in the negative reality or dwelling group, participants mentally elaborated only the negative aspects of impeding reality. When participants' commitment toward the goal of improving in mathematics was assessed (in terms of effort in class and course grades as rated by the teacher), strength of goal commitment was in line with perceived feasibility in the mental contrast group but not in the indulging and dwelling groups. No matter whether perceived feasibility was low or high, goal commitment was at a medium level in the latter two groups. Apparently, mental contrasting makes people set binding goals for themselves if expectations of success are high but refrain from setting binding goals if expectations of success are low. Indulging and dwelling, however, cause people to be weakly pulled by the positive future or pushed by the negative reality, respectively, independent of expectations.

A series of further experiments using fantasy themes of different life domains replicated this pattern of results (Oettingen, 2000, Study 2; Oettingen, Hönig, & Gollwitzer, 2000; Oettingen et al., 2001, Studies 1–4). For instance, in young adults, mental contrasting has been found to create expectancy-dependent goals to solve interpersonal conflicts, to get to know an attractive person, to combine work and family life, and to study abroad, whereas indulging and dwelling failed to do so. In school settings, mental contrasting facilitated the expectancy-dependent setting of goals to excel in learning a foreign language. In all of these studies, cognitive, affective, and behavioral aspects of goal commitment were measured by means of self-report or observations by independent raters. Mental contrasting created expectancy-dependent goal commitments, irrespective of whether the desired future was self-set or assigned, and related to short-term or long-term projects (up to 6 months). Moreover, mental contrasting turned out to be an easy-to-apply self-regulatory strategy, as described effects were obtained even when participants elaborated the desired future and current impeding reality only very briefly (i.e., were asked to imagine only one positive aspect of the desired future and just one respective obstacle; Oettingen et al., 2000, Study 1). In all of these studies, indulging in a positive future or dwelling on the negative reality created goal commitments of only medium strength that were independent of perceived feasibility.

Mental Contrasting Changes Health Behavior

Mental contrasting has also succeeded in creating strong health-promoting goals, for example, the goal of reducing cigarette consumption in college students who smoke (Oettingen, Mayer, & Thorpe, 2006). To measure expectations, research participants were first asked to indicate how likely it is that they will reduce their cigarette consumption. Thereafter, they listed positive aspects of a future of reduced smoking (e.g., pretty skin, increased physical fitness, heightened self-respect) and aspects of present reality that stand in the way of attaining such a positive future (e.g., peer pressure, parties, stress). Like in the study on improving in mathematics, participants in the mental contrast group had to alternate in their mental elaborations between two positive aspects of a future with less smoking and two negative aspects of impeding reality. In the positive future-only control group, participants had to only mentally elaborate four positive aspects of the future, and in the negative reality control group, participants had to only mentally elaborate four negative aspects of impeding reality.

After participants had completed these different types of mental elaboration, they were handed a diary containing an hourly calendar for the next 14 days in which they were requested to record each cigarette smoked. Contrasting participants with high expectations smoked less than 7 cigarettes per day, whereas comparable high expectations control participants (those who elaborated only the future or elaborated only the negative reality) smoked more than 10 cigarettes per day. This finding implies that in light of high expectations of success, mental contrasting is a very useful self-regulatory tool to set strong goals. Physicians or health care providers who opt to maximize medical adherence (e.g., to eat low-fat foods) in their patients should therefore try to follow a two-step strategy. First, they should attempt to enhance feasibility-related beliefs by strengthening their relevant determinants (e.g., pointing to successful past performances or to successful performances of similar others, providing easy-to-process and useful information on how to successfully select low-fat food). Second, to make such feasibility-focused interventions behaviorally relevant, physicians should ask their patients to mentally contrast positive aspects of a desired future (e.g., slim and healthy body, looking nice and feeling well) with present impeding reality (e.g., old habits of eating foods high in fat, loving tasty foods, higher costs of low-fat foods), so that present reality is experienced as an obstacle to the desired future, thus creating a necessity to act. It is not enough to put participants' minds on positive consequences of adherence only or solely on obstacles of present reality. The latter two strategies instill goal commitment of just moderate strength by a pull or push mechanism, respectively. They do not capitalize on the induction of high expectations of success.

Mental Contrasting Changes Patient–Provider Communication

The importance of mental contrasting in medical contexts has also been demonstrated in a study geared at setting goals to improve the quality of patient–provider communication (Oettingen, Hagenah, et al., 2006, Study 1). More specifically, pediatric nurses had to indicate their expectations that they would be able to improve the way they interacted with their patients' relatives. In the contrast group, the nurses alternated in their mental elaborations between positive aspects of a future in which they improved the relationships with the relatives (e.g., contentment, affection, evenness of temper) and negative aspects of reality that impeded such a future (e.g., lack of time, too many patients, lack of patience). In the positive fantasy group, the nurses mentally elaborated only positive aspects of improved communication, and in the negative reality group, they elaborated only negative aspects of impeding reality. Two weeks later, all participating nurses were asked how hard they had tried to improve their relations with patients' relatives and to indicate their interest in participating in a workshop on improving communication with patients' relatives. Again, high-expectancy participants in the mental contrast group showed the strongest commitment to improve communication with patients' relatives. They reported having tried harder, and they were more interested in participating in the workshop than were participants in the control groups (the elaboration of the future-only and the reality-only groups).

Mental Contrasting and Efficiency in Health Service Managers

In an intervention study, personnel managers of four different large hospitals (Oettingen, Hagenah, et al., 2006, Study 5) were trained in using the self-regulatory strategy of mental contrasting and were asked to apply it to their pressing everyday problems. A control group was trained in using and applying the strategy of thinking only about positive aspects of having solved such problems. Two weeks later, all of the participants were asked how successful they were over the last 2 weeks in organizing their time, making decisions, completing overdue projects, and relinquishing futile projects. Participants in the mental contrast group reported having organized their time better, having made decisions with greater ease, having completed more overdue projects, and having relinquished more futile projects as compared with participants in the positive future-only control group. These findings suggest that mental contrasting of everyday problems forces managers in the health care domain to take a more decisive stand with respect to approaching and solving their daily tasks. The present study also indicates that the self-regulatory strategy of mental contrasting can be easily learned and successfully applied to all kinds of everyday problems, not just the ones that were used to acquire the technique.

Summary

The determinants of goal setting (high perceived feasibility and desirability) do not necessarily guarantee that people will commit themselves strongly to attaining a positive future (e.g., reducing cigarette consumption, obtaining physical fitness). It takes the application of the self-regulatory tool of mental contrasting (i.e., juxtaposing the positive future with relevant hindrances and obstacles posed by present reality) to make people act on their high expectations of success (feasibility). But the presented research suggests that mental contrasting not only benefits patients in setting strong health-promoting and disease-preventing goals but also can be used by health care providers to help them set binding goals to improve their communication with patients. Finally, the self-regulatory strategy of mental contrasting can be easily taught and learned. As it is a general cognitive procedure, once acquired, it may be applied to any health-related problem or concern patients, providers, or managers in the medical setting might have.

IMPLEMENTING MEDICAL ADHERENCE GOALS

In traditional theories on goal striving, the intention to achieve a certain goal is seen as an immediate determinant (or at least predictor) of goal-directed action, and a strong intention is expected to facilitate goal attainment more than a weak intention (Ajzen, 1991; Ajzen & Fishbein, 1980; Sheeran, 2002). Over time, evidence has accumulated showing that forming strong intentions was only a prerequisite for successful goal attainment as there are a host of subsequent implemental problems that need to be solved successfully (Gollwitzer, 1996). For instance, after having set a goal (e.g., to reduce smoking), people may procrastinate in acting on their intentions and thus fail to initiate goal-directed behavior. Moreover, in everyday life people normally strive for multiple, often even competing goals, many of which are not simple short-term but long-term projects that require repeated efforts (e.g., to lose weight). Goal pursuit may come to an early halt because competing projects have temporarily gained priority and the individual fails to successfully resume the original project. Also, to meet their goals, people have to seize viable opportunities to act, a task that becomes particularly difficult when attention is directed elsewhere (e.g., one is absorbed by competing goal pursuits, wrapped up in ruminations, gripped by intense emotional experiences, or simply tired) and when these opportunities are not obvious at first sight or only present themselves briefly.

In an attempt to find a self-regulatory tool for effective goal implementation, Gollwitzer (1993, 1996, 1999) distinguished between goal intentions and implementation intentions. Goal intentions (goals) have the structure of "I intend to reach Z," whereby Z may relate to a certain outcome or behavior to which the individual feels committed. Implementation intentions (plans) have the structure of "If situation X is encountered, then I will perform the goal-directed response Y." Holding an implementation intention commits an individual to perform the specified goal-directed response once the critical situation is encountered. Both goal intentions and implementation intentions are set in an act of will, whereby the first specifies the intention to meet a goal or standard, and the second refers to the intention to perform a plan. Commonly, implementation intentions are formed in the service of goal intentions as they specify the where, when, and how of goal-directed responses. For instance, a possible implementation intention in the service of the goal intention to eat healthful food would link a suitable situational context (e.g., one's order taken at a restaurant) to an appropriate behavior (e.g., asking for a low-fat meal). As a consequence, a strong mental link is formed between the situation of the waiter taking an order and the goal-directed response of asking for a low-fat meal.

Why Implementation Intentions Are Expected to Facilitate Goal Implementation

The mental links created by implementation intentions are expected to facilitate goal attainment on the basis of psychological processes that relate to both the anticipated situation and the specified response. Because forming implementation intentions implies the selection of a critical future situation, it is assumed that the mental representation of the situation becomes highly activated, hence is more accessible. This heightened accessibility should make it easier for one to detect the critical situation and readily attend to it even when one is busy with other things. Moreover, this heightened accessibility should facilitate the recall of the critical situation. As forming implementation intentions involves first a selection of an effective goal-directed behavior that is then linked to the selected critical situation, initiation of the intended response should become automated. Initiation should be swift and efficient and should not require conscious intent once the critical situation is encountered.

The Specified Situation

The accessibility hypothesis with respect to the specified situation was tested in studies measuring how well participants holding implementation intentions attended to, detected, and recalled the critical situation as compared with participants who had formed only goal intentions (Gollwitzer, Bayer, Steller, & Bargh, 2002). In a study using a dichotic listening paradigm (i.e., different information is presented simultaneously to research participants' left and right ears and participants have to repeat, or shadow, the information presented to the ear to which the experimenter asks them to attend), it was observed that words describing the anticipated critical situation were highly disruptive to focused attention in participants in the implementation intention group as compared with participants in the goal intention group (i.e., the shadowing performance of the attended materials decreased). In a study using the embedded figures test (Gottschaldt, 1926), in which smaller a-figures are hidden within larger b-figures, enhanced detection of the hidden a-figures was observed when participants had specified the a-figure in the *if*-part of an implementation intention (i.e., had made plans on how to create a traffic sign from the a-figure). In a cued-recall experiment, participants in the implementation intention group recalled the situational options to attain a given goal more effectively than participants in the goal intention group. Finally, Aarts, Dijksterhuis, and Midden (1999) using a lexical decision task observed faster lexical decision times (i.e., recognizing presented stimuli as words vs. nonwords) for those words that described critical cues specified in implementation intentions. It is important to note that the faster lexical responses to these critical words (i.e., their heightened accessibility) mediated the beneficial effects of implementation intentions on goal attainment. The latter result implies that the goal-promoting effects of implementation intentions are based on the heightened accessibility of selected critical situational cues.

The Specified Goal-Directed Behavior

The postulated automation of action initiation (also described as *strategic delegation of control to situational cues*; Gollwitzer, 1993, p. 173) has been supported by the results of various experiments that tested immediacy, efficiency, and the presence or absence of conscious intent. Gollwitzer and Brandstätter (1997, Study 3) demonstrated the immediacy of action initiation in a study wherein participants had been induced to form implementation intentions that specified viable opportunities for presenting counterarguments to a series of racist remarks made by a confederate. Participants with implementation intentions initiated the counterarguments more quickly than the participants who had formed the mere goal intention to counterargue.

In further experiments (Brandstätter, Lengfelder, & Gollwitzer, 2001, Studies 3 and 4), the efficiency of action initiation was explored. Participants formed the goal intention to press a button as fast as possible if numbers appeared on the computer screen, but not if letters were presented (go/no-go task). Participants in the implementation intention condition also made the plan to press the response button particularly fast if the number 3 was presented. This go/no-go task was then embedded as a secondary task in a dual-task paradigm. Participants in the implementation intention group showed a substantial increase in speed of responding to the number 3 compared with the control group, regardless of whether the simultaneously demanded primary task (a memorization task in Study 3 and a tracking task in Study 4) was either easy or difficult to perform. Apparently, the immediacy of responding induced by implementation intentions is also efficient in the sense that it does not require much in the way of cognitive resources (i.e., can be performed even when dual tasks have to be performed at the same time).

In a final set of two priming experiments, Bayer, Achtziger, Gollwitzer, Malzacher, and Moskowitz (2006) tested whether implementation intentions led to action initiation without conscious intent once the critical situation was encountered. In these experiments, the critical situation was presented subliminally, and its facilitating influence on initiating the goal-directed behavior was assessed. Results indicated that subliminal presentation of the critical primes led to a speed-up in responding in participants with implementation intentions but not in participants with mere goal intentions. These subliminal priming effects suggest that when planned through implementation intentions, the initiation of goal-directed behavior becomes triggered by the anticipated situational cue, without the need for further conscious intent.

There might be additional or even alternative process mechanisms to the stimulus perception and response initiation processes described earlier. For example, furnishing goals with implementation intentions might produce an increase in goal commitment, which in turn causes heightened goal attainment. However, this hypothesis has not received any empirical support. For instance, when Brandstätter et al. (2001, Study 1) analyzed whether heroin addicts under withdrawal benefit from forming implementation intentions in handing in a newly composed curriculum vitae before the end of the day, they also measured participants' commitment to do so. Although the majority of the participants in the implementation intention group succeeded in handing in the curriculum vitae on time, none of the participants in the goal intention group succeeded in this task. These two groups, however, did not differ in terms of their goal commitment ("I feel committed to compose a curriculum vitae" and "I have to complete this task") measured after the goal intention and implementation intention instructions had been administered. This finding was replicated with young adults who participated in a professional development workshop (Oettingen et al., 2000, Study 2), and analogous results are reported in research on the effects of implementation intentions on meeting health promotion and disease prevention goals (e.g., Orbell, Hodgkins, & Sheeran, 1997).

Implementation Intentions and Their Effects on Performing Wanted Behaviors

Given that implementation intentions facilitate attending to, detecting, and recalling viable opportunities to act toward goal attainment and, in addition, automate action initiation in the presence of such opportunities, people who form implementation intentions should show higher goal attainment rates as compared with people who do not furnish their goal intentions with implementation intentions. This hypothesis is supported by the results of a host of studies examining the attainment of various types of goal intentions (a recent meta-analysis by Gollwitzer & Sheeran, 2006, listed more than 90 studies demonstrating implementation intention effects). Many of the goals analyzed in these studies related to health protection and disease prevention (e.g., resisting taking up smoking, taking up regular exercise, performing breast self-examination, preventing binge drinking, eating a low-fat diet, using vitamin supplements regularly, flossing, and reducing snack food consumption).

Types of Goals

Gollwitzer and Brandstätter (1997) analyzed the attainment of a goal intention that had to be acted on at an inconvenient time (e.g., writing a report about Christmas Eve during the subsequent Christmas holiday). Other studies have examined the effects of implementation intentions on goal attainment rates with goal intentions that are somewhat unpleasant to perform. For instance, the goal intentions to perform health-protecting and health-enhancing behaviors such as regular breast examination (Orbell et al., 1997), cervical cancer screening (Sheeran & Orbell, 2000), resumption of functional activity after joint replacement surgery (Orbell & Sheeran, 2000), and engaging in physical exercise (Milne, Orbell, & Sheeran, 2002) were all more frequently acted on when people had furnished these goals with implementation intentions. Finally, implementation intentions were found to facilitate the attainment of goal intentions when it was easy to forget to act on them (e.g., regular intake of vitamin pills, Sheeran & Orbell, 1999; the signing of worksheets with the elderly, Chasteen, Park, & Schwarz, 2001).

Potential Moderators

The strength of the beneficial effects of implementation intentions depends on the presence or absence of several moderators. First, implementation intention effects are more apparent the more difficult it is to initiate the goal-directed behavior. For instance, implementation intentions were more effective in completing goals that research participants perceived to be difficult as compared with easy to implement (Gollwitzer & Brandstätter, 1997, Study 1). Moreover, forming implementation intentions was more beneficial to patients with frontal lobe impairment, who typically have problems with executive control, than to college students (Lengfelder & Gollwitzer, 2001, Study 2).

Second, the strength of commitment to the respective goal intention also matters. Orbell et al. (1997) reported that the beneficial effects of implementation intentions on compliance in performing a breast examination were observed only in those women who strongly intended to perform a breast self-examination. This finding suggests that implementation intentions do not work when the respective goal intention is weak. In line with this conclusion, the beneficial effects of implementation intentions on a person's recall of the specified situations (Gollwitzer, Bayer, et al., 2002, Study 3) can no longer be observed when the respective goal intention has been abandoned (i.e., the research participants were told that the assigned goal intention need no longer be reached as it had been performed by some other person). Third, the strength of the commitment to the formed implementation intention makes a difference, too. In Gollwitzer, Bayer, et al.'s (2002) Study 3, the strength of the commitment to the implementation intention was varied by telling the participants (after an extensive personality testing session) that they were the kind of people who would benefit from either rigidly adhering to their plans (i.e., high commitment) or staying flexible (i.e., low commitment). The latter group showed lower implementation intention effects (i.e., cued-recall performance for selected opportunities) than the former. Finally, the strength of the mental link between the *if*-part and the *then*-part of an implementation intention should also affect how beneficial forming implementation intentions turns out to be. For example, if a person takes much time and concentration encoding the if–then plan or keeps repeating a formed if–then plan by using inner speech, stronger mental links should emerge, which in turn should produce stronger implementation intention effects (Steller, 1992).

Applying these findings to the health domain, a health care provider who is concerned about maximizing the implementation of health goals in his or her patients should ask them to form respective implementation intentions. This is particularly true when the patients regard the implementation of the goal to be difficult (e.g., has to be acted on at inconvenient times, is unpleasant to perform, or is easy to forget). However, health care providers first need to be sure that the patients are highly committed to the health goal at hand. If this is not the case, measures to raise the perceived feasibility and desirability should be taken, and the mental contrasting procedure should be applied to achieve strong goal commitments. Moreover, implementation intentions should be suggested in a way so that patients find it easy to strongly commit to the plans made (e.g., patients are allowed to fill the *if*-parts and *then*-parts of implementation intentions with what they feel fit best to their daily lives and behavioral capabilities; Murgraff, White, & Phillips, 1996). Finally, physicians or other health care providers may want to motivate patients to mentally repeat the formed implementation plans to strengthen the links between the situations specified in the *if*-part and the goal-directed responses selected for the *then*-part.

Implementation Intentions and the Control of Unwanted Intrusions

Research on implementation intentions has focused mostly on the self-regulatory issue of getting started with goals that one wants to achieve, that is, doing more good (e.g., engaging in regular physical exercise) and less bad (e.g., avoiding unhealthful foods). However, once a person has initiated goal pursuit, he or she still needs to bring it to a successful ending. People need to protect an ongoing goal from being thwarted by attending to attractive distractions or by falling prey to conflicting bad habits (e.g., the goal of eating less fatty foods may conflict with the habit of snacking). There are two major strategies in which implementation intentions can be used to control unwanted intrusions that potentially hamper the successful pursuit of wanted goals: (a) directing one's implementation intentions toward the suppression of anticipated unwanted responses to disruptive stimuli and (b) blocking all (even nonanticipated) kinds of unwanted influences from inside or outside the person by directing one's implementation intentions toward spelling out the wanted goal pursuit (Gollwitzer, Bayer, & McCulloch, 2005).

Responding to Unwanted Intrusions With Suppression

If, for instance, a person wants to eat healthfully and not fall prey to tempting foods (such as chocolate bars), the person can protect him- or herself from snacking on tempting chocolate bars by furnishing the goal of not falling prey to temptations with suppression-oriented implementation intentions. Suppression-oriented implementation intentions can take different forms. They may focus on reducing the intensity of the unwanted response (i.e., falling for the temptation) by intending not to show the unwanted response: "And if my friend offers me chocolate, then I will not long for it and take it!" But they may also try to reduce the intensity of the unwanted response by specifying the initiation of the respective antagonistic response: "And if my friend offers me chocolate, then I will think of fruits and ask for them!" Finally, suppression-oriented implementation intentions may focus a person away from the critical situation: "And if my friend offers me chocolate, then I'll simply ignore his offer and my cravings!"

Two lines of experiments analyzed the effects of suppression-oriented implementation intentions. The first line analyzed the control of unwanted spontaneous attentional responses to tempting distractions (Gollwitzer & Schaal, 1998). Participants had to perform a boring task (i.e., perform a series of simple arithmetic tasks) while being bombarded with attractive distractive stimuli (e.g., clips of award-winning commercials). Whereas control participants were asked to form a mere goal intention ("I will not let myself get distracted!"), experimental participants in addition formed one of the following two implementation intentions: "And if a distraction arises, then I'll ignore it!" or "And if a distraction arises, then I will increase my effort at the task at hand!" The "ignore" implementation intention always helped participants to ward off the distractions (as assessed by their task performance), no matter whether the motivation to perform the tedious task (assessed at the beginning of the task) was low or high. The "effort increase" implementation intention, however, could only achieve this when motivation to perform the tedious task was low. Possibly, when motivation is high to begin with, effort increase implementation intentions may create overmotivation that hampers task performance. It seems appropriate therefore to advise highly motivated individuals who experience temptations (e.g., a person who is extremely motivated to reduce fat intake) to resort to implementation intentions that ignore the temptation rather than to implementation intentions that focus on the strengthening of efforts.

The second line of experiments analyzing suppression-oriented implementation intentions studied the control of the activation of stereotypical beliefs and prejudicial evaluations (Gollwitzer & Schaal, 1998). In various priming studies using short stimulus onset asynchronies (less than 300 ms), research participants with implementation intentions indeed managed to inhibit the automatic activation of stereotypical beliefs and prejudicial evaluations about women, the elderly, the homeless, and soccer fans. The implementation intentions used specified being confronted with a member of the critical group in the *if*-part, and a "then I won't stereotype" (alternatively: "then I won't evaluate negatively") or a "then I will ignore the group membership" response in the *then*-part. No matter which of the two formats was used, both types of suppression-oriented implementation intentions were effective.

Blocking Detrimental Self-States

In the research presented in the last paragraph, implementation intentions specified a critical situation or problem in the *if*-part that was linked to a *then*-part describing an attempt to suppress the unwanted response to an intrusive or tempting stimulus. This type of self-regulation by implementation intentions requires that the person correctly anticipate potential hindrances to achieving the goal and what kind of unwanted responses these hindrances elicit. However, implementation intentions can also be used to protect oneself from responding to unwanted intrusions by taking a different approach. Instead of gearing one's implementation intentions toward anticipated potential hindrances (or temptations) and the unwanted responses triggered thereof, the person may form implementation intentions geared to stabilizing the goal pursuit at hand. For instance, if a person who has the goal of eating low-fat foods stipulates in advance how he or she will go about having dinner (i.e., "When the waiter asks my order for the dessert, then I will request the berries"), internal distractions or interferences from inside (e.g., being hungry, tired, nervous) should not show any effect. The critical interaction with the waiter should simply run off as planned, and the intrusive self-states of being hungry or tired should not succeed in affecting the critical goal-directed behavior of ordering a low-fat dessert.

As is evident from this example, the present self-regulatory strategy should be of special value whenever the influence of detrimental self-states (e.g., being upset) on derailing one's goal-directed behavior has to be controlled. This should be true no matter whether such self-states and their influence on behavior reside in the person's consciousness or not. Gollwitzer and Bayer (2000) tested this hypothesis in a series of experiments in which participants were asked to make or not make plans (i.e., form implementation intentions) regarding their performance on an assigned task. Prior to beginning the task, participants' self-states were manipulated in such a way that performing the task at hand became more difficult (e.g., a state of self-definitional incompleteness prior to a task that required perspective taking, Gollwitzer & Wicklund, 1985; a good mood prior to a task that required evaluating others nonstereotypically, Bless & Fiedler, 1995; a state of ego depletion prior to a task that required persistence, Baumeister, 2000; Muraven, Tice, & Baumeister, 1998). It was observed that the induced critical self-states negatively affected task performance only for those participants who had not planned out working on the task at hand through implementation intentions (i.e., had only set themselves the goal of coming up with a great performance). In other words, successful task performance depended on additional implementation intentions that spelled out how to perform the task at hand to block the effects of these detrimental self-states.

This research provides a new perspective on the psychology of self-regulation. Effective self-regulation is commonly understood in terms of strengthening the self, so that the self can meet the challenge of being a powerful executive agent (Baumeister, Heatherton, & Tice, 1994). Therefore, most research on goal-directed self-regulation focuses on strengthening the self in such a way that threats and irritations become less likely, or on restoring an already threatened or irritated self. Instead, Gollwitzer and Bayer's (2000) research introduced a perspective on goal-directed self-regulation that focuses on facilitating action control without changing the self. It is assumed that action control becomes easy if a person's behavior is directly controlled by situational cues and that forming implementation intentions achieves such direct action control. As this mode of action control circumvents the self, it does not matter whether the self is threatened or secure, agitated or calm, because the self is effectively disconnected from its influence on behavior.

The research by Gollwitzer and Bayer (2000) supports this line of reasoning by demonstrating that task performance (e.g., taking the perspective of another person, judging people in a nonstereotypical manner, and solving difficult anagrams) is not impaired by the respective detrimental self-states (e.g., self-definitional incompleteness, mood, and ego depletion) if performing these tasks has been planned in advance through implementation intentions. Support for this line of reasoning also comes from studies that analyze special groups of individuals who are known to have problems with action control because of various attention, memory, and executive function deficits. For instance, Brandstätter et al. (2001, Studies 1 and 2) demonstrated that patients with schizophrenia and individuals addicted to heroine under withdrawal benefited greatly from forming implementation intentions when it came to performing an experimental go/no-go task or the real-life task of composing a curriculum vitae, respectively. Moreover, Lengfelder and Gollwitzer (2001) observed improved task performance on a go/no-go task in patients with frontal lobe impairment who had formed respective implementation intentions, even under conditions of high cognitive load created by a difficult dual task. Finally, Park and collaborators (Chasteen et al., 2001; Liu & Park, 2004) reported research with older adults indicating that implementation intentions facilitated the performance of experimental tasks (i.e., signing one's name on each worksheet) and real-life tasks (i.e., performing regular blood glucose tests) that engage prospective memory processes known to decline in older adults.

The studies with special samples suggest that implementation intentions block not only the negative effects of variable detrimental self-states (e.g., irritation) on goal attainment (task performance) but also the negative effects of more stable deficits in the cognitive functioning underlying effective action control. As implementation intentions are known to automate the implementation of the goal or task, the cognitive deficits overcome by implementation intentions should be of the more effortful type. The self-regulatory strategy of planning out goal striving through implementation intentions therefore is an easy-to-use and cheap alternative to training individuals who show deficits in effortful cognitive functioning.

Blocking Adverse Situational Influences

People's goal pursuits are threatened not only by detrimental self-states (e.g., being tired) or stable aspects of the self (e.g., lacking certain executive functions) but also by adverse situational contexts (e.g., peer pressure).

There are many situations that have negative effects on goal attainment unbeknownst to the person who is striving for a goal. A prime example is the *social loafing* phenomenon in which people show reduced effort in the face of work settings that produce a reduction of accountability (i.e., performance outcomes can no longer be checked at an individual level). As people are commonly not aware of this phenomenon, they cannot form implementation intentions that specify a social loafing situation as a critical situation, thereby rendering an implementation intention that focuses on suppressing the social loafing response as an unviable self-regulatory strategy. As an alternative, however, people may resort to forming implementation intentions that stipulate how the intended task is to be performed and thus effectively block any negative situational influences.

Indeed, when Endress (2001) ran a social loafing experiment that used a brainstorming task (i.e., participants had to find as many different uses for a common knife as possible), she observed that participants with an implementation intention ("And if I have found one solution, then I will immediately try to find a different solution!") but not participants with a mere goal intention ("I will try to find as many different solutions as possible!") were protected from social loafing effects. Further studies that support the idea that implementation intentions make a goal pursuit invulnerable to adverse situational influences are reported by Trötschel and Gollwitzer (in press). In their experiments on the self-regulation of negotiation behavior, loss-framed negotiation settings (i.e., the negotiation goal is framed in terms of avoiding losses) failed to unfold their negative effects on fair and cooperative negotiation outcomes when the negotiators had planned out their goal intentions to be fair and cooperative in terms of if–then plans. In a similar vein, Gollwitzer (1998) reported experiments in which ongoing goal pursuits (e.g., to drive safely, to concentrate on a given math task) that had been planned out in advance by implementation intentions were protected from intrusive influences of competing goals (e.g., to be fast and to attend to a person asking for help, respectively) activated outside of awareness by using classic goal-priming procedures (Bargh, 1990; Bargh, Gollwitzer, Lee-Chai, Barndollar, & Trötschel, 2001).

These findings suggest that the self-regulatory strategy of planning out goal pursuit in advance places a person in the position of reaping positive outcomes without having to change the environment from an adverse to a facilitative one. This is very convenient, as such environmental change is often cumbersome or not under the person's control (e.g., a person with the goal of reducing fat intake cannot easily change the menu at a favorite restaurant). Also, often people are not aware of the adverse influences of the current environment (e.g., the automatic activation of bad eating habits in situations in which the person has sinned repeatedly and consistently in the past). In such situations, implementation intentions that specify critical situations in the *if*-part and a coping response in the *then*-part do not qualify as a viable alternative self-regulatory tool. Rather, people need to resort to the strategy of planning the ongoing goal pursuit (e.g., eating healthfully) through implementation intentions, thereby protecting it from all kinds of expected and unexpected adverse situational influences.

Potential Costs of Using Implementation Intentions

Given the many benefits of forming implementation intentions, one wonders about the possible costs, if any. Three issues come to mind when considering this possibility. First, action control by implementation intentions may be characterized by rigidity and thus may hurt performance that requires flexibility. Second, forming implementation intentions may be a costly self-regulatory strategy in terms of producing a high degree of ego depletion and consequently handicap needed self-regulatory resources. Third, even though implementation intentions successfully suppress unwanted thoughts, feelings, and actions in a given context, these very thoughts, feelings, and actions may rebound in a subsequent different context.

With respect to rigidity, it is still an open question whether participants with implementation intentions refrain from using alternative good opportunities to act toward the goal by insisting on only acting when the critical situation specified in the *if*-part of the implementation intention is encountered. Even though these participants may feel that they have to stick to their plans, they may very well be faster in recognizing such alternative opportunities. The strategic automaticity created by implementation intentions should free cognitive capacities and thus allow for effective processing of information about alternative opportunities.

The assumption that implementation intentions delegate the control of behavior to situational cues implies that the self is not implicated when behavior is controlled through implementation intentions. As a consequence, the self should not become depleted when a self-regulation task is regulated by implementation intentions. This has been observed not only in a study by Gollwitzer and Bayer (2000) using a classic ego-depletion paradigm that required participants to control their emotions while watching a humorous movie but also in a recent experiment by Webb and Sheeran (2003, Study 1) in which participants had to perform the Stroop task as an initial task. Indeed, when participants had to perform a subsequent difficult self-regulation task (i.e., anagrams or puzzles) that required sustained effort, participants who had performed the initial task with the help of implementation intentions showed greater persistence than participants who had performed the initial task without implementation intentions.

Gollwitzer, Bayer, Trötschel, and Sumner (2006) ran two rebound experiments following research paradigms developed by Macrae, Bodenhausen, Milne, and Jetten (1994). In both studies participants first had to suppress the expression of stereotypes in a first-impression formation task that focused on a particular member of a stereotyped group (i.e., homeless people). Rebound was measured in terms of subsequent expression of stereotypes in either a subsequent task that demanded the evaluation of the group of homeless people in general (Study 1) or a lexical decision task that assessed the accessibility of homeless stereotypes (Study 2). Participants who had been assigned the mere goal of controlling stereotypic thoughts while forming an impression of the given homeless person were more stereotypical in their judgments of homeless people in general (Study 1) and showed a higher accessibility of homeless stereotypes (Study 2) than participants who had been asked to furnish this lofty goal with relevant if–then plans.

The ego-depletion and rebound studies on implementation intentions imply that a person who has set him- or herself the goal to adhere to certain medical instructions and furnished this goal with respective implementation intentions should experience less ego depletion and rebound effects. Accordingly, a person whose goal is to eat less fatty food should not be ego depleted after a tempting situation has been resisted, and thus should not be handicapped in performing subsequent tasks that require much self-regulation (e.g., dealing with problems at work or at home in a calm and emotionally controlled manner). Moreover, there should not be any rebound in the sense that having escaped one tempting situation (e.g., being offered a chocolate bar) will make the person more ready to succumb to a subsequent temptation (e.g., a German bratwurst).

Even though implementation intentions seem to achieve their effects without costs in terms of ego depletion or rebound, this does not mean that forming implementation intentions is a foolproof self-regulatory strategy. In everyday life, people may not succeed in using implementation intentions effectively for various reasons. First, a person may start forming implementation intentions even though he or she has not set a strong health goal yet. Before people start forming implementation intentions, it is important that they strengthen perceived feasibility and desirability and apply the self-regulatory strategy of mental contrasting. Second, a person may link a critical situation to a behavior or outcome that turns out to be outside of his or her control (e.g., if a person whose goal is to eat healthfully plans to ask for a vegetarian meal but the restaurant he or she frequents does not offer such meals). A similar problem arises with implementation intentions that specify opportunities that hardly ever arise (e.g., if a person who plans to ask for a vegetarian meal in his or her favorite restaurant mostly cooks for him- or herself at home) or implementation intentions that specify behaviors that have zero instrumentality with respect to reaching the goal (e.g., if a person with the goal of eating healthfully plans to ask for a vegetarian meal not knowing that most restaurants add fatty cheese to make it tasty).

Finally, there is the question of how concretely people should specify the *if*-parts and *then*-parts of their implementation intentions. If the goal is to eat healthfully, one can form an implementation intention that holds either this very behavior in the then-part or a more concrete operationalization of it. The latter seems appropriate whenever a whole array of specific operationalizations is possible, as planning in advance which type of goal-directed behavior is to be executed once the critical situation is encountered prevents disruptive deliberation in situ (with respect to choosing one behavior over another). An analogous argument applies to the specification of situations in the *if*-part of an implementation intention. People should specify the situation in the *if*-part to such a degree that a given situation will no longer raise the question of whether it qualifies as the critical situation or not.

SUMMARY

People can use implementation intentions not only to promote the initiation of goal-directed actions but also to protect their ongoing goal pursuits from being thwarted. The latter can be achieved in two different ways. As long as one is in a position to anticipate what could potentially make one stray off course (the relevant hindrances, barriers, distractions, and temptations), one can specify these critical situations in the *if*-part of an implementation intention and link it to a response that facilitates goal attainment. The response specified in the *then*-part of an implementation intention can then be geared to ignoring disruptive stimuli, suppressing the impeding responses to them, or overcoming obstructions to goal pursuit by engaging in it all the more.

This way of using implementation intentions to protect goal pursuit from straying off course necessitates that people know what kind of obstacles and distractions need to be watched for. Moreover, people need to know what kind of unwanted responses are potentially triggered (so that they can attempt to suppress them) and what kind of goal-directed responses are particularly effective in suppressing these unwanted responses (so that they can engage in these goal-directed activities). Consequently, much social, clinical, and cognitive psychological knowledge is required to be in a position to come up with effective *if*- and *then*-components of such implementation intentions.

However, an easier solution is available. Instead of concentrating on potential obstacles and various ways of effectively dealing with them, people may exclusively concern themselves with the intricacies of implementing the goal pursuit at hand. People can plan out the goal pursuit by forming implementation intentions that determine how the various steps of goal attainment are to be executed. Such careful planning encapsulates goal pursuit, protecting it from the adverse influence of potential obstacles and distractions, whether internal or external. This self-regulatory strategy of goal pursuit permits attaining goals without having to change a noncooperative self or an unfavorable environment.

Implementation intentions create cognitive links between select situational cues and intended goal-directed behaviors. The effectiveness of implementation intentions lies in the fact that after generation, the mental representation of the specified situational cue becomes highly activated. Once this cue is actually encountered, the planned behavior runs off automatically, overriding and defying any habits or divisive spontaneous attentional responses. Given people's limited resources for conscious and effortful self-regulation, delegating control to situational cues by one express act of fiat is an effective way to bridge the gap that exists between their best intentions and the successful attainment of their goals.

CONCLUSION

Classic motivational approaches to behavior change focus on increasing the target behavior's desirability and feasibility. It is assumed that such interventions strengthen a person's intention (goal) to perform the respective behavior, which in turn guides a person's actions. Recent research on action control observed, however, that high perceived feasibility (high expectation of success) is not necessarily translated into strong goal intentions and that strong goal intentions do not necessarily lead to the initiation of the respective behavior. With respect to translating high expectations of success into strong intentions, Oettingen (1996, 1999; Oettingen et al., 2001) reported that people with high expectations of success will only then form strong intentions if they have contrasted the positive aspects of the desired behavioral change with the obstacles they see in the way of achieving this change. With respect to translating strong intentions into behavior, Gollwitzer (1993, 1996, 1999) observed that furnishing this intention with if–then plans that specify when and where one wants to act drastically increases attainment rates. It is argued therefore that physicians' or other health care providers' instructions to patients should not only focus on enhancing the perceived desirability and feasibility of health-promoting and disease-preventing and -reducing behaviors (motivational intervention) but also be geared to teaching their patients the relevant skills of mental contrasting and planning (self-regulation intervention).

REFERENCES

Aarts, H., Dijksterhuis, A., & Midden, C. (1999). To plan or not to plan? Goal achievement or interrupting the performance of mundane behaviors. *European Journal of Social Psychology, 29*, 971–979.

Ajzen, I. (1991). The theory of planned behavior. *Organizational Behavior and Human Decision Processes, 50*, 179–211.

Ajzen, I., & Fishbein, M. (1980). *Understanding attitudes and predicting social behavior.* Englewood-Cliffs, NJ: Prentice Hall.

Atkinson, J. W. (1957). Motivational determinants of risk taking behavior. *Psychological Review, 64*, 359–372.

Bandura, A. (1997). *Self-efficacy: The exercise of control.* New York: Freeman.

Bargh, J. A. (1990). Auto-motives: Preconscious determinants of social interaction. In E. T. Higgins & R. M. Sorrentino (Eds.), *Handbook of motivation and cognition: Foundations of social behavior* (Vol. 2, pp. 93–130). New York: Guilford Press.

Bargh, J. A., Gollwitzer, P. M., Lee-Chai, A., Barndollar, K., & Trötschel, R. (2001). The automated will: Nonconscious activation and pursuit of behavioral goals. *Journal of Personality and Social Psychology, 81*, 1014–1027.

Baumeister, R. F. (2000). Ego-depletion and the self's executive function. In A. Tesser, R. B. Felson, & J. M. Suls (Eds.), *Psychological perspectives on self and identity* (pp. 9–33). Washington, DC: American Psychological Association.

Baumeister, R. F., Heatherton, T. F., & Tice, D. M. (1994). *Losing control: How and why people fail at self-regulation.* San Diego, CA: Academic Press.

Bayer, U. C., Achtziger, A., Gollwitzer, P. M., Malzacher, J., & Moskowitz, G. B. (2006). *Strategic automaticity by implementation intentions: Action initiation without conscious intent.* Manuscript under review.

Bless, H., & Fiedler, K. (1995). Affective states and the influence of activated general knowledge. *Personality and Social Psychology Bulletin, 21*, 766–778.

Brandstätter, V., Lengfelder, A., & Gollwitzer, P. M. (2001). Implementation intentions and efficient action initiation. *Journal of Personality and Social Psychology, 81*, 946–960.

Brehm, J. W., & Self, E. (1989). The intensity of motivation. *Annual Review of Psychology, 40*, 109–131.

Brownlee, S., Leventhal, H., & Leventhal, E. A. (2000). Regulation, self-regulation, and construction of the self in the maintenance of physical health. In M. Boekaerts, P. R. Pintrich, & M. Zeidner (Eds.), *Handbook of self-regulation* (pp. 369–416). San Diego, CA: Academic Press.

Carver, C. S., & Scheier, M. F. (1998). *On the self-regulation of behavior.* Cambridge, England: Cambridge University Press.

Chasteen, A. L., Park, D. C., & Schwarz, N. (2001). Implementation intentions and facilitation of prospective memory. *Psychological Science, 12*, 457–461.

Endress, H. (2001). *Die Wirksamkeit von Vorsätzen auf Gruppenleistungen. Eine empiri-sche Untersuchung anhand von Brainstorming* [Implementation intentions and the reduction of social loafing in a brain storming task]. Unpublished master's thesis, University of Konstanz, Konstanz, Germany.

Gollwitzer, P. M. (1990). Action phases and mind-sets. In T. E. Higgins & R. M. Sorrentino (Eds.), *Handbook of motivation and cognition: Foundations of social behavior* (Vol. 2, pp. 53–92). New York: Guilford Press.

Gollwitzer, P. M. (1993). Goal achievement: The role of intentions. *European Review of Social Psychology, 4,* 141–185.

Gollwitzer, P. M. (1996). The volitional benefits of planning. In P. M. Gollwitzer & J. A. Bargh (Eds.), *The psychology of action: Linking cognition and motivation to behavior* (pp. 287–312). New York: Guilford Press.

Gollwitzer, P. M. (1998, October). *Implicit versus explicit processes in goal pursuit.* Paper presented at the annual meeting of the Society of Experimental Social Psychology, Lexington, KY.

Gollwitzer, P. M. (1999). Implementation intentions: Strong effects of simple plans. *American Psychologist, 54,* 493–503.

Gollwitzer, P. M., & Bayer, U. C. (2000, October). *Becoming a better person without changing the self.* Paper presented at the annual meeting of the Society of Experimental Social Psychology, Atlanta, GA.

Gollwitzer, P. M., Bayer, U. C., & McCulloch, K. (2005). The control of the unwanted. In R. Hassin, J. Uleman, & J. A. Bargh (Eds.), *The new unconscious* (pp. 485–515). New York: Oxford University Press.

Gollwitzer, P. M., Bayer, U. C., Steller, B., & Bargh, J. A. (2002). *Delegating control to the environment: Perception, attention, and memory for pre-selected behavioral cues.* Unpublished manuscript, University of Konstanz, Konstanz, Germany.

Gollwitzer, P. M., Bayer, U. C., Trötschel, R., & Sumner, M. (2006). *Self-regulation by implementation intentions entails no costs: Ego-depletion and rebound effects.* Manuscript under review.

Gollwitzer, P. M., & Brandstätter, V. (1997). Implementation intentions and effec-tive goal pursuit. *Journal of Personality and Social Psychology, 73,* 186–199.

Gollwitzer, P. M., & Moskowitz, G. B. (1996). Goal effects on action and cognition. In E. T. Higgins & A. W. Kruglanski (Eds.), *Social psychology: Handbook of basic principles* (pp. 361–399). New York: Guilford Press.

Gollwitzer, P. M., & Schaal, B. (1998). Metacognition in action: The importance of implementation intentions. *Personality and Social Psychology Review, 2,* 124–136.

Gollwitzer, P. M., & Sheeran, P. (2006). Implementation intentions and goal achievement: A meta-analysis of effects and processes. *Advances in Experimental Social Psychology, 38,* 69–119.

Gollwitzer, P. M., & Wicklund, R. A. (1985). Self-symbolizing and the neglect of others' perspectives. *Journal of Personality and Social Psychology, 56,* 702–715.

Gottschaldt, K. (1926). Über den Einfluß der Erfahrung auf die Wahrnehmung von Figuren [The effects of familiarity on the perception of figures]. *Psychologische Forschung, 8,* 261–317.

Heckhausen, H. (1977). Achievement motivation and its constructs: A cognitive model. *Motivation and Emotion, 1,* 283–329.

Hochbaum, G. (1958). *Public participation in medical screening programs* (DHEW Publication No. 572). Washington, DC: U.S. Government Printing Office.

Lengfelder, A., & Gollwitzer, P. M. (2001). Reflective and reflexive action control in patients with frontal brain lesions. *Neuropsychology, 15,* 80–100.

Liu, L., & Park, D. C. (2004). Aging and medical adherence: The use of automatic processes to achieve effortful things. *Psychology and Aging, 19,* 318–325.

Locke, E. A., & Latham, G. P. (1990). *A theory of goal setting and task performance.* Englewood Cliffs, NJ: Prentice Hall.

Macrae, C. N., Bodenhausen, G. V., Milne, A. B., & Jetten, J. (1994). Out of mind but back in sight: Stereotypes on the rebound. *Journal of Personality and Social Psychology, 67,* 808–817.

Milne, S., Orbell, S., & Sheeran, P. (2002). Combining motivational and volitional interventions to promote exercise participation: Protection motivation theory and implementation intentions. *British Journal of Health Psychology, 7,* 163–184.

Morrell, R. W., Park, D. C., & Poon, L. W. (1990). Effects of labeling techniques on memory and comprehension of prescription information in young and old adults. *Journal of Gerontology, 45,* P166–P172.

Muraven, M., Tice, D. M., & Baumeister, R. F. (1998). Self-control as a limited resource: Regulatory depletion pattern. *Journal of Personality and Social Psychology, 74,* 774–789.

Murgraff, V., White, D., & Phillips, K. (1996). Moderating binge drinking: It is possible to change behavior if you plan it in advance. *Alcohol and Alcoholism, 31,* 577–582.

Oettingen, G. (1996). Positive fantasy and motivation. In P. M. Gollwitzer & J. A. Bargh (Eds.), *The psychology of action: Linking cognition and motivation to behavior* (pp. 236–259). New York: Guilford Press.

Oettingen, G. (1999). Free fantasies about the future and the emergence of developmental goals. In J. Brandtstädter & R. M. Lerner (Eds.), *Action and self-development: Theory and research through the life span* (pp. 315–342). Thousand Oaks, CA: Sage.

Oettingen, G. (2000). Expectancy effects on behavior depend on self-regulatory thought. *Social Cognition, 18,* 101–129.

Oettingen, G., & Gollwitzer, P. M. (2001). Goal setting and goal striving. In A. Tesser & N. Schwarz (Vol. Eds.), *Blackwell handbook of social psychology: Vol. 1. Intraindividual processes* (pp. 329–347). Oxford, England: Blackwell.

Oettingen, G., Hagenah, M., Mayer, D., Brinkmann, B., Pak, H., & Schmidt, L. (2006). *Mental contrasting and goal striving: Effects and mechanisms.* Manuscript under review.

Oettingen, G., Hönig, G., & Gollwitzer, P. M. (2000). Effective self-regulation of goal attainment. *International Journal of Educational Research, 33,* 705–732.

Oettingen, G., Mayer, D., & Thorpe, J. S. (2006). *Mental contrasting and smoking secession.* Unpublished manuscript, University of Hamburg, Hamburg, Germany.

Oettingen, G., Pak, H., & Schnetter, K. (2001). Self-regulation of goal setting: Turning free fantasies about the future into binding goals. *Journal of Personality and Social Psychology, 80,* 736–753.

Orbell, S., Hodgkins, S., & Sheeran, P. (1997). Implementation intentions and the theory of planned behavior. *Personality and Social Psychology Bulletin, 23,* 945–954.

Orbell, S., & Sheeran, P. (2000). Motivational and volitional processes in action initiation: A field study of the role of implementation intentions. *Journal of Applied Social Psychology, 30,* 780–797.

Rogers, R. W. (1983). Cognitive and physiological processes in fear appeals and attitude change: A revised theory of protection motivation. In J. T. Cacioppo & R. E. Petty (Eds.), *Social psychophysiology* (pp. 153–176). New York: Guilford Press.

Rosenstock, I. M. (1974). The health belief model and preventive health behavior. *Health Education Monographs, 2,* 354–386.

Scheier, M. F., & Carver, C. S. (1987). Dispositional optimism and physical well-being: The influence of generalized outcome expectancies on health. *Journal of Personality, 55,* 169–210.

Sheeran, P. (2002). Intention–behaviour relations: A conceptual and empirical review. In M. Hewstone & W. Stroebe (Eds.), *European review of social psychology* (Vol. 12, pp. 1–36). Chichester, England: Wiley.

Sheeran, P., & Orbell, S. (1999). Implementation intentions and repeated behavior: Augmenting the predictive validity of the theory of planned behavior. *European Journal of Social Psychology, 29,* 349–369.

Sheeran, P., & Orbell, S. (2000). Using implementation intentions to increase attendance for cervical cancer screening. *Health Psychology, 19,* 283–289.

Steller, B. (1992). *Vorsätze und die Wahrnehmung günstiger Gelegenheiten* [Implementation intentions and the detection of opportunities to act]. Munich, Germany: Tuduv-Studien.

Trötschel, R., & Gollwitzer, P. M. (in press). Implementation intentions and the willful pursuit of prosocial goals in negotiations. *Journal of Experimental Social Psychology.*

Vroom, V. H. (1964). *Work and motivation.* New York: Wiley.

Webb, T. L., & Sheeran, P. (2003). Can implementation intentions help to overcome ego-depletion? *Journal of Experimental Social Psychology, 39,* 279–286.

Wicklund, R. A., & Gollwitzer, P. M. (1982). *Symbolic self-completion.* Hillsdale, NJ: Erlbaum.

3

PROSPECTIVE MEMORY COMPONENTS MOST AT RISK FOR OLDER ADULTS AND IMPLICATIONS FOR MEDICATION ADHERENCE

MARK A. McDANIEL AND GILLES O. EINSTEIN

One aspect of following doctors' orders is to remember to implement prescribed actions, for example taking medication, at an appropriate moment in the future. In the basic memory literature this type of memory task has been termed *prospective memory*. With advancing age, health-related prospective memory demands accelerate because many diseases are associated with aging, thereby increasing requisite behaviors to treat and monitor those diseases. For instance, approximately half of all prescription medication is taken by older adults. A central issue regarding the impact of aging on remembering to follow medical instructions, remembering to take medication, and remembering to engage in health-monitoring behavior is the extent to which there are age-related declines in prospective memory.

Both authors contributed equally to this chapter and thus order of authorship is arbitrary.
Preparation of the chapter was supported by National Aeronautics and Space Administration Grant NCC-2-1085. The imagination inflation study was supported by National Institute on Aging Grant AG17481.

The initial theoretical speculation, as well as an intuitive orientation, has been that prospective memory tasks should be especially problematic for older adults. A seminal theoretical framework proposed by Craik (1986) reflects this expectation. In this view, a major determinant of age-related deficits in memory relates to the degree of self-initiated retrieval required by the memory task. For instance, a memory task such as recognition provides many environmental cues; in fact, a recognition task provides the target item itself on the test. Therefore, this kind of memory test would require low self-initiated retrieval processes. Instead, retrieval would be prompted by the cues provided on the test. Craik (1986) placed prospective memory at the end of this continuum of self-initiated retrieval requirements. The idea here is that prospective memory demands not only that people remember the particular action that is to be performed but also that they remember to perform that action when it is appropriate to do so. Such "remembering to remember" must be accomplished without an explicit request to remember at the appropriate moment (McDaniel & Einstein, 2000). So, in prospective memory the retrieval processes appear to be highly self-initiated. Consequently, on the basis of this framework, one would expect the most robust age-related deficits on a prospective memory task (relative to other kinds of memory tasks).

In this chapter our objective is to develop a more extended analysis of prospective memory that delineates among prospective memory tasks. This delineation of prospective memory tasks will be directly stimulated by considerations of the contexts related to following doctors' or other health care providers' instructions. Within the delineation, we characterize more precisely the prospective memory situations in which older adults are especially at risk for prospective memory failure. We also identify prospective memory situations and components that tend not to produce age differences.

To preview, we first distinguish event-based versus time-based prospective memory, noting that time-based prospective memory seems to parallel the everyday task of remembering to take medication. Our experimental results show prominent age-related deficits in time-based tasks more so than in event-based tasks. Yet, retrieval of the intention to take one's medication may not be as problematic as the single-trial prospective memory task typically studied in the laboratory because medication taking for older adults likely becomes habitual. However, habitual prospective memory tasks may create other memory challenges. After retrieving the intention to perform an action, one also has to assess whether that action has already been performed. Frequent thoughts about taking medication combined with the frequent actual taking of the medication (as is the case with a long-term prescription schedule) create great potential for reality confusions concerning whether one has recently taken the medication or simply thought about taking it. This kind of confusion can lead to failing to take a dose or repeating a dose. We describe our experimental research on habitual prospective memory that suggests that these kinds of reality-monitoring errors are more likely for older adults.

We next present some of our recent research suggesting that medication adherence in older adults may be especially susceptible to memory problems occurring after initial retrieval. Specifically, older adults seem to be particularly sensitive to distractions. Thus, after retrieving the intention to perform an action, distractions for periods as brief as 5 seconds dramatically decrease remembering. The chapter additionally offers some guidelines for how older adults might minimize their failures in medication-taking prospective memory tasks.

EVENT- VERSUS TIME-BASED PROSPECTIVE MEMORY

The first distinction that we think is important concerns a distinction between event-based prospective memory and time-based prospective memory (see Einstein & McDaniel, 1990). In an event-based prospective memory task, the occurrence of an environmental event signals the appropriateness of performing the intended action. For example, I may form the intention to take my blood pressure medicine when I have my cereal and juice in the morning. At breakfast the next morning, my cereal and juice can act as environmental cues or signals for triggering my memory to take my medication. To the extent that these cues do stimulate remembering of the intention, they reduce the self-initiated retrieval processing required for prospective memory. In contrast, for other prospective memory tasks it is appropriate to execute the action at a certain time or after a certain period of time has elapsed. For example, it may be appropriate to measure one's blood glucose level at a certain time of day. In terms of medication taking, the medication-taking regimen may require remembering after specified periods of elapsed time—say after every 4 or 5 hours if one is on a three-times-a-day regimen. For time-based tasks, there is no obvious and specific external cue that might help stimulate prospective remembering. Instead, for time-based tasks (in which no external reminding device like an alarm has been used) retrieval of the prospective memory intention should require high degrees of self-initiated processing. Thus, in accordance with Craik's (1986) framework, time-based tasks should show prominent age-related declines, whereas event-based prospective memory tasks may show much reduced, if any, age-related decline.

To test these predictions, we conducted a study with younger adults (18–22 years of age) and older adults (61–76 years of age) to examine performance on both event-based and time-based prospective memory tasks (Einstein, McDaniel, Richardson, Guynn, & Cunfer, 1995, Experiment 3).

TABLE 3.1
Proportion of Correct Prospective Memory Responses
(Out of 6 Possible)

Group	Event-based	Time-based
Younger		
Prop. correct	.93	.65
n	18	18
Older		
Prop. correct	.86	.32
n	13	13
Middle age		
Prop. correct	.93	.82
n	14	14

Note. Data from Einstein, McDaniel, Richardson, Guynn, and Cunfer (1995, Experiment 3).
Prop. = proportion.

Both types of prospective memory tasks were embedded in an identical ongoing activity. In one experiment the ongoing activity was a set of trivia questions for which participants were given four possible choices. Participants were asked to read the trivia questions and select the particular response that they thought was correct. Each response was then followed by 3 seconds of feedback. Both older and younger participants found this to be an engaging ongoing activity. In addition to this activity, participants were instructed that we had a secondary interest in their ability to remember to do something on their own. In the event-based prospective memory task, participants were instructed to press a designated key on the keyboard whenever they encountered a question about a U.S. president. The questions about the presidents were programmed to occur approximately every 5 minutes. On the parallel time-based prospective memory task, other participants were instructed that they should try to remember to press the designated key every 5 minutes. Participants in the time-based condition could assess the elapsed time by pressing the F1 key, which then briefly displayed the elapsed time on the monitor. On a vocabulary test, older participants performed slightly better than younger participants, so these were able and normally functioning older adults. In addition to the younger and older adult groups, in this experiment we included a middle-aged group (35–49 years of age) to provide information about where in the adult life span prospective memory decline might begin.

Table 3.1 displays the proportion of trials on which participants remembered to perform the prospective memory action. For the time-based task, correct responses were defined as those that occurred within a minute after the designated time. In addition, responses that were 15 seconds early or less before the designated elapsed time were counted as correct. As can be seen in Table 3.1, for event-based prospective memory there were virtually no differences in performance as a function of age group. Performance was relatively high for the younger, middle-aged, and older adults. In contrast, for the time-based prospective memory task, older adults showed a substantial and significant decline in prospective memory compared with the younger adults. In addition, middle-aged adults showed intact prospective memory performance, as good as that of the young and better than that of the older adults. This pattern of little or minimal age-related decline on event-based prospective memory and robust decline on time-based prospective memory appears to be reliable. The same pattern was found in two other experiments in this study using a different ongoing activity. In addition, Park, Hertzog, Kidder, Morrell, and Mayhorn (1997) reported the same pattern with yet another cover task and with somewhat different event-based prospective memory cues. They reported large age-related differences on the time-based task but small age-related differences on the event-based task (cf. d'Ydewalle, Luwel, & Brunfaut, 1999).

Thus, the time-based prospective memory task appears to be more problematic for older adults, and we suggest that the time-based prospective memory task is the one that most parallels the everyday task of remembering to take medication or remembering a doctor's appointment. That is, following doctors' instructions frequently involves a prospective memory task that appears to be especially challenging for older adults. Accordingly, we suggest that older adults might be apprised of the difficulty that they may encounter in remembering to take medication at certain times of the day or in remembering to take medication after a certain number of hours have elapsed since last taking the medication. Older adults might profit from external strategies such as using alarm clocks or watches with beepers to remind them to take medication. Perhaps even more useful from a practical standpoint would be to encourage older adults to convert their time-based medication-taking prospective memory tasks into event-based tasks. The idea here is that they integrate the medication-taking task into a prominent daily event. For example, one might remember to take medication while drinking juice at breakfast. One of the authors of this chapter has successfully used this strategy to help him to remember to take a newly prescribed medication. He decided to link taking the medication to eating dinner, so now the event "dinner" serves as a cue to stimulate remembering of the prospective memory medication activity.

HABITUAL PROSPECTIVE MEMORY

The results just reviewed may hold for temporary and ad hoc medication regimes, but they may not completely capture the age-related difficulties or absence of difficulties in an ongoing or extended medication-taking situation. Especially for older adults, medication regimens may be relatively chronic, even extending throughout the remainder of the individual's lifetime. Thus, for older adults the medication-taking task is something that is performed habitually over many days. We speculate that the habitual nature of the task likely minimizes the difficulties with remembering to perform the task (other than perhaps the first several days of being on the medication). However, the habitual nature of the task may introduce new problems for older adults. For instance, memories of taking the medication on previous days may make it difficult for older adults to remember whether or not they took the medication on that particular day (Park & Kidder, 1996). That is, older adults may forget the particular spatial–temporal context associated with their memory for taking the medication and thus have problems determining whether they took the medication that particular day. Another kind of source-monitoring problem that may occur with habitual prospective memory tasks is that there may be, over the course of the regimen, many times when the older adults think about taking the medication and many times when they actually take the medication. Thus, there may be problems differentiating doing the task from simply thinking about it.

We tested these possibilities in a paradigm that we developed to explore habitual prospective memory in the laboratory (Einstein, McDaniel, Smith, & Shaw, 1998). In our study, participants performed 11 different cover tasks with each task lasting 3 minutes. The cover tasks were designed to measure various cognitive and perceptual abilities and included things such as a perceptual speed task, a vocabulary task, and so on. The prospective memory task required participants to press a designated key during each cover task. The time-based component involved requiring participants to wait 30 seconds into each task before they were allowed to implement the prospective memory action. After each cover task we inserted a brief questionnaire that asked participants whether they had performed the prospective memory task during the preceding cover activity.

Age was one variable; half of the participants were older adults with a mean age of 70.3 years and half were younger adults with a mean age of 19.8 years. In addition, we manipulated the ongoing demands. For half of the participants in each age group, attention was divided with a digit detection task. So, half of the participants simply performed the cover activity and tried to remember the prospective memory action, whereas the other half of the participants had to perform a digit-monitoring activity in addition to the other tasks. We reasoned that the addition of the digit-monitoring activity would help approximate older adults' performance during times when they were especially busy.

Figure 3.1 shows the proportion of omission errors on the prospective memory task as a function of age and attention condition. Inspection of

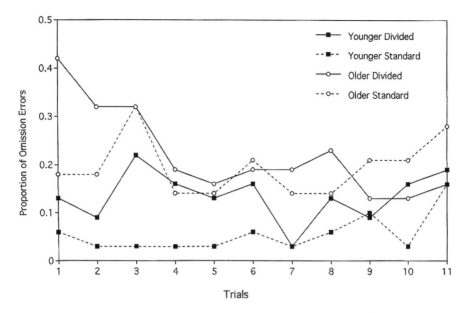

Figure 3.1. Mean proportion of omission errors. From "Habitual Prospective Memory and Aging: Remembering Intentions and Forgetting Actions," by G. O. Einstein, M. A. McDaniel, R. E. Smith, and P. Shaw, 1998, *Psychological Science, 9*, p. 287. Copyright 1998 by Blackwell Publishing. Reprinted with permission.

Figure 3.1 shows that on Trial 1 older adults, especially those in the divided attention (i.e., busy) condition, were more likely to forget to perform the prospective memory activity than younger adults were. This finding parallels the earlier findings that we discussed showing age-related declines on time-based prospective memory. However, as the trials proceeded so that the prospective memory task presumably became more habitual, older and younger adults quickly performed well on this task. Both age groups, regardless of the presence of a divided attention task, achieved performance that was 80% or better.

Figure 3.2 displays the proportion of repetition errors. These are the trials on which participants performed the prospective memory task more than once. As can be seen from Figure 3.2, the pattern of repetition errors is very different. On initial trials there were very few repetition errors and no differences between older and younger adults. But, by about the 4th trial and continuing on through the 11th trial, older adults in the divided attention condition showed a marked increase in repetition errors. By the 11th trial older adults in the divided attention condition were repeating the prospective memory activity nearly half of the time. Relating this to a medication-taking task, such behavior would represent overmedicating, presumably because of a failure to correctly remember that the action (taking

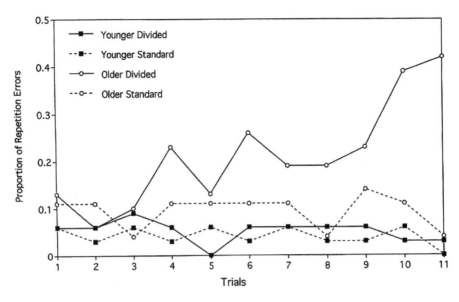

Figure 3.2. Mean proportion of repetition errors. From "Habitual Prospective Memory and Aging: Remembering Intentions and Forgetting Actions," by G. O. Einstein, M. A. McDaniel, R. E. Smith, and P. Shaw, 1998, *Psychological Science, 9*, p. 286. Copyright 1998 by Blackwell Publishing. Reprinted with permission.

medication) had been performed during the prescribed interval and consequently performing it again.

Further analyses revealed yet a different kind of error: trials for which an omission error occurred and for which participants reported in the questionnaire that they remembered pressing the key. Compared with younger adults, older adults in both the standard and divided attention condition showed an increase on the proportion of trials on which they made this kind of omission error (standard, .07; divided, .08), with younger adults rarely displaying this type of error (standard, .02; divided, .02). Relating such errors to the medication-taking situation would reflect instances in which older adults believed that they took the medication during the preceding interval and as a consequence omitted the behavior, thereby undermedicating.

These initial results show that the mnemonic challenges of a habitual prospective memory task change qualitatively over trials, and age-related decrements are not captured by a single type of failure. Further, difficulties for older adults are dramatically amplified under demanding attentional conditions. We believe that these demanding attentional conditions might be reflective of everyday circumstances in which the person is busily engaged in the activities of the day. We must caution, however, that the present results may not be entirely accurate estimates of the different kinds of difficulties and memory errors displayed by older adults in medically related habitual tasks. In everyday memory situations it may be that older adults, as well as younger adults, take a more conservative approach, which would lead to greater errors in undermedicating.

In addition, in the real world, medication-taking tasks for older adults are more complicated than simply taking one medication or remembering to perform one prospective memory activity. Park and Kidder (1996) reported 1981 World Health Organization data indicating that 34% of older adults take three or more medications daily. At the conference on which the chapters in this volume are based,[1] there were numerous examples of the complexity of the medication-taking demands for older adults. One example was a situation in which an older adult needed to remember to begin tapering a medication over the course of 2 weeks while at the same time maintaining other medications, and perhaps initiating a new medication as well. In this situation one might imagine that the types of memory illusions that were hinted at in the Einstein et al. (1998) results would become even more exaggerated. In these situations, one has numerous medications that are being taken, with these demands perhaps prompting more thoughts about taking the medication, and taking one medication might prompt thinking about other medications that need to be started or need to be related to the present medication.

IMAGINATION INFLATION AND AGING

To more closely approximate this scenario in which several medical actions are being performed, of which some are being thought about and some are both being performed and thought about, McDaniel, Butler, and Dornburg (2006) recently conducted an experiment patterned on the Goff and Roediger (1998) paradigm in which participants are given a list of action events. For example, the event statement might be "roll the toy car across the desk" or "tug your ear lobe" (Cohen, 1981). Some of the action events were performed by the participant. For other action phrases, participants were instructed to think about or imagine performing that action. And for still another set of action phrases, participants both performed and imagined the event. Two weeks later, participants returned to the laboratory and were given a list of action statements, some of which were not previously presented in the experiment and others were previously presented in the experiment. Participants were asked to report whether they initially imagined

---

[1] As noted in the preface, this volume is the result of a conference sponsored by the Roybal Center for Aging and Cognition: Health, Education, and Training (sponsored by the National Institute on Aging).

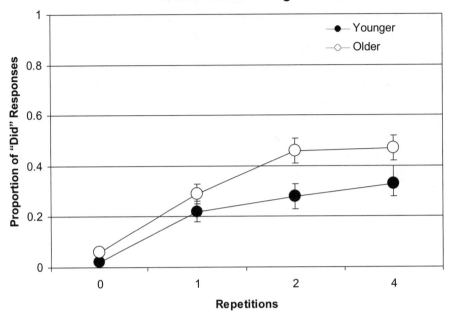

Source Errors - Imagined Items

Figure 3.3. Proportion of only-imagined action phrases that were remembered as having been performed by the participant.

performing the action, performed the action, or both. Although this research was not conducted in medication contexts, it is plausible to assume that people often think about (perhaps even imagine) taking their medication throughout the day, and these thoughts could potentially create confusions for the person regarding whether he or she only thought about taking the medication or actually took it.

Figure 3.3 shows a portion of these data. In the figure, we present the proportion of times younger and older participants indicated that they performed a particular stated action as a function of the number of times that they only imagined this action. In other words, these responses represent the memory illusion of performing an action that was only imagined. For younger adults, Figure 3.3 shows the typical imagination inflation effect reported by Goff and Roediger (1998). In this effect, participants increasingly report that they did in fact perform the action as they more often imagine performing the action. The important and new finding for present purposes is that this imagination inflation effect is significantly greater for older adults than for younger adults. When the action was never presented, younger and older adults were not likely to indicate that they performed the action. However, if the action was previously imagined as few as two times, over half of the time older adults reported that they actually performed the action. This is a substantial increase over the 30% rate reported by younger adults.

The foregoing finding relates to our report from Einstein et al. (1998) on the habitual prospective memory experiment in which older adults were more likely to omit a response because they reported that they had remembered performing it. The present results suggest that such difficulties for older adults may be more exaggerated in an everyday context in which many medication tasks are being performed and thought about. In these situations older adults may have profound difficulties in remembering whether they actually took medication or simply imagined doing so. In cases in which older adults just think about taking medication on a particular day, they may frequently believe that they took the medication and thus mistakenly omit taking the medication for the day.

TECHNIQUES TO AVOID CONFUSING "DOING" WITH "IMAGINING"

Though preliminary, we believe that these data may signal to health practitioners that there is a concern about possible source illusions leading to either under- or overmedication for older adults taking numerous medications on a habitual basis. Accordingly, we suggest that older adults should be encouraged to adopt techniques that would help them avoid confusions between doing and imagining in everyday health-related memory activities. Along these lines, external aids can be quite helpful. These aids might include a tear-off calendar with daily pages. When the person has performed the medication task, he or she can record it on the page or tear out the page. Either of these actions provides an external record that the task was either completed or not. A related technique might be to use a check-off chart or a daily log for each medication. When the medication has been taken, one can check off that fact and thereby provide an external record. Park reported (at the conference on which this volume is based; see Footnote 1) that the chart technique is especially effective for the oldest adults (over age 80). Another popular external aid is the medication-taking organizers in which medication or vitamins are put into separate compartments for each day of the week and for each time of the day (see chap. 1, this volume). One point emphasized during the conference was that when medication has to be repeatedly taken through various times of the day, these organizers seem to be especially helpful in preventing confusions.

Sometimes external aids are not available, and in these cases it would be useful to alert older adults to other techniques. These techniques generally force the individual to pay full attention to the medication-taking activity while doing it. Such a strategy conforms well to our data showing that when older adults are not especially busy and thus presumably can pay attention to performing the prospective memory task, there appear to be minimal problems with remembering whether or not they performed the task during a particular interval (Einstein et al., 1998). The following are some recommended techniques and instructions that would force older adults to not be distracted while performing the task:

1. Focus on the task while doing it, perhaps by paying attention to exaggerated or particular sensory and/or motor experiences. For example, you could swirl the pill around in your mouth and think about the swirling of the pill.

2. Say the task aloud while doing it. This verbalization provides additional sensory information to produce a distinctive memory record (see Bahrick & Boucher, 1968) that is discriminable from just thinking about doing the task. In addition, saying the task out loud as you are doing it focuses attention on the task.

3. Perform the task in an unusual or maybe a silly way; for instance, you might cross your arms to place the medication into your mouth. Or you might place your hand on your head as you put the medication in your mouth (see Ramuschkat, McDaniel, Kliegel, & Einstein, 2006, for data supporting the effectiveness of this technique). These unusual postures should help you distinguish taking the medication from intruding memories from other days in which you took the medication or from thinking about taking the medication. In addition, they also require you to pay more attention to performing the task.

4. Try to integrate the task into a more complex event that itself is likely not to be forgotten. For example, integrate taking the morning medication with taking the juice out of the refrigerator, pouring the juice, and then taking the medication with the first sip. You are likely to remember executing this extended routine and consequently can remember that you have taken the medication for the day.

THE EFFECTS OF DELAYS AND INTERRUPTIONS ON REMEMBERING TO PERFORM AN ACTION

An important aspect of effective medication adherence is remembering to take one's medication at the appropriate point in time. Much experimental research investigating performance on prospective memory tasks resembles medication adherence conditions (e.g., the event- and time-based prospective memory research described earlier), and this research along with our intuition about the nature of medication adherence suggests that initial retrieval of the intention to take one's medication at the appropriate point in time may not be the most severe problem in the real world. Real-world medication-taking is often prompted by external support. As described earlier, to the extent that we associate an external event with a time-based task (e.g., convert the task of taking a pill at 8:00 a.m. to taking a pill at breakfast), prospective memory will improve and show minimal age differences. Moreover, in everyday life, people use calendars, pillboxes, and notes; respond to signals from aches and pains; and finally many tasks become habitual. Recently, we have begun to wonder whether the more problematic aspect of accurately following a medication regimen might not occur after retrieval. In this section, we develop some of our recent work indicating that successful prospective memory is not assured just because the intention to remember is consciously retrieved at the appropriate moment.

A feature of event-based prospective memory tasks that have thus far been studied in the laboratory is that participants are asked to perform an action as soon as a target event occurs. For example, in the event-based task that we discussed earlier in which participants were asked to answer trivia questions and at the same time to press a designated key on the keyboard when they saw a question about a president, participants were allowed to respond immediately after seeing the word *president*. We believe that there are many real-world analogs of this kind of prospective memory task. For example, one's task might be to give a colleague a message, and on seeing the colleague, often you can deliver the message immediately. In terms of medication adherence, your task might be to take a pill with breakfast, and on getting to the breakfast table, you think about taking your pill and often you can act on that intention immediately.

However, in prospective remembering situations in everyday life, frequently after retrieving an intention people have to delay an action until the conditions are appropriate for performing it. To continue the previous example, on seeing your colleague, he or she may be busily involved in a conversation, and thus you might need to maintain the intention for a period of time until there is a pause in the conversation. Or, you might retrieve the thought to take your medication when you are in the bedroom, but then have to keep the thought activated until you get to the kitchen where you keep you pills. Another likely event is that after remembering to take your pill with breakfast, the phone rings or you are interrupted with a question, and thus you must remember to take your pill after the interruption.

A story that is currently making the rounds over e-mail among elderly people captures the prevalence of delays and interruptions and their effects on everyday life. A portion of this story is as follows:

> They have finally found a diagnosis for my condition. Hooray!! I have recently been diagnosed with AAADD, which is Age Activated Attention Deficit Disorder. This is how it goes: I decide to wash the car; I start toward the garage and notice mail on the table. OK, I'm going to wash the car. But first I am going to go through the mail. I lay the car keys down on the desk, discard the junk mail, and I notice the trashcan is full. OK, I will just put the bills on my desk and take the trashcan out, but since I'm going to be near the mailbox anyway, I'll pay these few bills first. Now, where is my checkbook? Oh, there is the Coke that I was drinking, I'm going to look for those checks. But first I need to put my Coke farther away from the computer . . .

It turns out that this person does not accomplish anything during the day because each intended action is interrupted by a new task. Stories of this type as well as reflection on our own lives suggest that delays and interruptions are common in the real world. The following research examines whether people have difficulty maintaining intentions over brief delays and whether this might be especially difficult for older adults.

It seemed to us that once an intention is retrieved and a delay is encountered, people try to actively maintain the intention in working memory through rehearsal. Given the well-documented age-related decrements in working memory resources (Craik & Jennings, 1992; Park et al., 2002), we expected large age differences in the ability to maintain intentions over brief delays. The basic idea here is that it would be difficult for older adults to actively rehearse an intention while also attending to the demands associated with the cover activities. Indeed, recent definitions of working memory conceptualize it as something that should be critical for maintaining intentions over brief delays. Engle, Tuholski, Laughlin, and Conway (1999) defined it as the ability to keep a representation active, particularly in the face of distraction. For Kimberg and Farah (1993), working memory reflects the ability to maintain an integrated representation of the task context or current task concerns. Maintaining current goals and keeping them activated while involved in other activities seems exactly what one does when an intended action is delayed, and thus from this prospective we expected to find significant age differences.

An alternative expectation rests on our procedure of using brief delays (5–30 seconds in length), with little activity going on during some of the delays. Under these conditions, rehearsal strategies would seem easy to initiate and maintain (see Reitman, 1971). From this perspective, one might expect that maintaining intentions during brief delays might not be problematic for either younger or older adults.

To examine this issue, we (Einstein, McDaniel, Manzi, Cochran, & Baker, 2000) involved people in a prospective memory task in which they had to delay an execution of a response after retrieving the intention (hereinafter we refer to this as a *delayed-execute task*). Participants in this experiment were told that our major goal was to examine their comprehension of three-sentence paragraphs. They were told that they would receive 20 trials of these paragraphs and on each trial they would (a) read three sentences about an event (presented one at a time), (b) experience a 10- to 30-second delay that was either filled with performing a synonym task or unfilled (i.e., simply a break), (c) answer two unrelated trivia questions, and (d) answer two multiple-choice comprehension questions about the sentences. Once participants understood the nature of this task, we told them that we had an additional interest in their ability to remember to perform an action in the future. Specifically, they were told that whenever they saw the words *TECHNIQUE* or *SYSTEM*, they were to press the F1 key on the keyboard, but not until they reached the trivia questions. Thus, when it occurred, the target word *TECHNIQUE* or *SYSTEM* was presented in the third sentence of a paragraph, and participants needed to maintain the intention over the 10- to 30-second delay period until they reached the trivia questions.

An important methodological point is that the word *TECHNIQUE* or *SYSTEM* was presented in uppercase letters, whereas the other words in the sentences were presented in lowercase letters. We purposely created distinctive target events because we wanted participants to retrieve the intention to perform the action to press the F1 key whenever these target events occurred. It is important to note that we tested younger and older immediate control groups to examine whether participants were indeed able to retrieve the intention when the target events occurred. In these groups, the participants were asked to press the key immediately on seeing the target events *TECHNIQUE* or *SYSTEM*. Except for one older participant who failed to press the key on nearly all trials, performance was virtually perfect for both younger and older adults (97% and 95% correct, respectively). This high performance indicates that participants were retrieving the intention to press the key when these very distinctive target events occurred, and thus we were assured that performance after the delay nearly always reflected the ability to maintain the intention over the delay rather than initial retrieval of the intention.

Our younger participants were traditional-age college students, and our older participants averaged 68.7 years of age and were very healthy community-dwelling older adults who significantly outperformed the younger participants on a vocabulary test. With unfilled intervals, our expectation was that both younger and older adults would have the resources needed to actively maintain the intention in working memory during these break periods. By contrast, we expected large age differences during filled

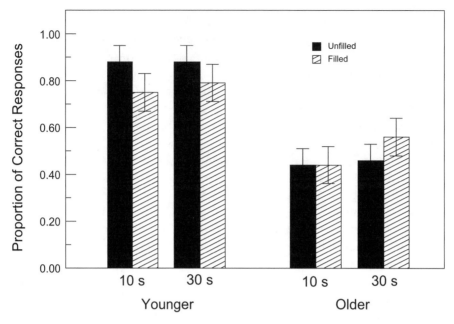

Figure 3.4. Mean proportion of delayed-execute responses. Error bars reflect the standard error of the mean. s = seconds. From "Prospective Memory and Aging: Forgetting Intentions Over Short Delays," by G. O. Einstein, M. A. McDaniel, M. Manzi, B. Cochran, and M. Baker, 2000, *Psychology and Aging, 15*, p. 678. Copyright 2000 by the American Psychological Association.

delays (i.e., when participants were performing the synonym task), mainly because it should be difficult for resource-limited older adults to actively rehearse the intention while also solving the synonym problems. As can be seen in Figure 3.4, younger participants tended to do very well on this task, as they remembered on about 82% of the trials. Older adults, by contrast, showed dramatic declines with performance averaging 44% (compared with 95% when they could respond immediately). Indeed, in what would seem the easiest condition, 10 seconds with unfilled delays, older adults remembered on only 47% of the trials. Thus, maintaining intentions over brief delay seems to be especially difficult for older adults.

Two other features of the data are worth noting. One is that there was not increased forgetting in the longer delay relative to the shorter delay. The other is that younger participants remembered more often with unfilled delays, whereas for the older participants prospective remembering was nominally better with filled delays. The fact that older adults did poorly in general, even with unfilled delays, suggests that the source of their memory problem may be more than resource limitations. Specifically, the poor retention of the intention even over unfilled delays suggests that older adults do not try to strategically maintain the intended action in working memory. It is possible that older adults, who are generally less aware of the appropriate memory strategy to use in different situations (i.e., metamemory), are less sensitive to the fleeting nature of passively stored information. The idea here is that on seeing one of the target items, older adults may find the retrieved intention very vivid in memory and unforgettable. Because of this, older adults may be unaware that the trace duration of unrehearsed information is around 2 seconds (Muter, 1980; Schweickert & Boruff, 1986) and that maintenance of the intention over the kinds of delays used in this research requires strategic rehearsal.

In the next experiment (McDaniel, Einstein, Stout, & Morgan, 2003, Experiment 1), we examined the effects of strong rehearsal instructions for older adults. This experiment was just like the previous one except for the fact that we used shorter delays (5 and 15 seconds) and included an older-adult rehearsal condition. Participants in the rehearsal group received strong instructions warning them of the fleeting nature of retrieved intentions. We also told them that after seeing a target item, they needed to actively rehearse the intended action "trivia press key" until they got to the trivia task. To help ensure that older participants activated this rehearsal strategy, we flashed the word REHEARSE three times in the last 4 seconds of the screen containing the sentence with the target word TECHNIQUE or SYSTEM.

As shown in Figure 3.5, the results for the younger-control and older-control conditions parallel closely the results in the previous experiment. That is, younger adults rarely forgot to perform the intended action (they remembered on 85% of the trials), there was no effect of the length of the delay, and performance was nominally higher with unfilled delays than with filled delays. For older adults, in the control condition, performance was quite low (46%), there was no effect of the length of the delay, and performance was mixed across filled and unfilled delays. Again, the dramatic nature of older adults' rapid loss of an intention is reinforced by performance at only 45% after a 5-second unfilled delay, presumably the easiest condition.

As can be seen in the bars on the right of Figure 3.5, rehearsal instructions had surprisingly modest effects in helping participants maintain an intention over delay. Although older rehearsal participants were nominally better than the older control participants at each of the four types of delays, they were significantly better only with 5-second unfilled delays. Moreover, strong rehearsal instructions did not bring the level performance of the older participants up to that of the younger participants.

The finding that rehearsal instructions improved remembering, at least with 5-second unfilled delays, suggests that older adults do not spontaneously rehearse an intended action after encountering a delay. As mentioned earlier, this could be due to a metamemory problem. But the age-associated problem

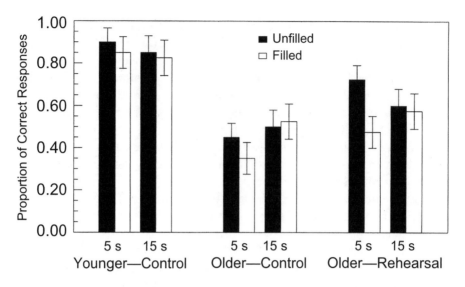

Figure 3.5. Mean proportion of delayed-execute responses for young and old control participants and rehearsal-instructed older adults. Error bars reflect the standard error of the mean. s = seconds. From "Aging and Maintaining Intentions Over Delays: Do It or Lose It," by M. A. McDaniel, G. O. Einstein, A. C. Stout, and Z. Morgan, 2003, *Psychology and Aging, 18*, p. 825. Copyright 2003 by the American Psychological Association.

appears to be more profound than this. Even when instructed to rehearse, older adults seem unable to sustain a strategic rehearsal process. This inability to maintain rehearsal could be due to working memory resource limitations (Craik & Jennings, 1992), which prevent older adults from actively rehearsing while also performing the cover activities (i.e., solving the synonym problems). It seems, however, that one needs to go beyond resource limitations and metamemory problems to explain the relatively poor performance of older rehearsal participants even with unfilled delays.

Perhaps difficulties in inhibiting irrelevant information (Hasher & Zacks, 1988; Hasher, Zacks, & May, 1999) make older adults generally more susceptible to distraction, and this interferes with a strategic rehearsal process. For example, older adults in the rehearsal condition might initiate a strategic rehearsal process during an unfilled delay and then happen to look around the room and outside through the window and see a bud growing on a tree. This might remind them that it is time to dig up their vegetable garden, and pretty soon they are thinking about their spring planting and no longer rehearsing. Similarly, during filled delays, after seeing the item *penurious* and realizing that it means *stingy*, older participants might begin to think of their stingy neighbor who never buys glasses of lemonade from their grandchildren. To the extent that older adults are easily distracted by these kinds of thoughts, it will be difficult to sustain an effective rehearsal strategy.

Regardless of which explanation is more accurate, it seems clear that older adults have real difficulty in keeping thoughts activated in working memory over brief delays. If this is a major problem for them, then their performance should be more dependent on favorable conditions present at encoding and retrieval. Our thinking here is that there are multiple ways to perform on a delayed-execute prospective memory task. One way is to actively maintain the intention over the delay, and younger adults seem to be able to do this effectively. The other is to retrieve the intention from long-term memory at the end of the delay (i.e., when the trivia task is encountered). So, in lieu of actively maintaining the intention over the delay in working memory, participants might do fairly well on this task by reformulating their intentions when the target event occurs. That is, on seeing the target word *TECHNIQUE* or *SYSTEM*, they could specifically form the intention to "press the key when the trivia task appears." Marsh, Hicks, and Landau (1998) showed that people frequently report reformulating their plans in real-world situations in response to new constraints. To the extent that participants tend to rely on reformulating their plans and retrieval from long-term memory, their performance should be highly sensitive to conditions at encoding and retrieval. Thus, in the next experiment, we varied the resources available at encoding and retrieval. Our expectation was that reducing attentional resources at encoding and retrieval should be more detrimental for older adults.

This experiment (McDaniel et al., 2003, Experiment 2) used the same three-sentence-paragraph comprehension task used in the previous two experiments. In this experiment, however, the delays on all trials consisted of 10 seconds of solving two synonym problems. Attention was divided at encoding on half of the trials by adding a digit detection task. The digits for this task were presented at the rate of one every 2 seconds, and the task of the participants was to press a lever on a handheld counter whenever they detected two consecutive odd-numbered digits. Resources at retrieval were manipulated by varying whether the prompt for performing the action was trivia questions or simply a break. The idea here was that presenting trivia items would capture the attention of participants and perhaps interfere with the retrieval of the intention from long-term memory.

As can be seen in Figure 3.6, the results were consistent with our expectations. Younger participants again performed at a higher level than older participants, but it is important to note that dividing attention had a smaller effect for younger participants (a reduction of 9%) than for older participants (a reduction of 24%). Also, presenting trivia items at the

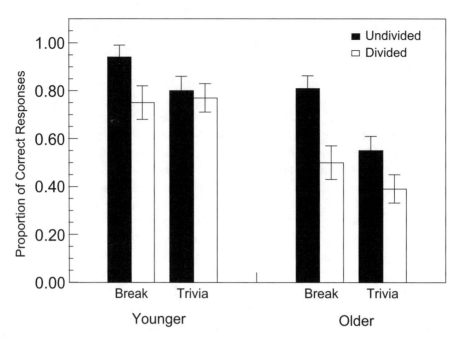

Figure 3.6. Mean proportion of delayed-execute responses for young and old adults as a function of resource demands at initial retrieval (encoding) and at execution. Error bars reflect the standard error of the mean. From "Aging and Maintaining Intentions Over Delays: Do It or Lose It," by M. A. McDaniel, G. O. Einstein, A. C. Stout, and Z. Morgan, 2003, *Psychology and Aging, 18*, p. 829. Copyright 2003 by the American Psychological Association.

execution relative to the break had a smaller effect for younger participants (average reduction of 6%) than for older participants (average reduction of 19%). It is also interesting to note that under the most favorable conditions, full attention at encoding and a break at retrieval, older adults did relatively well (on average they remembered on 81% of the trials).

In summary, there seem to be multiple ways to remember after encountering a delay. One can rely on working memory resources to actively maintain the intention. Our results showing that dividing attention during the delay period (with synonym problems relative to a break period) decreased performance more for younger adults than for older adults support the view that younger people seem to rely on the strategy. One can also rely on retrieval of the intention from long-term memory when one reaches the appropriate point for executing the action. Our findings that older adults were less affected by the division of attention during the delay phase and yet more affected by the availability of resources at encoding and retrieval suggest that they were more dependent on plan reformulation and retrieval from long-term memory.

Fundamental Age-Related Decrements in Keeping Goals Activated

Our empirical results converge with a number of theoretical views that suggest that older adults should have fundamental problems in keeping goals activated. As noted earlier, recent views of working memory define it as the ability to maintain the representation of information in the face of distraction. In more specific terms, Kane, Bleckley, Conway, and Engle (2001) suggested that working memory reflects the general "ability to effectively maintain stimulus, goal, or context information in an active, easily accessible state in the face of interference" (p. 180). Hasher and Zacks (1988; see also Hasher et al., 1999) believe that older adults are highly susceptible to distraction from internal (one's own thoughts) and external (events in the environment) sources. Problems of this type would surely affect the ability to maintain the activation of intentions. Further, Johnson, Reeder, Raye, and Mitchell (2002) believed that there are age-related deficits "in a specific reflective process, refresh, which operates during ongoing cognition to prolong or increase activation of information that is potentially relevant to task goals" (p. 67). All of these views converge on the idea that older adults have a core problem in keeping representation activated, and we believe that delayed prospective memory tasks are examples of highly prevalent, real-world tasks that depend heavily on this core ability.

PRESCRIPTIONS FOR OVERCOMING THE EFFECTS OF DELAYS AND INTERRUPTIONS

What can older adults do to minimize the forgetting that results from delays and interruptions? At a general level, it seems that lists of planned activities will be useful. Because it is difficult for older adults to maintain current intentions in the face of distraction, it is useful to have external support or cuing to keep one on task. For the older adult described earlier who believes that he has age-activated attention-deficit disorder, frequently consulting a list of the day's plans will help keep him on task.

For overcoming those momentary delays and unpredictable interruptions that invariably occur in people's daily lives, we suggest that it may be useful to develop a physical cue of some type. Participants in our experiments sometimes develop a physical cue such as crossing their fingers until the end of the delay. We prevent them from using these strategies in our studies, but our impression is that they are very useful, an impression consistent with findings using the paradigm described earlier (Rendell, Ozgis, & Wallis, 2004). The idea is that this physical cue will serve as an external reminder and after the delay or interruption can cue a person to remember that there is an uncompleted task that needs to be finished. Given the difficulties that older adults have in cognitively maintaining an intention, this external physical cue should be quite effective.

Another technique may be somewhat difficult to implement in busy situations but is likely to be very effective. Following from the impressive research of Gollwitzer (1999; see also chap. 2, this volume), forming a detailed implementation intention at the time of the delay or interruption should be very effective. Implementation intentions involve forming detailed plans of how and when one will perform an action. Thus, if the goal is to remember to stop and pick up a book at the library, rather than just forming a general intention, Gollwitzer has shown that people can greatly improve their chances of following through on that intention by imagining the visual scene of walking to the library and then imagining walking in the library and checking out the book. According to Gollwitzer, when one forms this kind of detailed implementation intention, one no longer needs to actively maintain the intention over the delay period and instead can rely on a relatively automatic retrieval process that is cued by seeing the library.

Research has shown that implementation intentions can increase the probability with which women actually carry out breast self-examination (Orbell, Hodgkins, & Sheeran, 1997), the likelihood that college students will follow through on plans to exercise (Milne, Orbell, & Sheeran, 2002), and the probability that people will eat healthful foods (Verplanken & Faes, 1999). In an experiment using a laboratory prospective memory paradigm with college-student participants (McDaniel, Howard, & Butler, 2006, Experiment 1), we found positive effects of implementation intentions for prospective memory. Participants given implementation intentions ($n = 18$) improved to an average of 92% correct compared with a control group ($n = 16$) performance of 64% correct. Further, half of the participants in the control group forgot the prospective memory task on at least one trial, whereas less than a quarter of the participants in the implementation-intention group showed forgetting. Liu and Park (2004) showed that older adults' prospective memory for a health behavior (checking blood glucose levels) also benefited from implementation intentions. Similary, Chasteen, Park, and Schwarz (2001) reported that older adults more than doubled the probability that they would carry out an action in the future when using an implementation intention.

Therefore, ideally, when a person is interrupted, what the person should do is to imagine where he or she will be after the interruption and imagine performing the interrupted activity at that point. For example, the person could say to himself or herself,

> If I remember to take my medication while I am in the bedroom but I anticipate a delay because my medication is in the kitchen, what I

should do is to imagine myself walking into the kitchen and then taking my medication.

Even though it will take a short while to get to the kitchen and even though the person may experience several interruptions during the delay (perhaps a conversation or two), entering the kitchen should now cue the thought to take the medication.

One problem with forming implementation intentions is that focused attention and ample time are needed to develop a specific plan of when and where the person will perform an action. In many cases, when one is interrupted, one simply does not have the time to form an implementation intention before dealing with the interruption. Also, depending on the demands of the interruption, one is unlikely to think of using an external physical cue or developing an implementation intention. In these cases, our recommendation is that people weigh the importance of the current task relative to the interruption. Whenever the current task is quite important, our recommendation is to be sensitive to the fact that delays cause a good deal of forgetting of intentions of older adults and thus to perform the action right away. In fact, our research suggests that one should "do it or lose it."

It is not often the case that your own research changes your behavior, but both of us have been impressed by the magnitude of the forgetting of the intentions over brief delays. Thus, whenever we can, we perform actions right away. For example, if our intention is to take our medication and the phone rings, rather than picking up the phone, we now take the medication and then listen to the message on our answering machine. As another example, when constructing an e-mail message and getting the thought to include an attachment, we attach the file as soon as we think of it rather than waiting until the end of the message. It is surprising to realize the number of e-mail messages that we have received (even from prospective memory researchers) in which the intended attached file was not appended. We think this is because our mental set is to append the file at the end of writing a note, and one can easily lose this intention over the course of writing a letter. The basic suggestion here is, whenever possible, all of us, but especially older adults, should act on an intention immediately.

SUMMARY

Although there have not been many studies examining medication adherence in older adults in natural contexts, those that have been conducted are very encouraging. Park et al. (1999) examined the ability of different age groups to follow a medication regimen for rheumatoid arthritis and found that older adults age 60 to 75 were the least likely (relative to other age groups) to make errors in medication taking even though all of them were taking four or more medications. Morrell, Park, Kidder, and Martin (1997) found similar results in a study examining medication adherence for hypertension. Although older adults show age-related declines on a variety of cognitive tests when tested in the laboratory (see chap. 1, this volume), in retrospect, the results of these studies are not completely surprising. The older adults tested in these studies were healthy and community dwelling, and they were likely to be highly motivated to perform well in the research. Also, compared with other cognitive demands such as comprehending and retaining the information in this volume, the amount of information in a medication regimen is not typically extensive (although it can get complex, especially with many medications, when the dosages change, and when there are complex dependencies among the medications). Moreover, the real world allows the use of a variety of external cues, such as pillboxes, and often there are physical symptoms (like aches) that can cue medication taking. Also, as found by Park and her colleagues, less frantic and busy lifestyles were associated with better medication adherence, and older adults tend to have less hectic daily demands in their lives. Thus, at least with the kinds of illnesses and populations used in existing studies, medication adherence does not seem to be especially difficult for community-dwelling older adults (see Wilson & Park, in press, for a recent review).

It should be recognized, however, that there is evidence that measures of cognitive functioning predict medication adherence in the real world (Hinkin et al., 2004; Insel, Morrow, Brewer, & Figueredo, 2006) and that older adults are at risk for cognitive decline. Also, when medication failures do occur, they may have more dire consequences for older adults, whose health is generally more fragile. Also, although older adults tend to outperform middle-aged adults in these studies, it is still the case that many medication errors occur. In Park et al.'s (1999) study, for example, 53% of the older adults made at least one error over the month-long study. The results described in this chapter, derived from highly controlled laboratory research, are useful for alerting us to the medication conditions that should be especially difficult for older adults and for suggesting remedies in these situations. Our results indicate that medication regimens that are strictly interpreted as time-based tasks may be particularly problematic for older adults because these kinds of tasks do not provide people with a good external cue that can prompt retrieval. We also believe the tasks that eventually become habitual cause problems for older adults, not because they fail to retrieve the intention to take their medication, but rather because confusion can arise about whether or not they have already performed the action. As described in this chapter, problems of this sort could lead to either undermedication or overmedication. Also, our recent research suggests that delays and interruptions, which are highly prevalent in the real world, can dramatically affect remembering when to perform an action.

These results articulate well with generally found age-associated problems in self-initiated retrieval, source monitoring, and working memory. We believe that awareness and understanding of the cognitive problems that are most affected by age and how these relate to the cognitive processes involved in medication adherence situations are useful for signaling those medication situations for which older adults are most at risk.

REFERENCES

Bahrick, H. P., & Boucher, B. (1968). Retention of visual and verbal codes of the same stimuli. *Journal of Experimental Psychology, 78*, 417–422.

Chasteen, A. L., Park, D. C., & Schwarz, N. (2001). Implementation intentions and facilitation of prospective memory. *Psychological Science, 12*, 457–461.

Cohen, R. L. (1981). On the generality of some memory laws. *Scandinavian Journal of Psychology, 22*, 267–281.

Craik, F. I. M. (1986). A functional account of age differences in memory. In F. Klix & H. Hangendorf (Eds.), *Human memory and cognitive capabilities: Mechanisms and performances* (pp. 409–422). Amsterdam: Elsevier.

Craik, F. I. M., & Jennings, J. M. (1992). Human memory. In F. I. M. Craik & T. A. Salthouse (Eds.), *The handbook of aging and cognition* (pp. 51–110). Hillsdale, NJ: Erlbaum.

d'Ydewalle, G., Luwel, K., & Brunfaut, E. (1999). The importance of on-going concurrent activities as a function of age in time- and event-based prospective memory. *European Journal of Cognitive Psychology, 11*, 219–237.

Einstein, G. O., & McDaniel, M. A. (1990). Normal aging and prospective memory. *Journal of Experimental Psychology: Learning, Memory, and Cognition, 16*, 717–726.

Einstein, G. O., McDaniel, M. A., Manzi, M., Cochran, B., & Baker, M. (2000). Prospective memory and aging: Forgetting intentions over short delays. *Psychology and Aging, 15*, 671–683.

Einstein, G. O., McDaniel, M. A., Richardson, S. L., Guynn, M. J., & Cunfer, A. R. (1995). Aging and prospective memory: Examining the influences of self-initiated retrieval processes. *Journal of Experimental Psychology: Learning, Memory, and Cognition, 21*, 996–1007.

Einstein, G. O., McDaniel, M. A., Smith, R. E., & Shaw, P. (1998). Habitual prospective memory and aging: Remembering intentions and forgetting actions. *Psychological Science, 9*, 284–288.

Engle, R. W., Tuholski, S. W., Laughlin, J. E., & Conway, A. R. A. (1999). Working memory, short-term memory, and general fluid intelligence: A latent variable approach. *Journal of Experimental Psychology: General, 128,* 309–331.

Goff, L. M., & Roediger, H. L., III (1998). Imagination inflation for action events: Repeated imagings lead to illusory recollections. *Memory & Cognition, 28,* 20–33.

Gollwitzer, P. M. (1999). Implementation intentions: Strong effects of simple plans. *American Psychologist, 54,* 493–503.

Hasher, L., & Zacks, R. T. (1988). Working memory, comprehension, and aging: A review and a new view. In G. H. Bower (Ed.), *The psychology of learning and motivation* (Vol. 22, pp. 193–225). New York: Academic Press.

Hasher, L., Zacks, R. T., & May, C. P. (1999). Inhibitory control, circadian arousal, and age. In D. Gopher & A. Koriat (Eds.), *Attention and performance: Vol. 17. Cognitive regulation of performance: Interaction of theory and application* (pp. 653–675). Cambridge, MA: MIT Press.

Hinkin, C. H., Hardy, D. J., Mason, K. I., Castellon, S. A., Durvasula, R. S., Lam, M. N., & Stefaniak, M. (2004). Medication adherence in HIV-infected adults: Effect of patient age, cognitive status, and substance abuse. *AIDS, 18*(Suppl. 1), 19–25.

Insel, K., Morrow, D., Brewer, B., & Figueredo, A. (2006). Executive function, working memory, and medication adherence among older adults. *Journal of Gerontology Series B: Psychological Sciences and Social Sciences, 61,* P102–P107.

Johnson, M. K., Reeder, J. A., Raye, C. L., & Mitchell, K. J. (2002). Second thoughts versus second looks: An age-related deficit in reflectively refreshing just-activated information. *Psychological Science, 13,* 64–67.

Kane, M. J., Bleckley, M. K., Conway, A. R., & Engle R. W. (2001). A controlled-attention view of working-memory capacity. *Journal of Experimental Psychology: General, 130,* 169–183.

Kimberg, D. Y., & Farah, M. J. (1993). A unified account of cognitive impairments following frontal lobe damage: The role of working memory in complex, organized behavior. *Journal of Experimental Psychology: General, 122,* 411–428.

Liu, L. L., & Park, D. C. (2004). Aging and medical adherence: The use of automatic processes to achieve effortful things. *Psychology and Aging, 19,* 318–325.

Marsh, R. L., Hicks, J. L., & Landau, J. D. (1998). An investigation of everyday prospective memory. *Memory & Cognition, 26,* 633–643.

McDaniel, M. A., Butler, K. M., & Dornburg, C. (2006). Binding of source and content: New directions revealed by neuropsychological and age-related effects. In H. D. Zimmer, A. Mecklinger, & U. Lindenberger (Eds.), *Binding in human memory: A neurocognitive approach* (pp. 657–675). New York: Oxford University Press.

McDaniel, M. A., & Einstein, G. O. (2000). Strategic and automatic processes in prospective memory retrieval: A multiprocess framework. *Applied Cognitive Psychology, 14,* S127–S144.

McDaniel, M. A., Einstein, G. O., Stout, A. C., & Morgan, Z. (2003). Aging and maintaining intentions over delays: Do it or lose it. *Psychology and Aging, 18,* 823–835.

McDaniel, M. A., Howard, D., & Butler, K. M. (2006). *Implementation intentions facilitate prospective memory: Immunity to high attention demands.* Manuscript in preparation.

Milne, S., Orbell, S., & Sheeran, P. (2002). Combining motivational and volitional interventions to promote exercise participation: Protection motivation theory and implementation intentions. *British Journal of Health Psychology, 7,* 163–184.

Morrell, R. W., Park, D. C., Kidder, D. P., & Martin, M. (1997). Adherence to anti-hypertensive medications across the life span. *The Gerontologist, 37,* 609–619.

Muter, P. (1980). Very rapid forgetting. *Memory & Cognition, 8,* 174–179.

Orbell, S., Hodgkins, S., & Sheeran, P. (1997). Implementation intentions and the theory of planned behavior. *Personality and Social Psychology Bulletin, 23,* 953–962

Park, D. C., Hertzog, C., Kidder, D. P., Morrell, R. W., & Mayhorn, C. B. (1997). Effect of age on event-based and time-based prospective memory. *Psychology and Aging, 12,* 314–327.

Park, D. C., Hertzog, C., Leventhal, H., Morrell, R. W., Leventhal, E., Birchmore, D., et al. (1999). Medication adherence in rheumatoid arthritis patients: Older is wiser. *Journal of American Geriatrics Society, 47,* 172–183.

Park, D. C., & Kidder, D. P. (1996). Prospective memory and medication adherence. In M. Brandimonte, G. O. Einstein, & M. A. McDaniel (Eds.), *Prospective memory: Theory and applications* (pp. 369–390). Mahwah, NJ: Erlbaum.

Park, D. C., Lautenschlager, G., Hedden, T., Davidson, N., Smith, A. D., & Smith, P. (2002). Models of visuospatial and verbal memory across the adult life span. *Psychology and Aging, 17,* 299–320.

Ramuschkat, G., McDaniel, M. A., Kliegel, M., & Einstein, G. O. (2006). *Habitual prospective memory and aging: Benefits of a complex motor action.* Manuscript submitted for publication.

Reitman, J. S. (1971). Mechanisms of forgetting in short-term memory. *Cognitive Psychology, 2,* 185–195.

Rendell, P. G., Ozgis, S., & Wallis, A. (2004, April). *Age-related effects in prospective remembering: The role of delaying execution of retrieved intentions.* Paper presented at the 10th biennial Cognitive Aging Conference, Atlanta, Georgia.

Schweikert, R., & Boruff, B. (1986). Short-term memory capacity: Magic number or magic spell? *Journal of Experimental Psychology: Learning, Memory, and Cognition, 12,* 419–425.

Verplanken, B., & Faes, S. (1999). Good intentions, bad habits, and effects of forming implementation intentions on healthy eating. *European Journal of Social Psychology, 29,* 591–604.

Wilson, A. H., & Park, D. C. (in press). Prospective memory and health behaviors: Context trumps cognition. In M. Kliegel, M. A. McDaniel, & G. O. Einstein (Eds.), *Prospective memory: Cognitive, neuroscience, developmental, and applied perspectives.* Mahwah, NJ: Erlbaum.

4

PATIENT–DOCTOR INTERACTIONS IN AN AGING SOCIETY: THE OPPORTUNITIES FOR BEHAVIORAL RESEARCH

ELAINE A. LEVENTHAL AND HOWARD LEVENTHAL

The primary goal of the doctor–patient relationship is to establish a "contract" that enables the patient to manage the burden of chronic illnesses in the most effective and efficient way to either slow or change the trajectory of those inexorable illnesses that accompany the older years. The contract implies that the physician or health care provider understands both the medical issues and the strategies that the patient must adopt (adherence) to maintain an optimal level of health. Also implicit are the expectations that patients have an idiosyncratic understanding of their body, its symptoms of both being ill and well, and how individuals manage and assess their physical condition. These patient-generated "commonsense" models may or may not be congruent with the physician's medical models. The degree of, or lack of, congruence may be critical to the patient's outcome because even a vigorous and healthy individual will eventually become frail with limited reserves in most physiological systems and increasing vulnerability to chronic illness if he or she lives long enough. The minimization of frailty and the preservation of functional independence is the goal of the physician–patient contract.

The main goal of our chapter is to describe five models or schemata of chronic conditions that underlie patient behavior, that is, the symptoms they treat as indicators of illness, their expected causes, duration and responsiveness to treatment, and their consequences. These models are experiential in nature; that is they organize somatic experience and shape the perception and interpretation of somatic experiences perceived to be a product of treatment. Because they are experiential they may be implicit and not fully conscious, though this does not seem to minimize their control of behavior and the meaning of symptom and functional experience. Thus, words alone may be insufficient to reshape them sufficiently to move a patient's behavior toward improved treatment outcomes.

Management of behavioral models in older adults is complicated by frailty. *Frailty* has been defined as functional impairment that is comorbid with and may be directly associated with a disease process. It is likely to be present when there is unintended weight loss of 10 pounds (4.54 kilos) or more in 1 year, self-reports of exhaustion, objective weakness measured by grip strength, slow walking speed, and low physical activity. It is associated with anorexia and a loss of muscle mass, because of the increased immobility that is directly related to the decrease in physical activity and impaired balance. All of these changes can result in depression. Frailty is closely associated with common conditions such as cardiovascular disease, diabetes, obstructive lung disease, and cognitive impairment. Frailty predicts falls, social isolation, hospitalization, and death. Thus, as people get older, frailty is anticipated as they accumulate more and more of the vicissitudes associated with age as well as the chronic illnesses that are the result of lifelong exposure to environmental and occupational stresses. Frailty complicates management in three ways. First, it can diminish the cognitive and behavioral competencies essential for understanding and implementing behavioral change. Second, it introduces a set of somatic and functional changes that overlap those produced by disease. From the practitioner's perspective, this complicates diagnosis and treatment. For patients, it presents an array of symptoms and functional changes that complicate their ability to discriminate between changes that are disease related and amenable to treatment and those that are not. Failure to make these differentiations can reduce motivation for adherence. Third, frailty complicates communication between practitioners and patients; patients may place greater emphasis on symptoms and changes that are not life-threatening and less amenable to treatment, underestimate treatment benefits, and become nonadherent.

The diminution in physiological reserves may be the result of not only accumulated insults from behavioral factors, exposure to environmental pathogens, injuries, and infections, but also, even in our society, occult

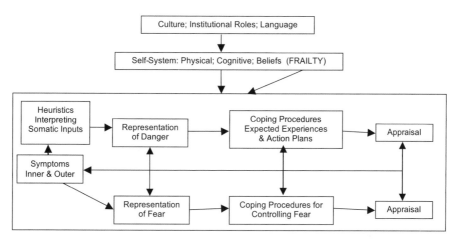

Figure 4.1. The commonsense self-regulatory model.

malnutrition. These can result in changes in somatic experiences and increased susceptibility to disease, slowed recovery from illness, and blunted symptom presentations. Diagnosing the older patient becomes increasingly complex and is dependent on understanding the superimposition of the pathological processes that produce disease effects on the normal processes of aging. Blunted and atypical symptoms can generate often ambiguous chief complaints from patients and can be difficult to interpret.

In the clinical encounter, the clinician or health care provider is confronted by a patient who is complaining of symptoms, either actually experienced or assumed to be present. The symptoms take on a representation from the self-system that is both concrete and abstract—concrete in, for example, their location, and abstract in that they generate an emotional response or fear state and may cause the patient to adopt concrete coping procedures. These can include seeking medical care to alleviate both the cognitive sense of threat and the emotional response. If seeking medical care, there is the assumption that the patient will be appraising the recommendations that are made by the clinician. In addition, the patient's self-system depends on his or her particular physical and cognitive ability, the concrete identities ascribed to the symptoms, and the individualized self-regulatory strategies. These are all nested within one's culture, institutional roles, language, and other factors. This is diagrammed in Figure 4.1.

The commonsense model describes how patients construct representations or mental models of the symptoms, signs, and dysfunctions associated with illness and age. Although the model is complex, it is based upon a set of quite simple propositions, the most elementary of which is the notion of symmetry; patients seek explanations or labels for somatic change and will seek somatic changes when labeled. The process of labeling, or more specifically the construction of a representation of an illness and a representation of treatment, involves heuristics, or simple, mental if–then rules that make sense of somatic experience. If the experience is breathlessness or swelling of the legs, the *location* heuristic helps to define its meaning; breathlessness is labeled as a lung problem and the swelling as a leg or foot problem. Though congestive heart failure may be the cause of both of these symptoms, neither is attributed to the heart, as the heart is in the chest, not in the lungs or legs. Other if–then rules that contribute to the symmetry or binding of somatic events to labels or models are *duration* (if it lasts long, it is serious), *trajectory* (Is it getting worse or improving?), *severity* (unbearable, seek help), *stress-illness* (if stress, do things to calm down), and so on. The *age-illness* heuristic is of special importance for elderly individuals' appraisals of somatic changes caused by chronic conditions; that is, if a change is a signal of aging, one must tolerate and live with it.

The clinician, in turn, generates a representation or model that fits the symptoms that have brought the patient in for care. This medical model incorporates any comorbidity that the elderly patient may have. These can include any of the following: cardiovascular disease, which is feared by the patient because of its significant morbidity and mortality; mental illness, which carries high morbidity and mortality and may or may not be feared by the patient; depression, which has moderate morbidity and mortality yet is assumed to be relatively innocuous by the lay public; alcohol use, which carries very high morbidity and mortality yet is assumed to be socially acceptable; stroke, which has high morbidity and mortality and is aptly feared by the patient; injuries and violence, which occur with increasing frequency in the elderly and are of significant morbidity and mortality and moderately feared by the patient; and cancer, which is tenfold less frequent than cardiovascular disease with high morbidity and mortality yet is greatly feared by the patient. Thus, these conditions carry different stigmas and life-threatening properties. Given that there may be disparate beliefs between physicians and patients about illness and symptom generation, we have begun to explore both patient self-management strategies and belief structures.

Because of our research findings, clinical experience, and the pressure we feel to better understand and more effectively teach clinical medicine, we have become interested in what happens in the doctor–patient interaction. What are the real-life scenarios at play as the patient seeks care (to conserve energy resources) by bringing self-perceptions of symptoms and the presumed disease labels into the medical setting? Given that there is a considerable body of research that reports great dissatisfaction with doctor–patient interactions, it is timely to explore this particular area.

First, it is necessary to look at what happens in an encounter between a doctor and a patient. The doctor sees a patient who has a variety of complaints, which represent symptoms that sometimes accompany physical findings that could be the signs of an illness. The doctor automatically assigns a disease name to this constellation of symptoms and signs, and by doing so registers the prognosis, complications, treatment, and appropriate assessment of the particular disease. The patient's perspective of the encounter follows the script of "I was okay; I was functional, I felt well. I don't feel okay now; I can't function; I have symptoms (pain or distress) and I see some sign of disease or a potential disease I can't explain." That patient wants to be listened to, wants to be told what is wrong, and wants to be given something to make the particular symptom or sign go away and be restored to health. The medical model follows a set of prototypic patterns in which signs and symptoms must represent a diagnosis that defines a set of prognoses, treatments, and outcome expectations, both short term and long term. If the symptoms are ambiguous, then the diagnosis becomes a set of *differential diagnoses* in which one diagnosis after another is systematically eliminated by a variety of examinations, assays, or behaviors, until only one remains and presumably explains the patient's problem.

In our model system, we are proposing that the traditional medical strategies are insufficient and the clinician also needs to make use of the patient's commonsense model (i.e., of the heuristics the patient is using in defining the perception of the illness). The physician's model should include the possibility that patients look for symmetry, either anatomic or symptomatic, or a relationship to stress, age, or illness. The patient's heuristic can also address prevalence (common or rare) and treatment responsiveness.

The first component of the patient's commonsense model defines the identity attached to the symptom, generating a label that is connected to the symptoms. It has a perception of a timeline measured in days or years. It has consequences, physical and social, that may generate fear. There is an automatic search for internal or external causality and evidence of controllability that may require self-management or the seeking of expert advice. Finally, there is always assessment of effectiveness of treatment and coping.

After describing some of our findings briefly, we discuss a set of models that offer opportunities for investigation and allow the construction of interventions that would readily translate into clinical practice. We have been able to show that elderly patients adopt strategies of risk aversion for purposes of energy conservation. They try to reduce risk to control the onset and sometimes worsening of often ambiguous and threatening symptoms that can lead to concerns about their overall health. This strategy of risk aversion underlies a variety of motivated actions, in particular swift seeking of health care, not replacing activities given up because of illness, and unwillingness to expend energy, such as exercising, one of the most frequent management strategies prescribed by the doctor. Elderly patients who think they might have a serious problem delay much less in calling for a medical appointment than do middle-age patients, who show significant delay in seeking health care if they think they are experiencing symptoms from what could be a serious disease (Cameron, Leventhal, & Leventhal, 1995; Leventhal, Easterling, Leventhal, & Cameron, 1995).

In Duke, Brownlee, Leventhal, and Leventhal (2002), we looked at the cessation of activities when older persons become ill and related activity replacement to both illness and psychological variables. In a sample of 177 individuals who had reduced their activities when they became sick, the severity and duration of the illness were important predictors for not returning to preillness functional levels, but psychological factors had the more significant relationships to activity replacement (Duke et al., 2002). Those individuals with satisfying social support and those who felt that they had someone depending on them were the ones who returned to a socially engaged level of function. Optimism also enhanced the resumption of activities. However, those who scored very highly on energy conservation did not replace activities because of concern about erosion of their energy reserve (Duke et al., 2002).

The evolution of the commonsense model represents a large body of work and is the model system on which we have structured our prototypic patterns of doctor–patient interactions. We believe these heuristics underlie most illness perceptions and have come from the studies that have asked patients about whether they feel an illness is acute or chronic, underlying etiologies, what the consequences are of having a disease, and whether the illness can be cured with treatment (see Figure 4.1). What clinicians find, consistently, is the lack of lay understanding of chronic disease and the assumption that a treatment "cures." For example, a significant proportion of patients believe that chronic illnesses such as cancer, hypertension, diabetes, coronary artery disease, and hyperlipidemia occur in acute episodes and are curable. If indeed patients believe that an illness is acute, then the way in which they self-manage may be quite different than if they accept that an illness is chronic. A label of chronicity accepts continuous treatment rather than intermittent urgent responses (Halm, Mora, & Leventhal, 2006). This is one of the clear sources of incongruity between the perceptions of illness that lay patients have and those held by the clinician. This lack in agreement can occur in the labeling, in the timeline, in the consequence of the illness, and clearly in the management and appraisal of the efficacy of treatment.

We have designed a research strategy by constructing a model set of five disease patterns that may help to describe what is seen in most clinical interactions. These disease patterns are dependent on the commonsense self-regulatory model that has been presented in Figure 4.1. The five prototypes are presented and illustrated in Exhibit 4.1, and in the following sections we discuss examples of patient–doctor models and types of doctor strategies to establish congruence to help describe these patterns.

EXHIBIT 4.1
Five Disease Patterns Giving Rise to Incongruities Between
Patient and Medical Models

1. Life-threatening, non-life-threatening with common symptoms.
2. Silent but life-threatening.
3. Chronic but experienced as episodic (acute).
4. Dysfunctional but not life-threatening.
5. Life-threatening and vigilance inducing.

Can the clinical practitioner identify the schemata underlying the patient's symptom presentations, coping efforts, and care seeking and negotiate a treatment plan?

Symptoms/ Function Behavior	Patient's Schemata	Medical Diagnosis	Practitioner's View Patient Model As
Episodes of restricted breathing	Acute asthma	Chronic asthma	Acute/chronic
Warm face, tense and stressed, headaches	Acute elevation of blood pressure	Asymptomatic chronic elevation	Acute symptomatic/ chronic asymptomatic
No symptoms Feel fine	No disease	Chronic diabetes, hypertension	Well/chronic illness
Chest pain	Life threatening cardiac attack	Benign costo-chondritis	Cardiac/benign
Anxious monitoring for breast, urinary, or colon symptoms	Cancer fear and hypervigilance	No clinical disease present	Cancer/healthy and accepts reassurance
Decreased mobility, stiffness, pain	Age related and unmanageable	Osteoarthritis: Manage with PT	Age, hopeless/PT and improved function

Note. PT = Physical therapy.

LIFE-THREATENING, NON-LIFE-THREATENING WITH COMMON SYMPTOMS

Chest pain is the classic example of the first disease pattern, common symptoms that can be either life-threatening or non-life-threatening. For the physician, chest pain has three possible origins, but for the patient there is only one (see Figure 4.2). The primary and most concerning presentation is cardiac or anginal pain, which for the patient immediately conjures up thoughts of morbidity and sudden death. This is in agreement with the physician model. But the symptoms can also come from gastroesophageal

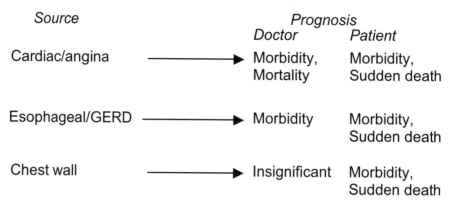

For doctor: Three possible origins
For patient: One possible origin

Source		Prognosis	
		Doctor	Patient
Cardiac/angina	⟶	Morbidity, Mortality	Morbidity, Sudden death
Esophageal/GERD	⟶	Morbidity	Morbidity, Sudden death
Chest wall	⟶	Insignificant	Morbidity, Sudden death

Figure 4.2. Chest pain: Life-threatening/non-life-threatening with common symptoms. GERD = gastroesophageal disease.

reflux disease, which carries morbidity but very rare mortality, yet the patient will frequently interpret these symptoms as cardiac. Finally, the pain can be in the chest wall or be muscular–skeletal, both medically insignificant, but for the patient, again, given its location, the pain still conjures up the fear of morbidity and sudden death.

The following are two contrasting clinical vignettes: A patient with chest pain, dyspnea, and diaphoresis came to the emergency room and had electrocardiographic changes compatible with myocardial ischemia and cardiac enzyme elevations, all part of the classic presentation of myocardial infarct requiring emergency management. Here the patient and doctor correctly interpreted the symptoms, and the patient was treated accordingly.

The second patient also came in with chest pain. The evaluation was negative. There were no electrocardiographic abnormalities and all the blood tests were negative. The patient was sent out, however, with the caveat that even though everything was negative, just to be on the safe side, the patient should have an outpatient exercise stress test. She was instructed to see a physician within the next 2 to 3 days. The patient came in for an urgent visit to the ambulatory clinic. She was observed to be sitting stiffly in a chair in the examination room with hand to chest, providing the aforementioned history. The physician listened carefully; asked to examine the patient; listened to the patient's lungs, anterior chest, and heart; and then pressed on the patient's chest wall at the junction of the ribs and the sternum. The patient responded, "That is my *pain*." Thus the chest wall pain was interpreted by the patient as cardiac in origin and was ambiguously diagnosed in the emergency room. It was only when objectified or concretized in the ambulatory setting that the appropriate noncardiac etiology could be ascribed. The incongruity was therefore dispensed with by objectifying the symptom for the patient by physical examination.

SILENT BUT LIFE THREATENING

In the second disease pattern of silent but life-threatening illnesses, asymptomatic chronic illnesses are particularity prone to the incongruities between patient and physician models specifically because of the lack of symptoms; there is nothing to remind the patient of the presence of the disease. Though the physician can generate disease *signs*, the symptoms remain silent until there is significant end organ damage. There are, however, ways in which the signs can be made salient or concretized for the patient by specific management strategies. Teaching the patient to self-monitor blood pressures on a prescribed schedule can concretize hypertension for the patient. Specifying routinized testing, rather than monitoring when the patient thinks his or her blood pressure is up, allows the patient to track variability and efficacy of treatment. The same strategy can work even more effectively for the diabetic patient trained to monitor blood sugars, again on a systematic prescribed schedule. The objective quantitative data generated by the ability to self-monitor blood sugars can lead to better control if the patient understands how to manipulate diet and medication and their relationship to blood sugar values.

When patients take a medication that stabilizes their condition, they may assume a cure has occurred. This is most likely the case if they have embedded in their illness representation the idea that the disease is episodic, not chronic. For example, hypertensive patients who take medications as directed and document normalization of the blood pressure readings assume that they are cured and therefore will stop taking the tablets. If patients only monitor blood pressures when they think there are symptoms of elevation (i.e., flushed face, headache, malaise) and then note that pressure is indeed high, they may take the tablets only when these symptoms are present.

In patients with diabetes, there is another avenue for incongruity. They may become more willing to pay attention to monitoring of blood glucose levels as the disease progresses, the end organ damage increases, and they become symptomatic. For example, peripheral neuropathy is frequently associated with significant pain and hyperesthesias. However, with further progression, patients become essentially insensate and think that they are better because they no longer feel pain. When this occurs, vigilant behaviors decrease or stop. Decreased vigilance, in the context of increased susceptibility to injury because of the lack of sensation, leads to infection, gangrene, and usually amputation. The strategies most likely to increase adherence rests with convincing the patient to routinely and consistently monitor blood glucose levels. Maintaining vigilance in the insensate diabetic depends on enhancing concern about amputation.

CHRONIC BUT EXPERIENCED AS EPISODIC

The third disease pattern examines chronic conditions that are mistaken as episodic. For intermittent episodes, the medical model anticipates that intermittent flares are the result of poor self-management of chronic illness, whereas the patient's model assumes the disease is acute and cyclical. The classic example is asthma. Although a chronic illness, asthma was thought in the past to be totally reversible, indeed intermittent, and patients only had to treat symptoms when they had an acute flare. Recent research has demonstrated that asthma is, in fact, not reversible but is instead a chronic inflammatory condition that must be prophylactically managed with maintenance medications to moderate the intensity of flares. This represents a recent change in management strategy, and patients who have had the disease for a long time and been coached in management by physicians trained before the introduction of current management recommendations may not be able to change their model to the more current model. If they reject it, there is incongruity between current management recommendations and their learned coping behaviors. Those patients who do not learn to monitor their respiratory status and use "preventors" on a consistent basis are the ones who end up with severe respiratory distress and potential emergency room intubation. This pattern also fits congestive heart failure. When patients do not watch salt intake, their weight, and proper titration of their medicines, they slowly can become dyspneic and edematous. After gaining a significant amount of weight and ignoring pedal edema, they arrive at the emergency room in respiratory distress instead of attending to the presence of early signs of decompensation and initiating a set of simple management steps that include alerting the physician, increasing diuretics, and cutting out all salt from their diet.

DYSFUNCTIONAL BUT NON-LIFE-THREATENING

The fourth disease pattern describes the highly dysfunctional state that generates severe functional discomfort and pain but is non-life-threatening. This pattern generates more hospital visits and disrupts more daily activities than other chronic illnesses. The classic example is osteoarthritis, which compromises mobility and function because of pain and stiffness. If the patient becomes immobilized, social isolation results and profoundly affects quality of life. Degenerative arthritis and joint pain are pathonomonic of aging in the lay mind. The pain and dysfunction also lead to significant drug seeking, frequently of over-the-counter drugs reported to have miraculous curative properties by the media. These drugs have high potential for severe adverse effects, and although the dysfunction may be non-life-threatening, the self-management strategies may result in life-threatening situations because there is a high incidence of gastrointestinal bleeding and renal failure associated with self-treatment without surveillance.

LIFE THREATENING AND VIGILANCE INDUCING

The last disease pattern represents life-threatening illness that, even when stable or in remission, induces hypervigilance by the patient. The incongruity seen in these situations occurs because of what the patient assumes that the experiential signs and symptoms represent and what is perceived by the clinician. A classic example is any cancer in remission, in which the patient assumes that all pain is cancer related and all functional decrement must be cancer related. The complete discrepancy in labeling the etiology of the symptoms between the doctor and the patient does not automatically occur in this situation because the clinician is compelled to expect to make sure that the presenting symptom is not, in fact, related to any recurrence of the malignancy despite its assumed quiescent state. However, the patient automatically assumes the cancer must be returning, and until there is concrete evidence produced by the physician that the symptom is not cancer related, that perception will persist.

In one example, a patient with bladder cancer, in remission, presented with severe back pain. The oncologist, who did some preliminary testing, could find no evidence of metastatic disease or recurrence and sent the patient to the internist. The patient was clearly not convinced that the reoccurrence of cancer was ruled out and had immobilizing pain. The clinician, therefore, had to perform a few additional diagnostic tests that would allow the clinician to assure the patient that the symptoms were generated by aging-related degenerative disease, that is, osteoarthritis plus some compression fractures secondary to osteoporosis. Once the studies with sufficient sensitivity and specificity had been completed and no evidence of metastatic involvement was found, the patient became more and more comfortable with a variety of conservative therapies, including physical therapy. The pain began to miraculously diminish and finally disappear. The patient has been essentially pain free for 2 years.

Another patient had cancer of the prostate and had chosen to have radiation therapy to preserve sexual function and avoid incontinence. The patient was in remission, was doing well, and had no evidence of disease for 5 years. He developed acute pain in the arm at the triceps insertion. The patient was seen in routine follow-ups by the oncologist and the radiation oncologist, and the oncologist was convinced this had to be a metastatic lesion. Although he took some X-rays and did not see anything, the oncologist remained convinced there was a recurrence and was insisting on irradiating the arm. The internist looked carefully at the studies, reviewed them with the radiologist, who did not see any evidence of malignancy, and, after examination and a very specific pinpointing of the particular symptom, made a diagnosis of bursitis, an inflammatory process that responds well to a short course of nonsteroidal medication or steroids and rest. The patient, meanwhile, was unable to keep from feeling the spot because of his worry, exacerbated by the oncologist, and was convinced this pain had to be from the malignancy. After discussion with the patient's wife, who was a nurse, it was decided that there could be a variety of strategies, and they agreed that they would try several to make him relax and decrease his opportunity to feel him arm. After a period of 4 days of rest induced with sedatives and with careful monitoring by the patient's wife, the symptoms disappeared and the patient was spared radiation to his arm for a phantom metastasis.

Malignancy is not the only condition generating hypervigilance. Hypervigilance can also be seen in patients who worry about other life-threatening illnesses such as stroke, myocardial infarct, and dementia. In addition, there are many who believe that they are more sensitive than most people to drugs (*sensitive soma*) and therefore must have only natural or homeopathic substances. The current escalation of hypervigilance may reflect significant recent changes in the U.S. health care delivery system. This past decade has seen the integration of informed consent and advance directives along with increased visibility of ethic committees in the hospital. In addition, there has been an explosion of print media, television, and information on the Web that have led to more shared decision making and an increase in self-care strategies. These are superimposed on the patterns previously discussed and lead to more complicated heuristics about patient care seeking or indulgence in self-care for energy conservation. Self-care and self-diagnosis fit into the general model and can lead either to inappropriate or appropriate management strategies that can have a profound effect on the patient's health.

SUMMARY

The newest challenge to patients, clinicians, and academics is how to understand what drives these health behaviors and how to meld them with what may be incongruous doctor–patient models of health and illness. This is also important for training health care professionals. These models may capture some of the elements of the art used by expert clinicians and other health care providers and may lay out some ground rules for making operational findings from such research. Introducing these concepts into the training of clinicians and other health care providers will allow them to better understand and also generate strategies for more effective clinical management.

Physicians and other health care providers can facilitate congruence by externalizing and objectifying the patient's idiosyncratic perceptions by listening, interpreting, and if possible eliciting symptoms and emotional responses from the patient. The *laying on of the hands* becomes very salient. This can allow the patient and the physician to generate mutual agreement about reasonable treatment, outcomes and action plans, outcome expectations, and appraisal procedures of treatment efficacy. The illness and behavioral models need to be shared by the clinician with the patient as well as key members of the patients' social network to support more effective management. This is important because incongruous models are also shared by family members and the social environment, thus the health care provider's ability to defuse inaccurate and confusing assumptions with the social milieu will help to define the most advantageous treatment plan for the patient.

It is important to understand what some of the logistics are for negotiating a treatment plan. The patient brings fear or distress that is problem based, is specific to the particular set of symptoms, and generates a specific identity label. The identity or label must be discussed, and the patient (and family members) need to believe that the clinician understands the patient's model, its inherent concept of timeline, consequences, cause, as well as controllability of the particular set of presenting symptoms. There then needs to be consensus on what the problem is, its etiology, timeline, and consequences, therefore, on its identity and cause, along with possibilities for control. This consensus will then allow for the development of the treatment procedures that become mutually generated. Therefore what the doctor will suggest will be something that the patient can do within his or her social environment. There will be a set of mutually agreed on procedures that allow for appraisal of the outcomes.

Health psychology has traditionally generated many models that purport to help in the understanding of health and illness behaviors, but most of these models are not readily applicable to the reality of the clinic. Damasio (1999) offered a useful model of mental processing, describing the prototypic autonomic processor, the perceptive mind, and the integrated cognitive mind in a healthy person. In this model the prototypic self is viewed as a system for maintaining homeostasis; it is a system that regulates physiological processes such as blood pressure and blood sugar control, and it does so without the participation of conscious awareness. Indeed, in this model there is an impenetrable barrier between these systems and consciousness. By contrast, the core conscious self is the self related to environmental objects and persons, and the autobiographical self is the source of the individual's history; it is the temporal integration of life experience. This model is interesting but is inadequate clinically. It must be adapted for the sick body as breakdowns in the homeostatic processes that operate outside of awareness during healthy times produce symptoms and functional change during sickness that bring information into consciousness from the automatic, nonconscious realm. The perceptive mind then becomes distressed and confused, the integrative mind looks for answers; "where" and "how" provide the challenge for the caregiver.

The model presented in this chapter provides an opportunity for the blending of behavioral and clinical medicine models, both practice and research. What forms the patients' models clearly is their personal experience, the observation of others, and their network—personal, communal, and social—based on anecdotes, testimonials, and credible media sources. Understanding the disease patterns that we have discussed, and how these patterns shape mental models and the rules and procedures that practitioners need to know, can create the expert diagnostician, who can then be an expert physician. This expert physician will work with patients and families to affect their mental models and optimize patient treatment. The challenge is to determine how and what the doctor and the patient need to teach each other. It is important to better understand how the physician or other health care provider can teach the patient to interpret body symptoms. A future direction for behavioral research should be how to teach the teacher to teach the patient how to interpret symptoms and design creative interventions.

REFERENCES

Cameron, L. D., Leventhal, E. A., & Leventhal, H. (1995). Seeking medical care in response to symptoms and life stress. *Psychosomatic Medicine, 57,* 37–47.

Damasio, A. (1999). *The feeling of what happens: Body and emotion in the making of consciousness.* Orlando, FL: Harcourt.

Duke, J., Brownlee, S., Leventhal, E. A., & Leventhal, H. (2002). Giving up and replacing activities in response to illness. *Journals of Gerontology Series B: Psychological Sciences and Social Sciences, 57,* P367–P376.

Halm, E. A., Mora, P., & Leventhal, H. (2006). No symptoms, no asthma: The acute episodic disease belief is associated with poor self-management among inner city adults with persistent asthma. *Chest, 129,* 573–580.

Leventhal, E. A., Easterling, D., Leventhal, H., & Cameron, L. (1995). Conservation of energy, uncertainty reduction, and swift utilization of medical care among the elderly: Study II. *Medical Care, 33,* 988–1000.

II

UNDERSTANDING DOCTORS' INSTRUCTIONS

5

HOW OLDER PATIENTS LEARN MEDICAL INFORMATION

SCOTT C. BROWN

Older adults experience more chronic illnesses than any other age group (Merck Research Laboratories, 1997) and thus are frequently exposed to several types of medical information, including treatment recommendations, medical advertisements, and instructions for using medications and home medical devices. The present chapter considers how older patients acquire and use medical information across a wide range of real-world contexts. Of particular interest is how older patients comprehend and remember complex dietary and drug regimens as well as medical claims and instructions for use of medical technologies, despite facing numerous challenges (i.e., sensory, cognitive, biomedical, and psychosocial) in processing this information. A more complete understanding of how older adults process health information should result in greater treatment compliance,

This work was supported by National Institute of Arthritis and Musculoskeletal Diseases Grant T32-AR07080 awarded to the Division of Rheumatology at the University of Michigan Medical Center, by National Institute of Aging (NIA) Grants P50-AG11715 and R01-AG09868 awarded to Denise C. Park and colleagues, and by NIA Grant T32-AG00017 awarded to Ruth Dunkle and Berit Ingersoll-Dayton at the University of Michigan. Preparation of this chapter was also supported by Department of Army Grant DAMD17-00-2-0018 awarded to Daniel Clauw and colleagues.

better informed decisions, and lower health care costs through reduced hospitalizations.

In this chapter, I first provide an overview of age-related sensory and cognitive changes that may affect older adults' ability to learn medical information. This is followed by a summary of key findings on aging and medical information processing, including the roles of age and prior knowledge in learning new health information and suggestions for overcoming older patients' inaccurate health beliefs. Next, I examine how medical conditions and medical treatments may themselves affect older patients' learning of medical information. This is followed by an examination of psychosocial issues in older patient–provider interactions, including the roles that the older patient, health care provider, and third parties play in the transmission of information during the medical encounter. Finally, I conclude by suggesting ways in which health care providers, policymakers, and designers of medical devices and Web sites might improve their delivery of health information to older adults.

BRIEF OVERVIEW OF SENSORY AND COGNITIVE AGING

Age-related sensory and cognitive changes may affect the ability of older adults to learn medical information. These changes are explored in the following sections.

Age-Related Sensory Changes

Age-related sensory changes are well documented (see, e.g., Fozard & Gordon-Salant, 2001) and can hinder older adults' ability to acquire new medical information. For example, hearing loss, particularly of the higher auditory frequencies (i.e., presbycusis), is common in older individuals and may make it more difficult for patients to understand information presented by health care providers, particularly in noisy environments such as hospitals. Therefore, health care providers should try to speak in a loud, clear, low tone when presenting information to older patients, and they should also encourage older patients with known hearing impairments to use their hearing aids during office visits. In addition, age-related changes in visual acuity and contrast sensitivity can make it more difficult for older adults to read the fine print in prescription drug inserts or drug advertisements. Therefore, providers of written health information should use a large font (i.e., at least 12-point) with a high degree of contrast for older readers to reduce the likelihood of older adults not understanding information because of difficulties in reading the text.

Age-Related Cognitive Changes

There are multiple age-related cognitive changes that could affect older adults' processing of health information (S. C. Brown & Park, 2003; Park, 2000; see also chaps. 1 and 3, this volume). For example, Park et al. (2002) examined the cognitive functioning of a life span sample of 345 adults and found that there were linear age declines from ages 20 to 90 on several effortful cognitive tasks, including speed of processing, working memory (i.e., the amount of information that can be simultaneously stored and processed in consciousness), and long-term episodic memory. Park and other researchers have theorized that decreases in information-processing speed and in working memory capacity place limits on long-term memory (Park et al., 1996), as well as other important mental activities such as comprehension of new materials, problem solving, and reasoning (Kemper, 1992; Salthouse, 1992). In addition, others have argued that there are age declines in *inhibition*, or the ability to direct attention away from irrelevant information, which is important for several cognitive tasks on which older adults are impaired (Hasher & Zacks, 1988; Zacks & Hasher, 1997). As a result of age declines in basic cognitive resources—such as speed of processing, working memory, and inhibition—older adults show deficits on types of memory that are effortful, such as recall tasks, which require the individual to remember information with few cues in the environment to support retrieval operations (Craik & McDowd, 1987; Park et al., 1996). In addition, explicitly remembering source information or the specific context in which information was presented is a resource-intensive activity that declines with age (Frieske & Park, 1999; Spencer & Raz, 1995).

In contrast to the aforementioned findings of age-related declines on effortful tasks requiring substantial cognitive resources, age sparing or even age gains in knowledge structures such as vocabulary and domain-specific expertise can also be present (Craik & Jennings, 1992; Park et al., 2002). Similarly, age differences are typically small or nonexistent on tasks requiring primarily automatic processes, which require little or no mental capacity to perform and which may develop as a result of experience (e.g., typing). For example, picture recognition is considered relatively automatic because it provides environmental supports or rich external cues for remembering (Craik, 1986) and therefore requires little in the way of deliberate retrieval. Thus, picture recognition shows small age differences compared with recall tasks (Park, Puglisi, & Smith, 1986). In addition, age differences are generally small on implicit or indirect memory tasks that do not require deliberate referencing of a prior study episode (e.g., having an increased likelihood of completing the word stem *SP____* with the word *SPEED* after reading about speed of processing earlier in this chapter) compared with traditional or "explicit" memory tasks that do directly reference a prior study episode

(La Voie & Light, 1994; Park & Shaw, 1992). Finally, some researchers have suggested that there is age invariance in the ability to use the automatically generated feeling of familiarity to distinguish previously seen items from new items on a memory task (Jacoby, Jennings, & Hay, 1996). *Familiarity* has been described as a feeling of déjà vu or a vague sense that information was encountered previously (Mandler, 1980) and is contrasted with *recollection*, or the retrieval of clear contextual details surrounding acquisition of information, which shows age declines (Jacoby et al., 1996). Jacoby et al. (1996) suggested that memory performance reflects a combination of familiarity (automatic) and recollection (effortful) components and that in the relative absence of effortful processes, older adults can come to be dominated more by automatic or habitual modes of responding (e.g., automatically reaching for one's osteoporosis medicine when climbing out of bed after several years of taking this medicine first thing in the morning).

Summary of Age-Related Cognitive Changes

The classic pattern of findings with regard to age and cognition is one of age declines in tasks requiring effortful processing versus age invariance in tasks relying primarily on automatic processes, with growth occurring in knowledge structures such as vocabulary and world knowledge (Craik & Jennings, 1992; Light, 1992). This pattern of results suggests specific hypotheses regarding the magnitude of age differences in learning of medical information. First, it would be expected that older adults would have particular difficulty with medical tasks requiring considerable cognitive resources, such as following a physician's rapid-fire presentation of medical jargon or recollecting whether a medical claim they remember came from a physician or from a drug advertisement. Second, older adults should show superior performance in situations that are relatively familiar or driven by external cues in the environment, such as learning about a disease that a close family member experienced or remembering to take a new medication when prompted by a pill organizer or a preset alarm. I review the evidence for each of these two hypotheses (i.e., age declines in cognitively effortful medical tasks vs. age invariance in relatively automatic medical tasks) in the sections that follow.

AGE DIFFERENCES IN LEARNING OF MEDICAL INFORMATION

Age-related cognitive changes may play a part in how people learn new health information. This section examines how older adults comprehend medical information and how they use external aids and medical devices.

Comprehension of Medical Information

Much research has indicated that older adults have difficulty comprehending and remembering several types of medical information because of age declines in basic cognitive abilities such as working memory. For example, Morrell, Park, and Poon (1989) found that older adults incorrectly comprehended 21% of the information on prescription labels as written by an actual pharmacist (e.g., "Take one capsule three times a day") when they were asked to use this information to develop a specific medication plan. Although Morrell et al. improved participants' comprehension of the pharmacist's instructions by using revised labels with well-structured verbal instructions (e.g., "Take one capsule at 8 a.m., 3 p.m., and 10 p.m."), the older adults consistently recalled less information than did young adults, regardless of the quality of the instructions or the amount of time they were given to study the materials.

In a follow-up study, Morrell, Park, and Poon (1990) attempted a further improvement over real-world prescription labels by using a mixed text-plus-pictures format (e.g., a picture of a milk carton, indicating that the drug should be taken with milk) based on the finding that memory for simple pictures is relatively intact in old age (Park et al., 1986). Although the text-plus-pictures format increased younger adults' recall of the information, this format actually reduced older adults' recall compared with standard, verbal instructions. Morrell et al. (1990) theorized that older adults' failure to benefit from the picture labels could reflect the high processing demands required to interpret these symbols (i.e., integrating both verbal and visual information). Alternatively, the older adults may have suffered in the mixed-instructions condition because this was not a familiar format that they had experienced in the past. It is therefore possible that the older adults may have shown a greater benefit if they had had more exposure and training with these symbols.

However, work by Hancock, Rogers, and Fisk (2001) has suggested that mere exposure to prescription symbols is not enough to reduce age differences in comprehension. These authors found that although older adults reported attending to warning information for household products and over-the-counter medications more often than younger adults, their comprehension of this information was significantly worse than that of younger adults for 6 out of the 12 common warning symbols examined in this study.

Taken together, the findings by Morrell et al. (1989, 1990) and by Hancock et al. (2001) suggest that older adults have particular difficulty in understanding information that is complex or requires making inferences, which is a resource-intensive process (Kemper, 1992; Rogers, Rousseau, & Lamson, 1999). Consistent with this view, Morrow and Leirer (1999) have suggested ways in which to structure medication instructions to improve older adults' comprehension, including presenting information in a streamlined list format with headers to indicate individual topics (e.g., dosage, times to take medicine), as well as ordering information in a manner consistent with the reader's existing knowledge structures or schemas for taking medicine (e.g., presenting dose and time information before side effects).

Use of External Aids to Support Adherence

Other research has considered the use of environmental supports or external aids to help older adults remember to take their medications. For example, Park, Morrell, Frieske, Blackburn, and Birchmore (1991) found that older arthritis patients made substantial numbers of errors in loading over-the-counter medication organizers except when using a 7-day medication organizer with several compartments per day. The authors theorized that the 7-day organizer with multiple compartments decreased comprehension errors compared with an hour-by-hour wheel and a 7-day organizer with one compartment, because it presented the most appropriate structure for organizing older patients' medication plans across the week and thus supported working memory function in these individuals. Later, Park, Morrell, Frieske, and Kincaid (1992) demonstrated that the use of this organizer in the field, in conjunction with an organizational chart, facilitated very accurate medication taking in very old adults (i.e., those over the age of 75) who were otherwise at high risk of medication errors due to age-related cognitive impairments. Finally, Park, Shifren, Morrell, Watkins, and Stuedemann (1997) showed that another type of cognitive aid—a triathlon watch with a preset alarm that beeps when it is time to take medicine—was an effective means of enhancing medication adherence in a nonadherent sample of older individuals with hypertension.

Thus, external reminders such as pillboxes or beeping wristwatches can facilitate older adults' medication adherence by supporting their prospective memory function (i.e., remembering to take medicine at a particular time) as well as providing relatively automatic cues for medication taking that increase the likelihood that this behavior will be repeated in the same environment in the future (see also chaps. 1 and 3, this volume). Similarly, other researchers have suggested that the formation of a detailed implementation plan for a future action can be an effective means of enhancing older patients' adherence (e.g., "I will monitor my blood glucose when I've finished eating dinner"), because the environmental cues generated in the plan (e.g., dirty dinner plates) will automatically trigger the desired behavior at the time that the plan is to be implemented (see Liu & Park, 2004; see also chaps. 2, 8, and 9, this volume).

Learning to Use Medical Devices

A related line of research by Rogers and colleagues (see, e.g., Fisk & Rogers, 2001; chap. 11, this volume) concerns whether older adults can learn to use medical devices and technologies for managing their chronic health conditions. An example is the use of blood-glucose meters by patients with diabetes, which allow patients to determine whether their blood sugar levels are within prescribed limits and to adjust their diet, exercise, and insulin accordingly. Although many manufacturers claim that their medical products are easy to use, there is evidence that some systems and technologies place unreasonable demands on even the most sophisticated user. For example, Rogers, Mykityshyn, Campbell, and Fisk (2001) performed a task analysis of one blood-glucose meter and determined that contrary to the manufacturer's claim that it was as "easy to use as 1-2-3" there were over 50 specific substeps involved in calibrating the meter. Thus, users of this device have multiple opportunities to make mistakes.

Rogers et al. (2001) also examined the manufacturer's instructional video for this particular blood-glucose meter and identified a number of problems for older users: For instance, the video failed to summarize main steps and omitted critical substeps, which created difficulties for older adults' cognitive systems because of age declines in comprehension, working memory, and long-term memory (e.g., Kemper, 1992; Park et al., 1996). Later, Mykityshyn, Fisk, and Rogers (2002) improved on the manufacturer's video training system by developing their own video that explicitly demonstrated and reviewed the task sequence for calibrating the meter, including all of the specific substeps. The redesigned system improved the accuracy of both older and younger adults to approximately 90%. This finding suggests that designers of medical devices and technologies can reduce errors by redesigning products in ways that take into account the needs and abilities of the user as well as developing adequate instructional materials, including numbered steps, warnings, and structured reviews.

Still other research suggests that older adults have difficulty in acquiring other types of health information. These have included studies on medical appointment messages (Morrow, Leirer, Carver, Tanke, & McNally, 1999), treatment recommendations (B. J. F. Meyer, Russo, & Talbot, 1995), and information presented during real and simulated medical encounters (McGuire, 1996; Rost & Roter, 1987).

Summary of Age Differences in Learning Health Information

Age-related cognitive declines may cause older adults to have difficulty in learning about complex medical topics or in using a medical device that requires them to hold several steps in mind. However, the good news is that a number of interventions are available to facilitate acquisition of medical information in older patients, such as designing well-structured instructions for use of medications and devices that do not require making inferences as well as providing external aids such as medication organizers or brochures that patients can refer to on an ongoing basis.

ROLES OF AGE AND PRIOR KNOWLEDGE IN MEDICAL INFORMATION PROCESSING

Thus far, this chapter has primarily discussed aspects of the outward environment, such as informational characteristics and external reminding devices, that may affect older adults' processing of medical information. This section considers the impacts of mechanisms that are internal to older adults—including existing knowledge structures and familiarity with medical topics—that may influence older patients' ability to acquire new health information. The section also provides a summary of key findings on aging and medical information processing and suggestions for overcoming older patients' inaccurate health beliefs.

Older Adults as "Medical Experts"?

In contrast to much research suggesting downward trends in multiple cognitive abilities with age (e.g., Park, 2000; chap. 1, this volume), other work suggests that aging can be accompanied by stability or even gains in knowledge and expertise that can allow older adults to compensate for declines in basic cognitive resources (Park & Hall Gutchess, 2000). For example, Long and Shaw (2000) reported that older adults were better at learning new vocabulary words from context than were younger adults, a finding that the authors attributed to older adults' greater existing vocabulary knowledge. Similarly, Park et al. (1999) showed that older patients with rheumatoid arthritis remembered to take their medicine more often than did middle-aged adults, despite the fact that the older patients performed less well on several laboratory measures of cognition. Park et al. attributed their result to the older adults' greater practice at taking medications; many had taken medicine for years and had arranged their schedules to fit their medication taking rather than the other way around. In addition, Park (1999) suggested that older adults have accumulated prior knowledge of certain medical conditions—through a lifetime of experience with the medical system—that may enable them to acquire new information with relatively few demands on their impaired working memory. She further suggested that older adults would have fewer difficulties in learning about a familiar disease, such as arthritis, as opposed to a disease with which they were completely unfamiliar.

Role of Prior Knowledge in Learning Medical Information

Denise C. Park and I conducted a study to assess the hypothesis that familiarity with a medical condition reduces age differences in learning of medical information (S. C. Brown & Park, 2002). In this study, a volunteer sample of 40 older adults (ages 60–84) and 40 younger adults (ages 18–28) received new information on either a familiar disease (i.e., breast cancer) or a disease about which they knew little (i.e., acromegaly, a rare pituitary disorder). None of the participants had directly experienced either disease, and we excluded both current and former health professionals because of the likelihood that they might have expert knowledge of both diseases. The two diseases were selected because they were similar to each other in severity level (i.e., both are potentially life-threatening diseases), in gross etiology (i.e., both are caused by a tumor), and in the complexity of treatments used (i.e., both diseases are often treated using a combination of surgery, drugs, and radiation). Moreover, the two diseases varied in their familiarity to the general public, as revealed by pilot testing: Almost all of the older and younger adults tested knew at least some facts about breast cancer, whereas almost no one had heard of acromegaly.

After reading a passage on one of the diseases, participants answered questions assessing their recollection of the information. A separate control group (i.e., a knowledge group) of 20 younger and 20 older adults received no new information but answered the same questions as participants in the recollection or experimental group, to assess prior knowledge. Participants' retention of the medical information was then assessed by two types of test: open-ended questions (i.e., recall), followed by multiple-choice questions (i.e., recognition). Similar questions were asked for the two diseases (e.g., "According to the passage, what type of treatment will nearly all patients with the disease undergo? A. Surgery; B. Radiation; C. Drug therapy; D. Hormone therapy; E. Gene therapy"). Learning was assessed for each retention test by subtracting from each recollection participant's score the knowledge participants' group mean for that age group and disease condition (i.e., recollection–knowledge). These corrected learning scores were critical for separating what participants in the recollection group actually learned from their existing knowledge. We assessed learning as the difference between the recollection and knowledge groups rather than as a pre- versus posttest comparison for each individual participant, because we wished to avoid a situation in which participants would develop a schema for an unfamiliar disease solely as a result of the questions asked in a pretest. Finally, participants' cognitive functioning was assessed.

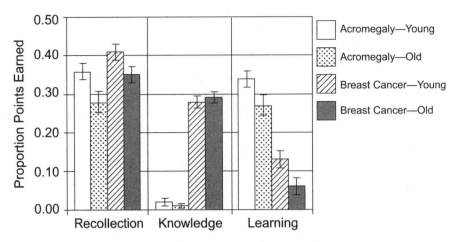

Figure 5.1. Mean recollection, knowledge, and learning (i.e., corrected recollection scores) by age group and disease condition for open-ended questions. Error bars indicate the standard error of the mean for each condition. From "Roles of Age and Familiarity in Learning Health Information," by S. C. Brown and D. C. Park, 2002, *Educational Gerontology, 28,* p. 703. Copyright 2002 by Taylor & Francis. Adapted with permission.

Figures 5.1 and 5.2 show participants' mean recollection, knowledge, and learning (i.e., corrected recollection) scores as a function of age group and disease condition for the open-ended and multiple-choice questions, respectively. The critical analyses focused on learning: As shown in the far-right columns in each of Figures 5.1 and 5.2, older adults learned less new information than younger adults, regardless of the familiarity of the information or the type of memory test used (i.e., open-ended or multiple-choice questions). This result runs counter to previously published findings suggesting that older adults can compensate for age declines in basic cognitive ability by relying on existing knowledge or experience (Long & Shaw, 2000; Park et al., 1999). However, it is possible that prior knowledge only minimizes age differences for tasks that are high in both ecological validity and environmental support, such as learning new words from a text providing many contextual cues (Long & Shaw, 2000) or remembering to take medicine by following a consistent daily routine that has been established over a period of months or years (Park et al., 1999). The ubiquity of age differences in acquisition of medical information in the present study suggests that older adults' capacity to consent to treatment may be impaired even for a familiar medical condition (in this case, breast cancer) and that physicians should give their older patients written health information for later consultation rather than having patients rely on their poor recollection of information presented during the office visit (see also, e.g., Marson & Harrell, 1999).

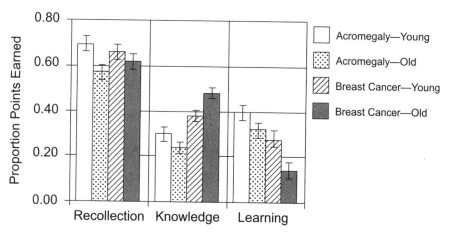

Figure 5.2. Mean recollection, knowledge, and learning (i.e., corrected recollection scores) by age group and disease condition for multiple-choice questions. Error bars indicate the standard error of the mean for each condition. From "Roles of Age and Familiarity in Learning Health Information," by S. C. Brown and D. C. Park, 2002, *Educational Gerontology, 28,* p. 705. Copyright 2002 by Taylor & Francis. Adapted with permission.

Figures 5.1 and 5.2 also show that both age groups actually learned *less* new information about a familiar disease than an unfamiliar disease. This result was somewhat surprising, given that there was substantial room for improvement in the breast cancer condition (i.e., both age groups were substantially below 100% performance). However, this lack of learning for a familiar disease is consistent with the view that prior knowledge of a topic can sometimes hinder additional learning of information on that topic. For example, the present results can be explained by a "schema-copy plus tag" model of text comprehension, in which a reader's representation of a passage contains much of his or her generic schema or knowledge relevant to the passage (e.g., Graesser & Nakamura, 1982). According to this model, information that is not typical of the schema is attached with a "tag" that decays over time, so that the reader's recall may revert to their existing schema rather than the new information presented in the passage. It is therefore possible that some of our new statements about breast cancer (which were selected so that they were not known by most participants) were perceived by our participants to be less typical of their breast cancer schema and therefore did not lead to an updating of their knowledge base.

Another possible explanation for the observed familiarity effect in the study by S. C. Brown and Park (2002) is that there is less room for growth of knowledge when more is already known about a topic. In other words, the rate of learning may be proportional to the amount of material yet to be learned (e.g., Sagiv, 1979). Consistent with this view, participants exhibited the greatest knowledge on the multiple-choice test if they were older adults answering questions about a familiar disease, but they also exhibited the least learning under these same conditions (see Figure 5.2). Although older adults' reduced rate of learning may seem to be of little importance for familiar medical topics because of their prior knowledge of these topics, even "minor" forgetting of medical information can have serious health consequences for older adults, whose diminished organ reserve or physiological capacity can make them more susceptible to mismanagement of health conditions caused by an incomplete illness representation (see Fries, 1990).

Overcoming Inaccurate Health Beliefs

S. C. Brown and Park's (2002) finding that participants learned little new information about a familiar illness is reminiscent of earlier work suggesting that older adults with chronic health conditions sometimes have existing, but inaccurate, beliefs about their conditions that can be difficult to revise (Okun & Rice, 1997, 2001). For example, a common misconception about hypertension is that patients can tell when their blood pressure is elevated by monitoring their symptoms (D. Meyer, Leventhal, & Gutmann, 1985). Similarly, some patients with osteoarthritis believe that hot, swollen joints improve with use, when in fact the opposite is true (Okun & Rice, 1997). Interestingly, Okun and Rice (2001) found that older adults with osteoarthritis were more likely than nonarthritic older adults to misinterpret a factual text on arthritis as confirming their false beliefs about the disease when in fact it disconfirmed these erroneous beliefs! Such false beliefs may arise through reliance on folk wisdom or illusory correlations (i.e., the appearance of a systematic relationship between two variables that is actually spurious) and likely have implications for participants' selection of treatments and subsequent compliance (e.g., decisions about taking medicines and exercising).

However, Okun and Rice (1997) have reported methods by which older adults' medical misconceptions may be overcome: These researchers assessed older osteoarthritis patients' beliefs about their disease and then subsequently presented each participant with a text about arthritis in which target items related to his or her misconceptions were embedded. Some of the target items that disconfirmed the participants' beliefs were explicitly signaled in the text through pointer phrases (e.g., "contrary to popular opinion" or "an important point is"), whereas some disconfirming statements were only implicitly signaled, without a pointer phrase. In addition, half of the participants were given the opportunity to restate their illness beliefs immediately after reading the text, and half were given a filler task. The authors found that the combined use of pointer words to signal important details in the text and having participants restate their beliefs led to the greatest changes in participants' false beliefs 2 weeks after testing.

Okun and Rice's (1997) finding suggests that when health professionals present new information to older adults on a familiar health topic, they should identify and understand the likely misconceptions that older patients may have about the topic as well as help the patient to recognize the contradiction between his or her misconceptions and the accurate information provided during the medical encounter. Health professionals should also ask patients to restate information in their own words to provide opportunities for the updating of beliefs. Finally, health care workers should be aware that individuals may vary greatly in their beliefs about a particular illness and that each individual's specific beliefs must be addressed (see also chaps. 4, 6, and 10, this volume).

Paradoxical Effects of Repeated Warnings

Recent work by Skurnik, Yoon, Park, and Schwarz (2005) suggests that health professionals may need to proceed somewhat cautiously when attempting to disconfirm patients' existing incorrect beliefs about medical conditions or treatments. More specifically, Skurnik et al. showed that repeated warnings to older adults that information is false can actually backfire and make the information seem all the more true later on. This is known as the *illusion of truth*, which is a memory distortion in which sheer repetition of statements causes people to believe the statements are true (e.g., Begg, Anas, & Farinacci, 1992). Older adults may be particularly vulnerable to this illusion because of the combination of age invariance in the automatically generated feeling of familiarity produced by viewing the statements presented during the experiment (e.g., Jacoby et al., 1996) and age declines in recollection or memory for detailed information about the source of this information (e.g., Spencer & Raz, 1995).

In other words, memories tend to become "decontextualized" in old age, so that if older adults think they have heard a piece of information before (i.e., it seems vaguely familiar to them) but cannot remember the specific source of the information (i.e., who said it or where it was learned), then they may use the heuristic or rule of thumb that if information seems familiar then it must be true. This type of memory distortion can be particularly problematic for older adults, given their greater consumption of medical services as well as their exposure to sometimes complex and unreliable medical claims from media reports as well as drug advertisements, supermarket tabloids, Web sites, friends, and family members.

In an initial study examining age differences in the illusion-of-truth effect, Skurnik et al. (2005) presented younger and older adults with a variety of health statements such as "DHEA supplements can lead to liver damage," which were labeled as either true or false and which were presented either once or three times. (For ethical reasons, all the statements were actually true.) Then, after a delay, participants saw these statements again and had to decide whether they were true. For both the older and younger adults, stating three times that a statement was false made it less likely to seem true immediately. That is, repeated warnings that a statement was false (e.g., "It is *not* true that shark cartilage cures cancer!") initially helped both age groups avoid the illusion-of-truth effect. However, after several days for older adults, the initially beneficial effect of repeated warnings backfired and paradoxically made false information seem all the more true. In other words, over time the older adults were *more* likely to believe that shark cartilage cures cancer if they were told repeatedly that the statement is false than if they were told just once! In contrast, the advantage of repetition stayed with younger adults after 3 days, and repeated warnings made them less likely to mistakenly remember a false statement as true.

An important implication of this line of research is that those who interact with older adults should state their instructions in positive terms rather than warning against negative results (e.g., "Take this medicine with food" rather than "Don't take this medicine on an empty stomach") to avoid producing memory distortions like the illusion of truth. A further suggestion is to provide additional elaborations for medical instructions and warnings, such as reasons for taking a drug with food (e.g., to prevent an upset stomach), which can also increase individuals' memory for this information. Finally, health professionals should provide older patients with reading materials that they can consult for future reference, which can strengthen memory for source information and hence reduce the likelihood of paradoxical memory illusions.

COGNITIVE EFFECTS OF MEDICAL CONDITIONS AND THEIR TREATMENTS

Medical conditions and their treatments may affect older patients' cognitive functioning and hence their ability to learn medical information. The cognitive impacts of medical conditions and their interventions are explored in the following section.

Cognitive Effects of Medical Conditions

Health professionals should be aware that in addition to age-related cognitive and sensory losses, many older patients have medical conditions and treatments that may limit their ability to process new medical information. For example, individuals experiencing high levels of physical pain or depression may show a reduction in the amount of basic mental resources that they have available to perform effortful cognitive tasks such as recall of information or decision making.

My colleagues and I assessed the relationship of pain and depression to cognitive function in patients with rheumatoid arthritis, a systemic illness characterized by chronic pain, stiffness, and swelling of joints (S. C. Brown, Glass, & Park, 2002). One hundred twenty-one community-dwelling rheumatoid arthritis patients (ages 34–84) completed a battery of cognitive tasks, including speed of processing, working memory, long-term memory, and reasoning (Park et al., 1999). Participants also completed multiple measures of pain and depression. Structural equation modeling techniques, which combine multiple regression with path-analytic procedures, were used to assess the relative contributions of pain, depression, and age to cognitive performance.

Statistical analyses revealed that individuals who performed poorly on the four effortful cognitive tasks reported more pain and depression and were older than those individuals who performed well on cognitive tasks. In addition, high levels of pain were associated with depression in this sample. Further analyses revealed that depression mediated the relationship between pain and cognition. That is, when depression was entered into the analyses after pain, there was no longer a significant direct effect of pain on cognition. It is interesting to note that when age was added as the final variable in the analyses, depression continued to mediate the pain–cognition relationship, and the effects of pain and depression on cognition were largely independent of age. Our hypothesized model of cognition in rheumatoid arthritis patients, shown in Figure 5.3, explained 55% of the variance in cognition.

Thus, rheumatoid arthritis patients with high levels of pain were at greater risk of cognitive impairment. However, pain's impact on cognition occurred indirectly, through pain's impact on depression, which in turn caused cognitive dysfunction. Perhaps high levels of rheumatoid arthritis pain cause patients to engage in self-destructive negative rumination that disrupts their performance on effortful cognitive tasks. These findings suggest that chronic pain, and more specifically psychological distress caused by pain, can deplete scarce cognitive resources that patients need to complete critical mental activities such as comprehending new medical information or deciding among treatment alternatives. However, these results do not rule out the possibility that pain and depression can exert independent effects on cognition in some patient populations: For example, pain but not depression is a predictor of cognitive problems in patients with

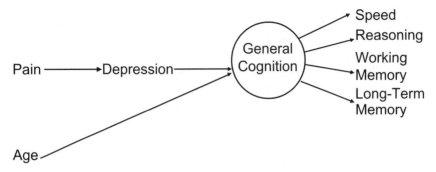

Figure 5.3. Final hypothesized model of the relations of age, pain, and depression to cognitive function in rheumatoid arthritis patients. From "The Relationship of Pain and Depression to Cognitive Function in Rheumatoid Arthritis Patients," by S. C. Brown, J. M. Glass, and D. C. Park, 2002, *Pain, 96,* p. 282. Copyright 2002 by Elsevier Science. Adapted with permission.

fibromyalgia, a puzzling rheumatologic disorder characterized by widespread musculoskeletal pain and fatigue (Park, Glass, Minear, & Crofford, 2001). Moreover, cognitive difficulties have been noted in patients with low back pain (Söderfjell et al., 2000) and in patients with depression but with no chronic pain (Christensen, Griffiths, MacKinnon, & Jacomb, 1997).

In addition to physical pain and depression, older patients may have any number of health problems or conditions that could negatively affect their cognitive functioning. These include cardiovascular disease and hypertension (Ylikoski et al., 2000), diabetes (Biessels, van der Heide, Kamal, Bleys, & Gispen, 2002), and long-term alcohol abuse (Glass, Park, & Zucker, 1999).

Cognitive Effects of Medical Treatments

Physicians should be aware that many individuals with the health problems previously described may not be properly diagnosed and may have cognitive deficits that reverse after adequate treatment: For example, patients with diabetes who were on a stable dose of an antihyperglycemic agent for 6 months showed improvements in fasting blood glucose and in multiple neuropsychological measures, including recall and reasoning (Meneilly, Cheung, Tessier, Yakura, & Tuokko, 1993).

On the other hand, cognitive functioning may also be adversely affected by the drugs many older patients take, including minor tranquilizers such as benzodiazepines (Sumner, 1998), pain medications such as opioids (Zacny, 1996), and chemotherapy treatments for cancer (Ahles & Saykin, 2001). The cognitive effects of such drugs may be even stronger in older patients because of age-related metabolic changes that may cause these drugs to remain active for longer periods of time (Halter, 1999). In addition, older adults may be at increased risk of cognitive problems because of the problem of *polypharmacy*, or the taking of several drugs at the same time that may interact with one another in unexpected ways to treat multiple conditions. For example, the Centers for Disease Control and Prevention (2002) estimated that over 51% of adults age 65 and older currently take two or more prescription drugs, and 12% take five drugs or more. Because many older adults take multiple drugs prescribed by different health specialists as well as over-the-counter drugs and herbal remedies not prescribed by physicians, it is imperative that health professionals get a complete listing of all medications and supplements taken by their older patients to avoid unanticipated drug interactions that could affect patients' mental and physical functioning.

Cognitive Impacts of Delirium and Dementia

Another important issue with implications for older patients' cognitive functioning concerns the distinction between delirium (i.e., acute brain syndromes resulting from drug toxicity, infections, and disturbances of mood or metabolism) and dementia (i.e., chronic brain syndromes involving a progressive deterioration of intelligence and cognitive ability over time). Although a thorough discussion of differences between delirium and dementia is beyond the scope of this chapter, delirium generally involves a sudden disorientation to one's surroundings and is reversible if the underlying causes are detected in time, whereas dementias such as those related to Alzheimer's disease have a slow onset and gradual intellectual deterioration over a period of months or years (for further discussion, see, e.g., Zarit & Zarit, 1998). However, both delirium and dementias can impair individuals' capacity to process medical information over and above the more benign effects of normal cognitive aging. Individuals with delirium or dementia may have a variety of information-processing deficits, depending on whether the individual is experiencing alterations in verbal knowledge, long-term memory, comprehension, or judgment (see also Marson & Harrell, 1999). Therefore, if a physician suspects that an older patient is showing signs of cognitive impairment, it may be necessary to perform a brief mental status examination as part of the initial session (Adelman, Greene, & Ory, 2000).

Summary of Cognitive Effects of Medical
Conditions and Treatments

Older patients may face a number of threats to their cognitive functioning as a result of medical conditions and their treatments as well as mood disorders and the effects of normal cognitive aging. It is important for health professionals to be aware of the distinction between the occasional memory lapses often experienced by older adults and the more severe alterations of mental functioning that are characteristic of either acute or chronic brain syndromes and to treat patients' cognitive difficulties accordingly.

PSYCHOSOCIAL ISSUES FACING OLDER PATIENTS

In addition to the impacts of normal aging and biomedical variables on older patients' processing of health information, several psychosocial issues can affect older patients' ability to learn about and comply with treatment programs. Some of these issues are explored in this section.

Older Patients' Behaviors in the Medical Encounter

There is evidence that older adults do not seek out medical information as actively as do younger adults. For example, B. J. F. Meyer et al. (1995) and Zwahr, Park, and Shifren (1999) both found that older adults who were asked to make hypothetical medical decisions considered fewer treatment options and made fewer comparisons among choices compared with younger adults. Similarly, several studies have shown that older adults are less active participants in the medical encounter compared with other age groups, and older patients exhibit fewer conversational behaviors such as asking questions, interrupting the physician, and asserting opinions (e.g., Kaplan, Gandek, Greenfield, Rogers, & Ware, 1995; Roter et al., 1997). Moreover, older patients may fail to ask for medical information from health professionals unless given enough time during the medical encounter to do so (Beisecker & Beisecker, 1990). However, older adults who have substantial experience with a chronic illness tend to participate more in the office visit, and they question physicians' treatment decisions more often than do younger or less experienced patients (Haug & Lavin, 1983).

Although older persons' more passive approach to information gathering could be partly the result of age-related cognitive impairments, it is also likely that many older adults, particularly those age 75 and older, have been socialized to defer to a physician's authority and judgment (Kaplan et al., 1995; Roter, 2000). Moreover, patients may draw comfort and support from a paternalistic doctor–patient relationship, particularly when they are very sick and thus at their most vulnerable (Roter, 2000). It is unclear whether the seeming passivity of older patients is a function of advanced chronological age or a cohort effect that will change as younger patients age. It is possible that the generation of baby boomers who are rapidly approaching retirement may be more active in their seeking of health care information and in their interactions with health professionals compared with previous generations of older adults (Kaplan et al., 1995).

The passivity of older patients in the medical encounter may be particularly problematic given findings that 56% of older patients failed to raise important medical problems with their physicians, and 60% neglected to discuss psychosocial issues that were important to them (Rost & Frankel, 1993). Moreover, other work suggests that older patients have less concordant medical encounters than do younger patients with regard to agreement with physicians on the main goal of the visit as well as the main medical topics, including symptoms, test results, medications, and prevention (Greene, Adelman, Charon, & Friedmann, 1989). This lack of agreement on health issues and unmet expectations may partly reflect the less complete information provided by older patients, which could lead to lower patient satisfaction and hence lower compliance with the physician's treatment plan (Stewart, Meredith, Brown, & Galajda, 2000). Moreover, other research suggests that patients who are not involved in treatment decisions or who do not ask questions have worse health outcomes than do patients who are more actively involved in the medical encounter (Stewart, 1995). However, the good news is that several studies have successfully coached patients to ask questions and to participate in medical decisions, and this has been associated with improved recall of information presented by the physician (Robinson & Whitfield, 1985) as well as objective changes in patients' communication behaviors and improvements in patients' functional and physiological status at the next office visit (Kaplan, Greenfield, & Ware, 1989).

Physicians' Behaviors Toward the Older Patient

A second but related set of issues concerns the physician's behaviors and attitudes toward the older patient. In particular, physicians' conversational behaviors, including the types and amounts of information that they provide, can affect older adults' processing of medical information. For example, several studies have shown that physicians ask older patients more questions than younger patients about their medications (Hall, Roter, & Katz, 1988) and give them more information, particularly biomedical information, compared with their younger counterparts (Kaplan et al., 1995; Roter et al., 1997). Although this increased informational exchange would appear to be helpful, other work has shown that as a physician gives more information and asks more questions, the percentage of information recalled by the patient decreases (Hall et al., 1988; Roter & Hall, 1989). Moreover, patients tend to be less satisfied with physicians who dominate the interview or who focus on biomedical issues to such a degree that they neglect the patient's emotional concerns (Roter et al., 1997). Still other work suggests that how physicians present treatment options to older patients has an impact on patients' treatment preferences. For example, Mazur and Merz (1993) reported that the manner in which physicians presented survival rate information to patients age 65 and older influenced the patients' treatment decisions (for further discussion of medical decisions in older patients, see also chap. 9, this volume).

Therefore, physicians may need to provide enough information to older patients to ensure understanding but not so much as to confuse them. Alternatively, health professionals can enhance a patient's recall of a complex medical regimen by blocking and simplifying instructions, prioritizing and stressing the most important messages, summarizing information, and soliciting feedback from the patient on his or her understanding of the information by asking closed-ended questions (Ley, 1979; Roter, 2000). In addition, physicians should consider providing take-home information to older patients in the form of either written pamphlets or an audiotape of the medical encounter, given the fact that older adults perform nearly as well as younger adults when they have materials that support memory at both encoding and retrieval (Craik & Jennings, 1992).

In addition, physicians' attitudes toward older patients can affect patients' ability to acquire new health information. For example, physicians may exhibit subtle forms of ageism during the medical encounter, including providing less preventive treatment information to older patients and treating their medical problems less aggressively because they believe that many health problems in older patients are the inevitable result of natural age-related processes or of long-standing lifestyle choices that are difficult to change (Cobbs, Duthie, & Murphy, 1999). Furthermore, physicians may dislike treating older patients because of their sometimes complex health problems, including multiple concurrent conditions, which may not be readily resolved within a single office visit. Consequently, physicians may rush through appointments with older patients or exhibit subtle negativity toward them in the form of negative voice tone or nonverbal behaviors, which may result in patients' not raising important medical and psychosocial issues with their physicians (Beisecker & Beisecker, 1990) or in the patients' placing little faith in the physician's treatment suggestions and hence not complying with the treatment plan (Linn, Linn, & Stein, 1982).

Providing more formal training in geriatrics may help physicians and other health professionals to address these challenges to informed care of older adults (Halter, 1999). In addition, physicians should encourage patients to ask questions and should incorporate their knowledge of the patient's daily life to determine the medication dosage schedule. Moreover, to the extent that the medical encounter is limited in time and physical space, physicians should consider giving patients the opportunity to phone a physician's assistant or contact the physician via e-mail to ask any questions that were not fully answered during the office visit. Alternatively, group care sessions, which enable patients to interact with a physician, nurse, and other patients with similar health conditions, can provide patients an opportunity to ask questions and gather information in an environment that allows peer support (Health Care Advisory Board, 1997).

Impact of a Third Person in the Medical Encounter

Another issue with implications for older patients' learning of medical information concerns the presence of a third person in the medical encounter. Various studies have estimated that between 20% and 57% of older patients bring a third person, such as a partner or adult child, with them to the doctor's office for emotional and informational support (Prohaska & Glasser, 1996).

The effects of this third person on older adults' medical information processing and health outcomes appear to be mixed. On the one hand, the involvement of a third person in the medical encounter has been shown to help older patients in their understanding of information provided by the physician (Prohaska & Glasser, 1996) as well as in their adherence to sometimes complex treatment regimens (Coe, Prendergast, & Psathas, 1984). A caregiver's assistance in remembering and implementing a medical regimen can be an important form of environmental support for an older patient, given findings that older patients may fail to recall up to 50% of the medications appearing on their medical charts (Rost & Roter, 1987). A caregiver may also act as an important advocate for the patient during the medical encounter by asking questions and providing helpful information to the physician on the patients' symptoms and responsiveness to treatments (Adelman et al., 2000).

On the other hand, the presence of a third person such as a caregiver has been shown to have some negative influences on the medical encounter, including fewer patient-initiated topics; less joint decision making and patient assertiveness; and more discussions about, and not with, the patient (Greene, Majerovitz, Adelman, & Rizzo, 1994). In addition, Adelman et al. (2000) have noted that caregivers who participate in medical encounters can sometimes work against the patient on either overt or covert levels— for example, by ignoring the patient's agenda or treating him or her as incompetent. However, one study of caregivers' participation in medical encounters revealed that physicians found the accompanying caregiver's behavior to be primarily supportive to both the patient and physician in the vast majority of cases (J. B. Brown, Brett, Stewart, & Marshall, 1998). Thus, conflicting data remain on the impact of a third person on the older patient–provider relationship and health outcomes (Stewart et al., 2000).

SUMMARY AND CONCLUSIONS

In summary, older patients have difficulties in learning several types of medical information because of age-related declines in sensory function and in basic cognitive abilities such as speed of processing and working memory. For example, older adults have difficulty comprehending and recalling instructions for use of medications and medical devices (Morrell et al., 1989, 1990; Mykityshyn et al., 2002) as well as treatment recommendations (B. J. F. Meyer et al., 1995) and information on advance medical directives (Zwahr et al., 1997). In contrast, older adults do relatively well in situations in which they can rely on environmental supports, such as medication organizers and preset alarms that automatically prompt them to take their medications (Park et al., 1992, 1997), as well as well-structured instructions that limit the need for making inferences (Morrow, Leirer, Andrassy, Hier, & Menard, 1998; Mykityshyn et al., 2002).

Some research suggests that older adults have substantial knowledge of certain medical topics that they could use to compensate for age-related declines in cognitive abilities when processing medical information (e.g., Park et al., 1999; Zwahr et al., 1999). For example, older patients have been found to be more adherent at taking their medications than younger patients, despite showing declines on laboratory tasks of cognition, which may reflect the older patients' greater experience with taking medicine (Park et al., 1999).

However, other research suggests that older adults appear to have only limited success in using their prior knowledge of medical topics as a "cognitive scaffolding" on which to hang additional medical information (S. C. Brown & Park, 2002). In addition, older patients may have false health beliefs (Okun & Rice, 1997, 2001) and a susceptibility to false medical claims because of age declines in detailed source memory (Skurnik et al., 2005; see also chap. 7, this volume).

Health care providers may be able to overcome older adults' false health beliefs by using language that helps individuals recognize the contradiction between their false beliefs and the new, accurate information that is presented to them and by having individuals restate their beliefs after the new information is presented (Okun & Rice, 1997). On the other hand, repeated warnings that medical claims are false can actually backfire and cause older adults to believe, later on, that the claims are true (Skurnik et al., 2005). Therefore, health professionals should try to (a) state instructions in positive, concrete terms (e.g., "Take three pills") rather than warning against more negative results (e.g., "Don't take too much medicine") and (b) provide older patients with take-home information to avoid paradoxical memory distortions such as the illusion of truth. Health professionals should also be aware that older adults may experience cognitive difficulties over and above the effects of normal aging due to the effects of some chronic medical conditions (e.g., Biessels et al., 2002; S. C. Brown et al., 2002; Ylikoski et al., 2000; Zarit & Zarit, 1998) and drug treatments (e.g., Sumner, 1998; Zacny, 1996).

Health care providers should also recognize that several psychosocial aspects of the doctor–patient interaction can affect older adults' ability to acquire new health information as well as their health outcomes. Some main points of research in this area are as follows:

- Older patients may not ask for health information unless there is sufficient time during the medical encounter (Beisecker & Beisecker, 1990);
- although older patients receive substantial medical information from their physician or other health care provider (Kaplan et al., 1995; Roter, 2000), patients' recall of information and satisfaction with the medical encounter have been shown to decrease as the health provider presents more information and dominates the medical interview (Hall et al., 1988; Roter et al., 1997); and
- many older patients report that they failed to discuss important psychosocial and biomedical issues with their physician or health care provider (Rost & Frankel, 1993).

Older adults have been successfully coached to ask questions and to participate more fully in medical decisions, with corresponding improvements in patients' conversational behaviors as well as in their understanding of health information and their health and functional status (Kaplan et al., 1989; Robinson & Whitfield, 1985). In addition, the presence of a third person such as a caregiver in the medical encounter can be a potentially important informational support for both the older patient and the health care provider (Adelman et al., 2000; J. B. Brown et al., 1998). Finally, health professionals can improve their communication of medical information to older patients by doing the following: (a) emphasizing and reviewing important points raised during the office visit; (b) providing take-home information; and (c) allowing for follow-up phone calls or e-mails, which may provide additional means for older patients to ask additional questions, as well as building trust in the older patient–provider relationship.

REFERENCES

Adelman, R., Greene, M., & Ory, M. (2000). Communication between older patients and their physicians. *Clinics in Geriatric Medicine, 16,* 1–36.

Ahles, T. A., & Saykin, A. (2001). Cognitive effects of standard-dose chemotherapy in patients with cancer. *Cancer Investigation, 19*, 812–820.

Begg, I. M., Anas, A., & Farinacci, S. (1992). Dissociation of processes in belief: Source recollection, statement familiarity, and the illusion of truth. *Journal of Experimental Psychology: General, 121*, 446–458.

Beisecker, A. E., & Beisecker, T. D. (1990). Patient information-seeking behaviors when communicating with their doctors. *Medical Care, 28*, 19–28.

Biessels, G. J., van der Heide, L. P., Kamal, A., Bleys, R. L., & Gispen, W. H. (2002). Ageing and diabetes: Implications for brain function. *European Journal of Pharmacology, 441*, 1–14.

Brown, J. B., Brett, P., Stewart, M., & Marshall, J. N. (1998). Roles and influence of people who accompany patients on visits to the doctor. *Canadian Family Physician, 44*, 1644–1650.

Brown, S. C., Glass, J. M., & Park, D. C. (2002). The relationship of pain and depression to cognitive function in rheumatoid arthritis patients. *Pain, 96*, 279–284.

Brown, S. C., & Park, D. C. (2002). Roles of age and familiarity in learning health information. *Educational Gerontology, 28*, 695–710.

Brown, S. C., & Park, D. C. (2003). Theoretical models of cognitive aging and implications for translational research in medicine. *The Gerontologist, 43*, 57–67.

Centers for Disease Control and Prevention. (2002). *National Health and Nutrition Examination Survey: Patterns of prescription drug use in the United States, 1988–94.* Retrieved July 27, 2006, from http://www.cdc.gov/nchs/data/nhanes/databriefs/preuse.pdf

Christensen, H., Griffiths, K., MacKinnon, A., & Jacomb, P. (1997). A quantitative review of cognitive deficits in depression and Alzheimer-type dementia. *Journal of the International Neuropsychological Society, 3*, 631–651.

Cobbs, E. L., Duthie, E. H., & Murphy, J. B. (1999). *Geriatrics review syllabus: A core curriculum in geriatric medicine* (4th ed.). Dubuque, IA: Kendall/Hunt.

Coe, R. M., Prendergast, C. G., & Psathas, G. (1984). Strategies for obtaining compliance with medications regimens. *Journal of the American Geriatrics Society, 32*, 589–594.

Craik, F. I. M. (1986). A functional account of age differences in memory. In F. Klix & H. Hagendorf (Eds.), *Human memory and cognitive capabilities, mechanisms, and performances* (pp. 409–422). North-Holland, Amsterdam: Elsevier Science.

Craik, F. I. M., & Jennings, J. M. (1992). Human memory. In F. I. M. Craik & T. A. Salthouse (Eds.), *The handbook of aging and cognition* (pp. 51–110). Hillsdale, NJ: Erlbaum.

Craik, F. I. M., & McDowd, J. M. (1987). Age differences in recall and recognition. *Journal of Experimental Psychology: Learning, Memory, and Cognition, 21*, 531–547.

Fisk, A. D., & Rogers, W. A. (2001). Health care of older adults: The promise of human factors research. In W. A. Rogers & A. D. Fisk (Eds.), *Human factors interventions for the health care of older adults* (pp. 1–12). Mahwah, NJ: Erlbaum.

Fozard, J. L., & Gordon-Salant, S. (2001). Changes in vision and hearing with aging. In J. E. Birren (Ed.), *Handbook of the psychology of aging* (5th ed., pp. 241–266). San Diego, CA: Academic Press.

Fries, J. F. (1990). Medical perspectives upon successful aging. In P. B. Baltes & M. M. Baltes (Eds.), *Successful aging* (pp. 35–49). New York: Cambridge University Press.

Frieske, D. A., & Park, D. C. (1999). Memory for news in young and old adults. *Psychology and Aging, 14,* 90–98.

Glass, J. M., Park, D. C., & Zucker, R. A. (1999). Alcoholism, aging, and cognition: A review of evidence for shared or independent impairments. *Aging, Neuropsychology, and Cognition, 6,* 157–178.

Graesser, A. C., & Nakamura, G. V. (1982). The impact of a schema on comprehension and memory. In G. H. Bower (Ed.), *The psychology of learning and motivation* (Vol. 16, pp. 59–109). New York: Academic Press.

Greene, M. G., Adelman, R. D., Charon, R., & Friedmann, E. (1989). Concordance between physicians and their older and younger patients in the primary care medical encounter. *Gerontologist, 29,* 808–813.

Greene, M. G., Majerovitz, S. D., Adelman, R. D., & Rizzo, C. (1994). The effects of the presence of a third person on the physician–older patient medical interview. *Journal of the American Geriatrics Society, 42,* 413–419.

Hall, J. A., Roter, D. L., & Katz, N. R. (1988). Meta-analysis of correlates of provider behavior in medical encounters. *Medical Care, 26,* 657–675.

Halter, J. B. (1999). The challenge of communicating health information to elderly patients: A view from geriatric medicine. In D. C. Park, R. W. Morrell, & K. Shifren (Eds.), *Processing of medical information in aging patients: Cognitive and human factors perspectives* (pp. 23–28). Mahwah, NJ: Erlbaum.

Hancock, H. E., Rogers, W. A., & Fisk, A. D. (2001). An evaluation of warning habits and beliefs across the adult life span. *Human Factors, 43,* 343–354.

Hasher, L., & Zacks, R. T. (1988). Working memory, comprehension, and aging: A review and a new view. In G. H. Bower (Ed.), *The psychology of learning and motivation* (Vol. 22, pp. 193–225). San Diego, CA: Academic Press.

Haug, M. R., & Lavin, B. (1983). *Consumerism in medicine: Challenging physician authority.* Beverly Hills, CA: Sage.

Health Care Advisory Board. (1997). *Innovations in eldercare: Managing senior care under risk.* Washington, DC: The Advisory Board Company.

Jacoby, L. L., Jennings, J. M., & Hay, J. F. (1996). Dissociating automatic and consciously-controlled processes: Implications for diagnosis and rehabilitation of memory deficits. In D. C. Hermann, C. L. McEvoy, C. Hertzog, P. Hertel, & M. K. Johnson (Eds.), *Basic and applied memory research: Theory in context* (Vol. 1, pp. 161–193). Hillsdale, NJ: Erlbaum.

Kaplan, S. H., Gandek, B., Greenfield, S., Rogers, W., & Ware, J. E. (1995). Patient and visit characteristics related to physicians' participatory decision-making style: Results from the Medical Outcomes Study. *Medical Care, 33,* 1176–1187.

Kaplan, S. H., Greenfield, S., & Ware, J. E., Jr. (1989). Assessing the effects of physician–patient interactions on the outcomes of chronic disease. *Medical Care, 27*(Suppl. 3), S110–S127.

Kemper, S. (1992). Language and aging. In F. I. M. Craik & T. A. Salthouse (Eds.), *The handbook of aging and cognition* (pp. 495–552). Hillsdale, NJ: Erlbaum.

La Voie, D., & Light, L. L. (1994). Adult age differences in repetition priming: A meta-analysis. *Psychology and Aging, 9,* 539–553.

Ley, P. (1979). Memory for medical information. *British Journal of Social and Clinical Psychology, 18,* 245–255.

Light, L. L. (1992). The organization of memory in old age. In F. I. M. Craik & T. A. Salthouse (Eds.), *The handbook of aging and cognition* (pp. 111–165). Hillsdale, NJ: Erlbaum.

Linn, M. W., Linn, B. S., & Stein, S. R. (1982). Satisfaction with ambulatory care and compliance in older patients. *Medical Care, 20,* 606–614.

Liu, L. L., & Park, D. C. (2004). Aging and medical adherence: The use of automatic processes to achieve effortful things. *Psychology and Aging, 19,* 318–325.

Long, L. L., & Shaw, R. J. (2000). Adult age differences in vocabulary acquisition. *Educational Gerontology, 26,* 651–664.

Mandler, G. M. (1980). Recognizing: The judgment of previous occurrence. *Psychological Review, 87,* 252–271.

Marson, D., & Harrell, L. (1999). Neurocognitive changes associated with loss of capacity to consent to medical treatment in patients with Alzheimer's disease. In D. C. Park, R. W. Morrell, & K. Shifren (Eds.), *Processing of medical information in aging patients: Cognitive and human factors perspectives* (pp. 109–126). Mahwah, NJ: Erlbaum.

Mazur, D. J., & Merz, J. F. (1993). How the manner of presentation of data influences older patients in determining their treatment preferences. *Journal of the American Geriatrics Society, 41,* 223–228.

McGuire, L. C. (1996). Remembering what the doctor said: Organization and adults' memory for medical information. *Experimental Aging Research, 22,* 403–428.

Meneilly, G. S., Cheung, E., Tessier, D., Yakura, C., & Tuokko, H. (1993). The effect of improved glycemic control on cognitive functions in the elderly patient with diabetes. *Journal of Gerontology, 48,* M117–M121.

Merck Research Laboratories. (1997). Drugs and aging. In R. Berkow (Ed.), *The Merck manual of medical information: Home edition* (pp. 39–41). Whitehouse Station, NJ: Author.

Meyer, B. J. F., Russo, C., & Talbot, A. (1995). Discourse comprehension and problem-solving: Decisions about the treatment of breast cancer by women across the life span. *Psychology and Aging, 10,* 84–103.

Meyer, D., Leventhal, H., & Gutmann, M. (1985). Common-sense models of illness: The example of hypertension. *Health Psychology, 4,* 115–135.

Morrell, R. W., Park, D. C., & Poon, L. W. (1989). Quality of instructions on prescription drug labels: Effects of memory and comprehension in young and old adults. *The Gerontologist, 29,* 345–354.

Morrell, R. W., Park, D. C., & Poon, L. W. (1990). Effects of labeling techniques on memory and comprehension of prescription information in young and old adults. *Journal of Gerontology, 45,* P166–P172.

Morrow, D. G., & Leirer, V. O. (1999). Designing medication instructions for older adults. In D. C. Park, R. W. Morrell, & K. Shifren (Eds.), *Processing of medical information in aging patients: Cognitive and human factors perspectives* (pp. 249–265). Mahwah, NJ: Erlbaum.

Morrow, D. G., Leirer, V. O., Andrassy, J. M., Hier, C. M., & Menard, W. E. (1998). The influence of list format and category headers on age differences in understanding medication instructions. *Experimental Aging Research, 24,* 231–256.

Morrow, D. G., Leirer, V. O., Carver, L. M., Tanke, E. D., & McNally, A. D. (1999). Effects of aging, message repetition, and note-taking on memory for health information. *Journals of Gerontology Series B: Psychological Sciences and Social Sciences, 54,* P369–P379.

Mykityshyn, A. L., Fisk, A. D., & Rogers, W. A. (2002). Learning to use a home medical device: Mediating age-related differences with training. *Human Factors, 44,* 354–364.

Okun, M. A., & Rice, G. E. (1997). Overcoming elders' misconceptions about accurate written medical information. *Journal of Applied Gerontology, 16,* 51–70.

Okun, M. A., & Rice, G. E. (2001). The effects of personal relevance of topic and information type on older adults' accurate recall of written medical passages about osteoarthritis. *Journal of Aging and Health, 13,* 410–429.

Park, D. C. (1999). Aging and the controlled and automatic processing of medical information and medical intentions. In D. C. Park, R. W. Morrell, & K. Shifren (Eds.), *Processing of medical information in aging patients: Cognitive and human factors perspectives* (pp. 3–22). Mahwah, NJ: Erlbaum.

Park, D. C. (2000). The basic mechanisms accounting for age-related decline in cognitive function. In D. C. Park & N. Schwarz (Eds.), *Cognitive aging: A primer* (pp. 3–21). Philadelphia: Psychology Press.

Park, D. C., Glass, J. M., Minear, M., & Crofford, L. J. (2001). Cognitive function in fibromyalgia patients. *Arthritis and Rheumatism, 44,* 2125–2133.

Park, D. C., & Hall Gutchess, A. (2000). Cognitive aging and everyday life. In D. C. Park & N. Schwarz (Eds.), *Cognitive aging: A primer* (pp. 217–232). Philadelphia: Psychology Press.

Park, D. C., Hertzog, C., Leventhal, H., Morrell, R. W., Leventhal, E., Birchmore, D., et al. (1999). Medication adherence in rheumatoid arthritis patients: Older is wiser. *Journal of the American Geriatrics Society, 47,* 172–183.

Park, D. C., Lautenschlager, G., Hedden, T., Davidson, N., Smith, A. D., & Smith, P. K. (2002). Models of visuospatial and verbal memory across the adult lifespan. *Psychology and Aging, 17,* 299–320.

Park, D. C., Morrell, R. W., Frieske, D., Blackburn, A. B., & Birchmore, D. (1991). Cognitive factors and the use of over-the-counter medication organizers by arthritis patients. *Human Factors, 31,* 57–67.

Park, D. C., Morrell, R. W., Frieske, D., & Kincaid, D. (1992). Medication adherence behaviors in older adults: Effects of external cognitive supports. *Psychology and Aging, 7,* 252–256.

Park, D. C., Puglisi, J. T., & Smith, A. D. (1986). Memory for pictures: Does an age-related decline exist? *Psychology and Aging, 1,* 11–17.

Park, D. C., & Shaw, R. J. (1992). Effect of environmental support on implicit and explicit memory in younger and older adults. *Psychology and Aging, 7,* 632–642.

Park, D. C., Shifren, K., Morrell, R. W., Watkins, K., & Stuedemann, T. (1997). Improving medication adherence in African-Americans with hypertension: A cognitive intervention strategy [Abstract]. *The Gerontologist, 37,* 330.

Park, D. C., Smith, A. D., Lautenschlager, G., Earles, J., Frieske, D., Zwahr, M., & Gaines, C. (1996). Mediators of long-term memory performance across the lifespan. *Psychology and Aging, 11,* 621–637.

Prohaska, T. R., & Glasser, M. (1996). Patients' views of family involvement in medical care decisions and medical encounters. *Research on Aging, 18,* 52–69.

Robinson, E. J., & Whitfield, M. J. (1985). Improving the efficiency of patients' comprehension monitoring: A way of increasing patients' participation in general practice consultations. *Social Science and Medicine, 21,* 915–919.

Rogers, W. A., Mykityshyn, A. L., Campbell, R. H., & Fisk, A. D. (2001). Only 3 easy steps? User-centered analysis of a "simple" medical device. *Ergonomics in Design, 9,* 6–14.

Rogers, W. A., Rousseau, G. K., & Lamson, N. (1999). Maximizing the effectiveness of the warning process: Understanding the variables that interact with age. In D. C. Park, R. W. Morrell, & K. Shifren (Eds.), *Processing of medical information in aging patients: Cognitive and human factors perspectives* (pp. 267–290). Mahwah, NJ: Erlbaum.

Rost, K., & Frankel, R. (1993). The introduction of the older patient's problem in the medical visit. *Journal of Aging and Health, 5,* 387–401.

Rost, K., & Roter, D. (1987). Predictors of recall of medication regimens and recommendations for lifestyle change in elderly patients. *The Gerontologist, 27,* 510–515.

Roter, D. L. (2000). The outpatient medical encounter and elderly patients. *Clinics in Geriatric Medicine, 16,* 95–107.

Roter, D. L., & Hall, J. A. (1989). Studies of physician–patient interaction. *Annual Review of Public Health, 10,* 163–180.

Roter, D. L., Stewart, M., Putnam, S. M., Lipkin, M., Jr., Stiles, W., & Inui, T. S. (1997). Communication patterns of primary care physicians. *Journal of the American Medical Association, 270,* 350–355.

Sagiv, A. (1979). General growth model for evaluation of an individual's progress in learning. *Journal of Educational Psychology, 71,* 866–881.

Salthouse, T. A. (1992). Reasoning and spatial abilities. In F. I. M. Craik & T. A. Salthouse (Eds.), *The handbook of aging and cognition* (pp. 167–211). Hillsdale, NJ: Erlbaum.

Skurnik, I., Yoon, C., Park, D. C., & Schwarz, N. (2005). How warnings about false claims become recommendations. *Journal of Consumer Research, 31,* 713–724.

Söderfjell, S., Molander, B., Barnekow-Bergkvist, M., Lyskov, E., Johansson, H., & Nilsson, L.-G. (2000, July). *Aging, stress, and musculoskeletal problems.* Poster presented at the International Congress of Psychology, Stockholm, Sweden.

Spencer, W. D., & Raz, N. (1995). Differential effects of aging on memory for content and context: A meta-analysis. *Psychology and Aging, 10,* 527–539.

Stewart, M. A. (1995). Effective physician–patient communication and health outcomes: A review. *Canadian Medical Association Journal, 152,* 1423–1433.

Stewart, M., Meredith, L., Brown, J. B., & Galajda, J. (2000). The influence of older patient–physician communication on health and health-related outcomes. *Clinics in Geriatric Medicine, 16,* 25–36.

Sumner, D. D. (1998). Benzodiazepine-induced persisting amnestic disorder: Are older adults at risk? *Archives of Psychiatric Nursing, 12,* 119–125.

Ylikoski, R., Ylikoski, A., Raininko, R., Keskivaara, P., Sulkava, R., Tilvis, R., & Erkinjuntti, T. (2000). Cardiovascular diseases, health status, brain imaging findings, and neuropsychological functioning in neurologically healthy elderly individuals. *Archives of Gerontology and Geriatrics, 30,* 115–130.

Zacks, R., & Hasher, L. (1997). Cognitive gerontology and attentional inhibition: A reply to Burke and McDowd. *Journals of Gerontology Series B: Psychological Sciences and Social Sciences, 52,* P274–P283.

Zacny, J. P. (1996). Should people taking opioids for medical reasons be allowed to work and drive? *Addiction, 91,* 1581–1584.

Zarit, S. H., & Zarit, J. M. (1998). *Mental disorders in older adults: Fundamentals of assessment and treatment.* New York: Guilford Press.

Zwahr, M. D., Park, D. C., Eaton, T. A., & Larson, E. (1997). Implementation of the Patient Self-Determination Act: A comparison of nursing homes to hospitals. *Journal of Applied Gerontology, 16,* 190–207.

Zwahr, M. D., Park, D. C., & Shifren, K. (1999). Judgment about estrogen replacement therapy: The roles of age, cognitive abilities and beliefs. *Psychology and Aging, 14,* 179–191.

6

REPRESENTATIONS OF SELF AND ILLNESS IN THE PATIENT–PHYSICIAN RELATIONSHIP

MANFRED DIEHL, ANGELENIA SEMEGON,
AND LISE M. YOUNGBLADE

Following a physician's instructions is part of the overall patient–physician relationship and is therefore subject to the interpersonal dynamics that govern this relationship. Although there is a large body of literature on patient–physician communication (Faulkner, 1998; Hinz, 2000; Ley, 1988; Pendleton & Hasler, 1983) and on the parameters that influence the patient–physician relationship (e.g., communication style and skills, expectations of help, beliefs and values), there are still a number of unresolved issues with regard to how this relationship can be improved so that an optimal therapeutic alliance can be achieved.

There are several reasons why increasing patients' adherence to their physicians' or other health care providers' instructions is of particular

Work on this chapter was supported in part by Grants AG 19328 and AG 21147 from the National Institute on Aging awarded to Manfred Diehl. We would like to thank Denise C. Park and Linda L. Liu for helpful comments on an earlier version of this chapter.

importance with regard to older adults. First, because of the age relatedness of most chronic diseases, older adults are most likely to receive medical treatment over long periods of time (Siegler, Bastian, & Bosworth, 2001). Second, because of conditions of comorbidity (Boult, Kane, Louis, Boult, & McCaffrey, 1994; Estes & Rundall, 1992), older adults are also more likely to receive treatment and instructions from multiple physicians or other health care providers (Anderson, 1991; Halter, 1999; Hinz, 2000). Thus, older adults need to understand the instructions of the different physicians or health care providers and need to integrate their understanding into a coherent action plan or behavioral script. If society assumes that physicians and other health care professionals (e.g., pharmacists, nurses, physical therapists, nutritionists) have the expert knowledge that is necessary to assure physical health and well-being, following their instructions is essential for achieving these goals.

The objective of this chapter is to focus on patients' self and illness representations as one avenue for increasing their adherence to their physicians' or other health care providers' instructions. First, we outline the basic assumptions that guide our theoretical reasoning. Second, we discuss the commonsense model of health and illness (H. Leventhal, Leventhal, & Cameron, 2001) that has greatly influenced our argument. Third, we present a model of self and illness representations that builds on the commonsense model of health and illness and explain its importance in the context of the patient–physician relationship. Fourth, we review the empirical evidence in support of the relevance of patients' representations of self and illness. In this section we also discuss the role of chronological age, because it is well documented that older adults' representations of self and illness tend to differ from the representations of younger individuals in important ways. Finally, we address how physicians and other health care providers may be able to assess their patients' representations of self and illness and how they may use the obtained information in their interactions with their patients.

BASIC ASSUMPTIONS GUIDING THE THEORETICAL ELABORATIONS

Researchers in health psychology and behavioral medicine have emphasized for a long time that the prevention and treatment of illness is critically dependent on individuals' willingness to modify and control their behavior (Baum, Revenson, & Singer, 2001; Shumaker, Schron, Ockene, & McBee, 1998). For example, current estimates from different sources suggest that between 60% and 70% of chronic illnesses are directly or indirectly related to lifestyle factors and therefore preventable or modifiable (e.g., U.S. Department of Health and Human Services, 2000). At the same time, health psychologists have documented that the amount of threat or fear associated with a symptom or an illness does not necessarily motivate individuals to seek medical care or to follow the treatment instructions of their physicians (H. Leventhal, Safer, & Panagis, 1983). Thus, more recent theoretical models in the study of communication and health behavior advocate a view of patients as active and self-regulating respondents (H. Leventhal et al., 2001; H. Leventhal & Nerenz, 1985; Zwahr, 1999). Thus, before we discuss the relevance of self and illness representations for the patient–physician relationship and for following physicians' instructions, we explicate the basic assumptions that guide these theoretical elaborations. In doing so, we draw on the work of several well-known health and cognitive psychologists, including the work of H. Leventhal and his colleagues (H. Leventhal et al., 2001), Carver and Scheier (1998), and Lazarus (Lazarus & Folkman, 1984).

Individuals as Active Problem Solvers

Consistent with the theorizing of George Kelly (1955), it is assumed that individuals act like "commonsense scientists." That is, it is assumed that individuals are active problem solvers who try to make sense of potential or actual changes in their physical health and try to control those changes that they perceive as signs of illness. In short, individuals are self-regulating systems, and their adaptation to an illness is the result of (a) their understanding of their symptoms or illness, (b) their available personal and social coping resources, and (c) their expectations regarding outcomes (see Carver & Scheier, 1998; H. Leventhal et al., 2001).

Representations of Self and Illness

Individuals' knowledge about their own person and about the world, including their knowledge about their illness, is organized as *cognitive schemas* or *representations* (Higgins, 1996; Markus & Wurf, 1987; Wyer & Srull, 1994). Cognitive representations can be expressed through language and are hierarchically organized. The position of a certain representation feature within the hierarchy (e.g., a certain self-attribute, such as "I am an optimistic person") determines how accessible and how important it is in the overall cognitive schema or representation. Representation features in higher, more primary positions within the hierarchy are more salient and more cognitively accessible, whereas those in lower, more subordinate positions are less salient and less accessible.

Basic Nature of the Patient–Physician Relationship

The relationship between patient and physician brings together the naive knowledge, attitudes, and expectations of the layperson and the knowledge and expertise of the biomedical professional. The knowledge of the patient regarding symptoms or illness reflects the sociocultural environment that influences his or her self and illness representations, whereas the knowledge of the biomedical expert reflects the established knowledge, current practices, and possibilities of the medical sciences. Several authors have argued that the long-term quality and effectiveness of the patient–physician relationship depend on the goodness of fit between the patient's knowledge, attitudes, values, and expectations and the physician's biomedical expertise. We would like to go even further and argue that a successful physician or health care provider is keenly aware that taking into account patients' self and illness representations is essential for creating a successful therapeutic alliance (Hinz, 2000). This is particularly the case with regard to the treatment of chronic illness conditions, in which the patient–physician relationship often extends over a long period of time and patient and physician get to know each other while the illness progresses through different stages.

In summary, consistent with the elaborations of a number of scholars, we assume that individuals are active, self-regulating problem solvers; that they use their self- and illness-related knowledge for self-regulatory purposes; and that the quality and success of the patient–physician relationship depends on the goodness of fit that is created between the patient's knowledge, attitudes, values, and expectations and the physician's biomedical expertise and interpersonal skills.

COMMONSENSE MODEL OF HEALTH AND ILLNESS

The notion that people's health behavior is influenced by representations of their symptoms and illness is not new. Indeed, this basic idea is inherent in several health behavior models, including the *commonsense model* proposed by Howard and Elaine Leventhal (H. Leventhal et al., 2001; see Figure 6.1).

For example, Figure 6.1 shows that the symptoms experienced by a person result in a specific illness representation that includes a label that encompasses the symptoms and the illness itself, assumptions about the temporal course (i.e., timeline) of the symptoms, their perceived cause, their severity and short- and long-term consequences, and their controllability. This illness representation, in turn, influences individuals' coping behaviors (e.g., problem-focused vs. emotion-focused coping; Lazarus & Folkman, 1984) and outcome appraisals (e.g., "With appropriate treatment and help

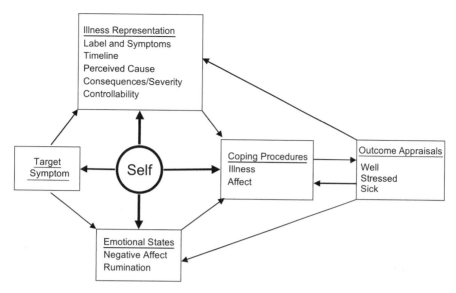

Figure 6.1. The self as a moderating factor in the commonsense model of health and illness. From "Are There Differences in Perceptions of Illness Across the Lifespan?" by E. A. Leventhal and M. Crouch, 1997. In K. J. Petrie and J. A. Weinman (Eds.), *Perceptions of Health and Illness: Current Research and Applications* (p. 79). Copyright 1997 by Harwood. Reprinted with permission.

from my physician, I will get well again" or "This is a chronic condition and I will have to learn to live with it"). In this model, the self is conceptualized as a factor that moderates the effects of symptoms, illness representation, and emotional states on coping behaviors and outcome appraisals (see also Figure 4.1 in chapter 4, this volume).

In general, models such as this one have been very helpful in guiding research on health behavior, and a considerable body of literature has accumulated elaborating the relevance of the different components of the models (see H. Leventhal et al., 2001). With regard to the focus of this volume, however, we argue that this model is limited in explicating the role of individuals' self-representations for improving their adherence with medical instructions. Thus, we propose a slightly different model that incorporates patients' representations about their own person more prominently and examines their relevance for the patient–physician relationship vis-à-vis patients' illness representations.

We refer to patients' *self-representations* as those "attributes or characteristics of the self that are consciously acknowledged by the individual through language—that is, how one describes oneself" (Harter, 1999, p. 3). Other terms that are often used interchangeably in the literature are *self-conceptions*, *self-descriptions*, or *self-perceptions*. We prefer the term *self-representations* as defined by Harter (1999) because it indicates that self-representations are a form of knowledge that the individual has about the own person and that can be accessed through self-report questionnaires or the clinical interview. Furthermore, we propose that adults' self-representations can be a source of either vulnerability and insecurity or resilience and personal strengths. Either way, we propose that physicians and other health care providers can benefit from learning about patients' general and health-related self-representations and from incorporating them into their clinical work. Thus, the main proposition of this chapter is that physicians who take into account their patients' self-representations and their illness representations will create a more effective therapeutic alliance. This therapeutic alliance will result in better adherence to treatment plans and instructions and ultimately in improved quality of life for the patients.[1]

A MODEL OF SELF AND ILLNESS REPRESENTATIONS IN THE CONTEXT OF THE PATIENT–PHYSICIAN RELATIONSHIP

Because most of our research over the past several years has focused on the content and structure of adults' role-specific self-representations (Diehl, Hastings, & Stanton, 2001; Diehl, Owen, & Youngblade, 2004), we have also started to think about the role of self-representations in the context of illness, and specifically in the context of chronic illness. Our current thinking about the role of self and illness representations in chronic illness and how they become important for the patient–physician relationship are illustrated in Figure 6.2. Several features of the model shown in Figure 6.2 are important and warrant a more detailed discussion.

Representations of Self

First, consistent with current theory and research, individuals' self-representations are conceptualized as dynamic cognitive structures that serve *adaptive and self-regulatory* functions (Baumeister, 1998; Harter, 1999; Higgins, 1996; Markus & Wurf, 1987; Showers, Abramson, & Hogan, 1998). That is, consistent with a large body of literature, it is assumed that knowledge about one's own person serves primarily self-regulatory and self-

---

[1] It is important to acknowledge that other authors have incorporated the notion of the self in their theoretical models (H. Leventhal, Idler, & Leventhal, 1999). For example, E. A. Leventhal, Leventhal, Robitaille, and Brownlee (1999) incorporated broad aspects of the self in their model of medication adherence. In particular, these authors emphasized that conceptions of the self play an important role in social comparison processes related to chronic illness. Although there is a good deal of common ground between these authors' deliberations and the propositions brought forward in this chapter, our propositions focus primarily on the specific *cognitive representations* of one's own person in the context of health and illness.

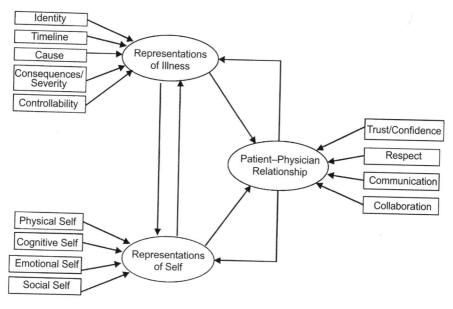

Figure 6.2. A model of self and illness representations in the context of the patient–physician relationship.

enhancing functions. For example, whether a person thinks of himself or herself as being resourceful, resilient, self-confident, and well liked by others will very likely result in a different coping behavior than if he or she thinks of himself or herself as being resource poor, vulnerable, self-doubting, and socially isolated. We propose that an individual's self-knowledge is also of importance in the adjustment to and management of a chronic illness.

Second, a large body of developmental research has documented that by late adolescence or early adulthood individuals have usually developed *role-* or *domain-specific* self-representations that influence their behavior (Damon & Hart, 1988; Harter, 1999; Harter & Monsour, 1992) and are the components of their overall self-concept. These domain-specific self-representations include (but are not limited to) a *physical self* (i.e., knowledge about one's physical attractiveness, physical abilities and limitations, and physical health), a *cognitive self* (i.e., knowledge about one's cognitive abilities or intelligence, interests, and values), an *emotional self* (i.e., knowledge about one's emotional states, emotional reactions to certain situations, and emotion regulation strategies), and a *social self* (i.e., knowledge about one's social network and available social support).

We suggest that it would be desirable for physicians or other health care providers to gain a detailed understanding of their patients' different self-representations for at least two reasons. First, a detailed understanding of patients' domain-specific self-representations and incorporation of this information into the treatment plan may be a promising way to improve patients' adherence to doctors' instructions and hence the effectiveness of the treatment (see chap. 8, this volume, on how individual differences produce differences in medical message processing). This seems to be particularly important for patients with chronic illnesses (e.g., cardiovascular disorders, cancer, diabetes, arthritis), because the treatment of chronic illness conditions extends, by definition, over long periods of time and therefore tends to lead to a long-term patient–physician relationship.

Third, paying attention to patients' domain-specific self-representations has probably become more important than ever, because there is clear evidence that medical decision making and treatment planning have increasingly moved from a paternalistic approach to a more collaborative approach (Hinz, 2000). For example, we suggest that with the aging of the baby boom generation—overall a fairly educated generation that is used to questioning authority and is familiar with the use of advanced information technologies—this issue will become even more relevant in the future.

Fourth, it is also important to note that self-representations possess certain organizational features. Three important features are *coherence, continuity,* and *meaningfulness* (Brandtstädter & Greve, 1994). That is, individuals construct their self-representations so that they are internally consistent (i.e., coherent), that they provide a sense of continuity over time, and that they organize their experiences in a meaningful way. Because of the very nature of chronic illness (i.e., being multiply determined, slowly developing, incurable, and degenerative), the diagnosis of such a condition challenges individuals' self-representations with regard to these three organizational features. For example, Taylor and her colleagues (Taylor, 1983; Taylor, Lichtman, & Wood, 1984) have shown that women who were treated for breast cancer engaged in an extensive search for meaning, including reevaluations of previously held self-representations.

Representations of Illness

Equally important in chronic illness are patients' illness representations. A review of the literature shows that representations of a wide variety of illnesses, ranging from the common cold to cancer, can be described with regard to five common attributes (H. Leventhal et al., 2001). First, patients interpret and label the symptoms that they experience, thus giving them an *identity* with regard to a suspected disease. Second, individuals hold certain assumptions about the onset and timing, development, duration, and recovery time of their illness and hence develop an implicit *timeline* for their symptoms and their disease (e.g., acute vs. chronic illness). Third, patients generate explanations in terms of the perceived *causes* of the disease (e.g., bacteria, virus, lifestyle factors such as stress, genetic disposition).

Fourth, patients develop expectations regarding the anticipated and experienced *consequences* and *severity* of the disease, which may involve physical, psychological, social, and economic outcomes. Finally, individuals develop personal expectations about the *controllability* of the disease that pertains to the anticipated and perceived responsiveness of the condition to self-treatment and treatment by biomedical experts.

The content and importance of these attributes may vary across individuals and within individuals over time as a function of the person's experience with the specific illness. However, what is probably most important about these representations is that physicians should address them explicitly to maximize patients' understanding of their illness and their adherence with the recommended treatment plan. In Figure 6.2, physicians' influences on the patients are expressed by the arrows that feed back from the patient–physician relationship to the representations of self and illness.

In agreement with other researchers, we argue that physicians who strive to gain a systematic understanding of their patients' illness representations can not only gain an insight into the patients' sociocultural understanding of their illness but also learn a great deal about some of the mechanisms that laypeople apply in self-managing their disease. For example, if a physician or health care provider knows that a patient with diabetes relies on the experience of symptoms to vary his or her insulin and food intake (Gonder-Frederick & Cox, 1991), then he or she may address this issue and may identify a major source of nonadherence to a prescribed medical regimen. Similarly, a physician or health care provider who learns that a patient has a completely erroneous understanding of the illness symptoms (e.g., acute vs. chronic illness) or the illness consequences (e.g., further progression, increased risk of mortality) may provide accurate information and real-life examples to illustrate the potentially devastating consequences of the false illness representations.

However, if a physician or health care provider realizes that a patient cooperates with his or her instructions; draws on supportive self-representations; and has appropriate representations of the causes, the course, and the outcomes of the illness, then he or she can use this knowledge to strengthen the patient–physician relationship and to optimize the adherence to the recommended treatment plan. Although this latter scenario is the therapeutically desirable one in chronic disease management, we are also aware that it may be the exception rather than the rule (H. Leventhal et al., 2001).

Linking Representations of Self and Illness

As Figure 6.2 shows, we propose a reciprocal relationship between individuals' self-representations and their representations of illness. That is, we propose that a person's self-representations affect his or her representations of illness, and that the representations of illness affect the person's representations of self. We briefly discuss this reciprocal relationship.

Consistent with the assumptions of other theorists, we propose that self-representations play an important role in a person's evaluation of his or her coping resources. For example, in terms of Lazarus and Folkman's (1984) theory of stress, appraisal, and coping, self-representations come into play during the processes of primary appraisal ("What are my personal resources? What can I do?") and secondary appraisal ("What are my social resources? Whom can I turn to for help?") and influence subsequent coping behavior. Moreover, self-representations play a role in the evaluation of illness symptoms and determine the personal relevance that symptoms are given. For example, individuals for whom physical health and a healthy lifestyle are central aspects of their self-conception are probably more likely to follow health care professionals' orders than individuals for whom this is not the case.

It is important to note that Figure 6.2 is only a snapshot of the complex and dynamic relationship between patient and physician, which is also greatly influenced by interpersonal variables such as mutual trust and confidence, mutual respect, styles of communication, and modes of collaboration. We clearly acknowledge that in real life this relationship is not necessarily a linearly progressive one but that the progression of an illness or the failure of a selected medical treatment can alter the importance of the different components. However, our basic assumption is that taking into account patients' illness and self-representations will result in an improved patient–physician relationship. In turn, an improved patient–physician relationship is expected to have positive effects on patients' treatment adherence and ultimately on their physical and psychological well-being. These assumptions are consistent with the observations of theorists who have pointed out that illness representations have "important implications for the physical, emotional, and functional integrity of the self, and the time frame (i.e., existence) of the self" (H. Leventhal et al., 2001, p. 28). Thus, by taking into account illness and self-representations, a "collision" between the two may be avoided to the overall benefit of the patient.

EMPIRICAL EVIDENCE FOR THE RELEVANCE OF SELF AND ILLNESS REPRESENTATIONS

So far, we have argued primarily from a conceptual point of view. The validity of the theoretical arguments, however, needs to be evaluated with regard to the available empirical evidence. Thus, in the following sections we review the available literature, suggesting that self and illness representations are relevant for improving patients' adherence to their physicians' instructions and treatment plans.

The Role of Illness Representations

In terms of illness representations, there is a solid body of research showing that the different attributes of the commonsense model are associated with adults' actual health behaviors and medical adherence (Park & Jones, 1997). Because this body of literature is quite extensive (for a comprehensive review, see H. Leventhal et al., 2001), we review only a select number of exemplary studies to illustrate the importance of illness representations. For example, Scharloo et al. (1998) showed in a study with adults from three chronic illness groups (i.e., rheumatoid arthritis, chronic pulmonary disease, and psoriasis) that the strength of patients' illness identity, their belief of extended illness duration, and their perceptions of more severe consequences were predictive of poorer treatment outcomes. In contrast, beliefs in controllability and curability of the disease were significantly related to better functioning. Similarly, in a British study of adolescents with diabetes, beliefs about the effectiveness of the treatment regimen predicted better dietary self-care (Skinner, John, & Hampson, 2000). Heijmans (1998) showed that patients with chronic fatigue syndrome who considered their illness to be a serious condition, who believed that they had no control over their illness, who saw little possibility for cure, and who believed that their illness would have serious consequences reported higher levels of impairment in physical and social functioning and reported greater problems in mental health and vitality. Moreover, illness representations were stronger predictors of outcomes than patients' actual coping behaviors (see also Heijmans & de Ridder, 1998). With regard to cancer patients, Heidrich, Forsthoff, and Ward (1994) showed that those individuals who perceived their cancer as a chronic rather than an acute disease exhibited poorer adjustment. Finally, Meyer, Leventhal, and Gutmann (1985) reported that patients with hypertension who believed that their treatment had beneficial effects on their symptoms also reported greater compliance with taking medications and were more likely to have their blood pressure controlled.

In summary, illness representations are related to how quickly individuals seek medical care, whether they are compliant with physicians' orders, and actual treatment outcomes. Results supporting this conclusion have been reported for chronic illnesses such as hypertension, cancer, diabetes, pulmonary disease, rheumatoid arthritis, and chronic fatigue syndrome. Moreover, the relevance of illness representations has also been documented in multiple age groups.

The Role of Self-Representations

With regard to the importance of patients' self-representations, the empirical evidence is not as well established as the role of illness representations. However, existing findings provide support for the importance of self-representations and discrepancies in self-representations in the adjustment to chronic illness. For example, Persson, Berglund, and Sahlberg (1996) drew on extensive interviews with patients treated for rheumatoid arthritis and examined whether their self-representations formed distinguishable factors. Their data revealed three positive factors, which they labeled Reevaluation, Acceptance, and Fighting Spirit, and three negative factors, which they labeled Deprivation of Life Values, Reserved, and Protest. A seventh factor was labeled Denial and indicated the extent to which patients denied the existence of their disease. Persson et al. (1996) also found that positive self-conceptions (e.g., "See my illness as a challenge" and "It is important to set up goals to fight for") showed significant negative associations with inflammatory activity of the disease, as judged by an independent rheumatologist. In contrast, negative self-representations (e.g., "I feel inferior to healthy people" and "It is hard not being able to be the one I was") were positively related to inflammatory activity. In addition, patients' assessment of pain showed significant positive associations with negative self-representations. Overall, this study showed that patients' self-representations with regard to their chronic illness could be reliably assessed and showed meaningful associations with clinically relevant markers such as inflammatory activity and experienced pain.

In another study, Heidrich et al. (1994) examined perceived self-discrepancies between cancer patients' actual and ideal self across 20 life domains and found that greater discrepancies between individuals' actual and ideal self-representations predicted poorer adjustment and poorer treatment outcomes. Moreover, self-discrepancy mediated the effects of illness representations (i.e., symptoms and timeline) on patients' emotional adjustment and psychological well-being.

Devins, Beanlands, Mandin, and Paul (1997) examined the role of self-representations in relation to illness intrusiveness in a sample of patients with end-stage renal disease. They hypothesized that self-conceptions that are highly similar to the representations of the chronic kidney patient would limit patients' potential for self-actualization and that this effect would be stronger for younger adults compared with older adults. Devins et al.'s study yielded several interesting findings. First, consistent with their hypothesis, patient self-representations that were similar to the representations of the chronic kidney patient correlated significantly with the occurrence of uremic symptoms, greater number of comorbid conditions, somatic symptoms of distress, higher number of hours required for weekly treatment, tiredness, and illness intrusiveness. Second, patients' self-conceptions moderated the effects of illness intrusiveness on measures of emotional stress and psychosocial well-being. Specifically, emotional distress increased with increasing illness intrusiveness among individuals whose self-conceptions were similar to the one of the chronic kidney patient, whereas emotional distress did not change appreciably among those patients who construed themselves as dissimilar. Age did not moderate this relationship.

In the case of psychosocial well-being, the deleterious effects of illness intrusiveness were moderated by self-concept and age. In particular, for young adults, illness intrusiveness compromised psychosocial well-being when individuals construed themselves as comparatively dissimilar to the chronic kidney patient, whereas well-being was not compromised by illness intrusiveness when self-conceptions were comparatively similar. For older adults, this pattern was reversed and mirrored the results that had been found for emotional distress. Thus, for older adults it was more beneficial with regard to their psychosocial well-being to construe themselves as dissimilar from the chronic kidney patient.

The findings from this study are relevant for several reasons. First, Devins et al. (1997) showed that patients with end-stage renal disease formed a self-concept as chronic kidney patient. Second, this self-concept was linked to objective symptoms and to the severity of the illness and moderated the effect of illness intrusiveness on emotional distress and psychosocial well-being. Third, some of the findings also suggest that the formation of an illness-related self-concept has different psychological benefits at different stages of the life span. For example, in younger adults a clearly defined illness-related self-concept may indicate a psychological acceptance of the chronic illness, whereas in older adults such a self-concept may indicate identification with the inevitable consequences of a chronic illness (Devins et al., 1997).

Finally, research with children and adolescents with diabetes has also shown that they hold illness-related self-representations (Wiebe et al., 2002). This study included 128 adolescents with Type 1 diabetes (mean age = 12.7 years; mean duration of illness = 4.6 years) and provided several interesting findings. First, adolescents' conceptions of the self in the context of diabetes were more negative than self-representations with family or friends, but they nevertheless were also a source for positive self-views. Second, a large number of the diabetes-related self-representations (42%) were rated as *most important* in defining the self, suggesting that they were not trivial aspects of adolescents' self-concept. Third, more negative self-concepts in the context of diabetes were associated with poorer adjustment (i.e., more depressive symptoms, poorer adherence). Finally, the data showed that the negativity of adolescents' diabetes-related self-representations had significantly stronger associations with depression when diabetes was psychologically central to the self-concept compared with when it was not central. Overall, Wiebe et al. (2002) concluded that a chronic illness such as diabetes presents a number of challenges for children's self-conceptions and that an understanding of the illness-related self-representations may be an important avenue to explore how individuals of different ages adjust to their chronic illness.

In summary, we believe that the presented empirical findings justify the recommendation that physicians and other health care providers pay attention to their patients' general and illness-related self-representations. Understanding the content, valence, and centrality of specific self-representations and drawing on the content of patients' self-conceptions may be a way for improving the patient–physician relationship and for optimizing the effectiveness of medical treatments.

The Role of Age in Self and Illness Representations

Because this volume addresses the patient–physician relationship with a particular emphasis on older adult patients, it is also important to attend to the role of chronological age in the context of self and illness representations. The main question in this context is, therefore, does age have an influence on patients' self and illness representations?

Effects of Age on Illness Representations

Unfortunately, there is not a great deal of research on the influence of age on adults' self and illness representations. For example, E. A. Leventhal and Crouch (1997) stated in a review chapter that

> because the investigation of the effects of age upon illness representations and self identity is in its infancy, we will be forced at times to engage in speculation about the ways in which these age-related changes may alter health and illness behaviors. (p. 80)

An extensive literature search confirmed this assessment and suggests that this statement is valid even almost 10 years later.

Because many chronic illnesses develop gradually and slowly and are in this way similar to the normal aging process, it is a great challenge for researchers to distinguish whether older adults attribute physical symptoms to illness or to normal aging. Although it is documented that older adults report more bodily symptoms than younger adults (Hale, Perkins, May, Marks, & Stewart, 1986; U.S. Department of Health and Human Services, 2000), they also tend to attribute physical symptoms more to normal aging rather than illness. This seems to be specifically the case for mild to moderate symptoms. Unfortunately, the tendency to assume that physical symptoms are due to the aging process tends to be associated with a delay in care seeking and may therefore put older adults at a particular risk (E. A. Leventhal &

Crouch, 1997, p. 83). However, E. A. Leventhal and her colleagues (E. A. Leventhal, Leventhal, Schaefer, & Easterling, 1993) showed that when older adult patients judged their symptoms to be serious they tended to report shorter total delays (i.e., the time from first noticing symptoms until calling for care) and significant shorter illness delays (i.e., decision one was ill until calling for care). What are needed are studies that investigate at a microlevel the appraisal processes and intraindividual symptom comparisons that influence when and why individuals seek medical care.

Other aspects of illness representations that seem to change systematically with age are perceptions of vulnerability and controllability. For example, a large body of research shows that there are important age differences in individuals' beliefs of control and self-efficacy with regard to health (for a review, see Lachman, Ziff, & Spiro, 1994; Rodin & Timko, 1992). In general, findings from this research show that older adults perceive having less control and feel less self-efficacious with regard to illness-preventing behaviors than younger age groups do. A study that illustrates this finding was reported by Prohaska, Leventhal, Leventhal, and Keller (1985). These researchers showed that although older adults reported higher frequencies of health-promoting activities than younger adults, they also considered themselves to be more vulnerable to disease, viewed their illness as more serious, and were less likely to view chronic mild symptoms as illness warnings.

In summary, although older adults seem to be more cautious and more concerned about their health than younger adults, they also may be at a greater risk for attributing the reasons for symptoms to aging rather than illness. In addition, older adults seem to have an increased sense of vulnerability and perceive having less control over their health than younger adults.

Effects of Age on Self-Representations

Findings with regard to the effects of age on adults' self-representations are equally sparse, because the overwhelming majority of studies in this area have been conducted with children and college students. The two types of studies that are relevant come from research on *possible selves* across adulthood (Cross & Markus, 1991; Hooker, 1992; Ryff, 1991; Smith & Freund, 2002) and from studies on the effects of self-concept differentiation on adults' psychological well-being (Diehl et al., 2001; Donahue, Robins, Roberts, & John, 1993).

Several studies have examined adults' possible selves across the adult life span. These studies have documented that health-related possible selves start to become salient in late midlife and increase in salience with age (Cross & Markus, 1991; Hooker, 1992; Hooker & Kaus, 1994). Moreover, perceived self-efficacy and number of goal-oriented activities to avoid feared health-related selves have been shown to be significant predictors of health behaviors.

A second type of study has examined the effect of self-concept differentiation and self-complexity on adults' psychological well-being and physical health. Findings from these studies suggest that domain-specific self-representations need to be integrated and coordinated into a coherent overall self-concept to be adaptive and a source of resilience (Showers, 2001). A second major finding in this area is that age seems to moderate the effects of self-concept differentiation on adults' psychological well-being. For example, Diehl et al. (2001) reported findings from an adult life span sample showing that age moderated the associations between self-concept differentiation and positive and negative psychological well-being. That is, a high level of self-concept differentiation was associated with lower positive and higher negative psychological well-being for both younger and older adults; however, this effect was significantly more pronounced in older adults (see Figure 6.3).

The findings by Devins et al. (1997) are also consistent with this literature. Recall that Devins et al. found that for young adults illness intrusiveness compromised psychosocial well-being when individuals construed themselves as comparatively dissimilar to the chronic kidney patient, whereas well-being was not compromised by illness intrusiveness when self-conceptions were comparatively similar. For older adults, however, this pattern was reversed, and it was more beneficial for them to construe themselves as dissimilar from the chronic kidney patient.

In conclusion, there is emergent evidence suggesting that health- and illness-related self-representations and their functions are not invariant across the adult life span. That means that physicians and health care providers need to be sensitive to age-related differences in their patients' self-representations and need to acknowledge that a one-size-fits-all approach may not be appropriate for improving the patient–physician relationship and medical adherence.

HOW CAN PHYSICIANS ASSESS THEIR PATIENTS' SELF-REPRESENTATIONS?

Interactions between patients and physicians or other health care professionals often occur under conditions of severe time constraints. Therefore, it is important to address how physicians or other health care providers can assess their patients' self-representations in a structured way so that they can incorporate this information into their treatment plan and therapeutic relationship.

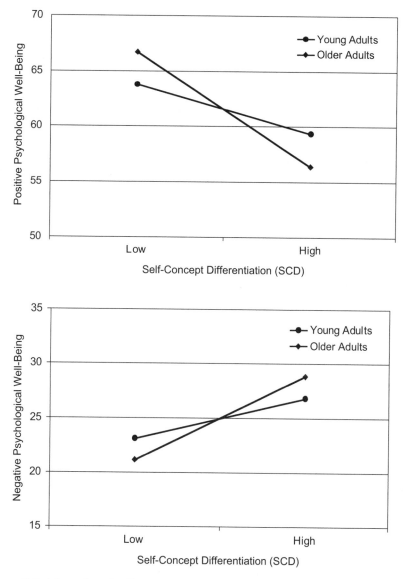

Figure 6.3. Interaction of self-concept differentiation and age for positive and negative psychological well-being. From "Self-Concept Differentiation Across the Adult Life Span," by M. Diehl, C. T. Hastings, and J. M. Stanton, 2001, *Psychology and Aging, 16,* p. 650. Copyright 2001 by the American Psychological Association.

One way of gathering information about patients' self-representations would be to include a brief list of positive and negative adjectives into the medical history questionnaire that patients often fill out while in the waiting room. Patients could be instructed to indicate on a rating scale (1 = *not very characteristic of me* to 6 = *very characteristic of me*) to what extent each adjective characterizes them as a person. The list of adjectives could easily be derived from well-established lists of adjectives (e.g., Goldberg, 1992) or from studies that have examined adults' self-representations in different social roles (e.g., Diehl et al., 2001; Donahue et al., 1993). From the ratings of the adjectives, physicians could easily glean what their patients perceive as their personal strengths and weaknesses and incorporate this information into their interactions with them.

Another way of obtaining information about patients' self-representations would be as part of the diagnostic interview or during regular office visits. In particular when a patient is diagnosed with or treated for a chronic illness, the physician will have to prepare the patient for the medically indicated treatment and will have to explain a great many things (e.g., type of treatment, objectives of the treatment, side effects, etc.). In the context of such conversations, physicians can explore what personal strengths and concerns patients have and how they may consider activating their personal and social resources to cope with their illness. Of course, this also gives patients the opportunity to mention what they see as their weak spots and vulnerabilities and where they may need the support from others to cope successfully with the different challenges of their illness. The bottom line of such patient–physician interactions is that the physician needs to be a careful and patient listener and needs to be open to the message that the patient is sending, because for every stated health complaint there may also be one unstated anxiety or an unstated hope (see Hinz, 2000).

Finally, physicians and health care providers also need to be sensitive to the fact that patients, especially when a treatment fails to produce the expected outcome, have their ups and downs and that self-representations reflect not only their stable self-concept but also their current mood states. Thus, physicians need to be prepared that different self-representations may be activated at different times and that their initial understanding may have to be reconstructed and integrated with new information. Like life and interpersonal relationships in general, the interactions between patients and physicians are highly dynamic and, therefore, are subject to reevaluations and reconstructions. Successful health care professionals embrace this aspect of their relationship with the patient and make it an integral part of the therapeutic alliance.

CONCLUSION

Despite all technological and medical advances, the patient–physician relationship remains an integral part of any medical treatment. This is particularly the case with regard to older adults who are more likely to be diagnosed with chronic diseases and are more likely to experience conditions of comorbidity. The objective of this chapter was to discuss the role of self and illness representations for the patient–physician relationship. Because the patient–physician relationship is a critical element for communicating effectively with patients and for achieving adherence with the medical regimen, we proposed a model in which individuals' representations of their symptoms and illness were complemented by domain-specific representations of their own person. We believe there is an emerging body of literature that shows that certain self-representations can represent a liability (e.g., highly discrepant self-conceptions) and can increase the psychological vulnerability of patients. However, there is also emerging evidence showing that self-representations can be a resource of resiliency and can be activated to facilitate the effectiveness of medical treatments. Overall, we argued that physicians and other health care providers should make every effort to gain an understanding of the content, valence, and centrality of their patients' self-representations and incorporate this information into their treatment plan. Using this information in constructive ways may increase patients' adherence to the medical treatment and may improve their overall quality of life.

REFERENCES

Anderson, E. (1991). Getting through to elderly patients. *Geriatrics, 46*(5), 74–76.

Baum, A., Revenson, T. A., & Singer, J. E. (2001). *Handbook of health psychology.* Mahwah, NJ: Erlbaum.

Baumeister, R. F. (1998). The self. In D. T. Gilbert, S. T. Fiske, & G. Lindzey (Eds.), *The handbook of social psychology* (4th ed., pp. 680–740). New York: McGraw-Hill.

Boult, C., Kane, R. L., Louis, T. A., Boult, L., & McCaffrey, D. (1994). Chronic conditions that lead to functional limitations in the elderly. *Journal of Gerontology, 49,* M28–M36.

Brandtstädter, J., & Greve, W. (1994). The aging self: Stabilizing and protective processes. *Developmental Review, 14,* 52–80.

Carver, C. S., & Scheier, M. F. (1998). *On the self-regulation of behavior.* New York: Cambridge University Press.

Cross, S., & Markus, H. (1991). Possible selves across the life span. *Human Development, 34,* 230–255.

Damon, W., & Hart, D. (1988). *Self-understanding in childhood and adolescence.* New York: Cambridge University Press.

Devins, G. M., Beanlands, H., Mandin, H., & Paul, L. C. (1997). Psychosocial impact of illness intrusiveness moderated by self-concept and age in end-stage renal disease. *Health Psychology, 16,* 529–538.

Diehl, M., Hastings, C. T., & Stanton, J. M. (2001). Self-concept differentiation across the adult life span. *Psychology and Aging, 16,* 643–654.

Diehl, M., Owen, S. K., & Youngblade, L. M. (2004). Agency and communion in adults' self-representations. *International Journal of Behavioral Development, 28,* 1–15.

Donahue, E. M., Robins, R. W., Roberts, B. W., & John, O. P. (1993). The divided self: Concurrent and longitudinal effects of psychological adjustment and social roles on self-concept differentiation. *Journal of Personality and Social Psychology, 64,* 834–846.

Estes, C. L., & Rundall, T. G. (1992). Social characteristics, social structure, and health in the aging population. In M. G. Ory, R. P. Abeles, & P. D. Lipman (Eds.), *Aging, health, and behavior* (pp. 299–326). Newbury Park, CA: Sage.

Faulkner, A. (1998). *Effective interaction with patients.* New York: Churchill Livingstone.

Goldberg, L. R. (1992). The development of markers for the big-five factor structure. *Psychological Assessment, 4,* 26–42.

Gonder-Frederick, L. A., & Cox, D. J. (1991). Symptom perception, symptom beliefs, and blood glucose discrimination in the self-treatment of insulin-dependent diabetes. In J. A. Skelton & R. T. Croyle (Eds.), *Mental representation in health and illness* (pp. 220–246). New York: Springer-Verlag.

Hale, W. E., Perkins, L. L., May, F. E., Marks, R. G., & Stewart, R. B. (1986). Symptom prevalence in the elderly: An evaluation of age, sex, disease, and medication use. *Journal of the American Geriatrics Society, 34,* 333–340.

Halter, J. B. (1999). The challenge of communicating health information to elderly patients: A view from geriatric medicine. In D. C. Park, R. W. Morrell, & K. Shifren (Eds.), *Processing of medical information in aging patients: Cognitive and human factors perspectives* (pp. 23–28). Mahwah, NJ: Erlbaum.

Harter, S. (1999). *The construction of the self: A developmental perspective.* New York: Guilford Press.

Harter, S., & Monsour, A. (1992). Developmental analysis of conflict caused by opposing attributes in the adolescent self-portrait. *Developmental Psychology, 28,* 251–260.

Heidrich, S. M., Forsthoff, C. A., & Ward, S. E. (1994). Psychological adjustment in adults with cancer: The self as mediator. *Health Psychology, 13,* 346–353.

Heijmans, M. (1998). Coping and adaptive outcome in chronic fatigue syndrome: Importance of illness cognitions. *Journal of Psychometric Research, 45,* 39–51.

Heijmans, M., & deRidder, D. (1998). Assessing illness representations of chronic illness: Explorations of their disease-specific nature. *Journal of Behavioral Medicine, 21,* 485–503.

Higgins, E. T. (1996). The "self digest": Self-knowledge serving self-regulatory functions. *Journal of Personality and Social Psychology, 71,* 1062–1083.

Hinz, C. A. (2000). *Communicating with your patients: Skills for building rapport.* Washington, DC: American Medical Association.

Hooker, K. (1992). Possible selves and perceived health in older adults and college students. *Journal of Gerontology, 47*, P85–P95.

Hooker, K., & Kaus, C. R. (1994). Health-related possible selves in young and middle adulthood. *Psychology and Aging, 9*, 126–133.

Kelly, G. (1955). *The psychology of personal constructs: Vol. 1. A theory of personality.* New York: Norton.

Lachman, M. E., Ziff, M. A., & Spiro, A. (1994). Maintaining a sense of control in later life. In R. P. Ables, H. C. Gift, & M. G. Ory (Eds.), *Aging and quality of life* (pp. 216–232). New York: Springer Publishing Company.

Lazarus, R. S., & Folkman, S. (1984). *Stress, appraisal, and coping.* New York: Springer Publishing Company.

Leventhal, E. A., & Crouch, M. (1997). Are there differences in perceptions of illness across the lifespan? In K. J. Petrie & J. A. Weinman (Eds.), *Perceptions of health and illness: Current research and applications* (pp. 77–102). Amsterdam, the Netherlands: Harwood.

Leventhal, E. A., Leventhal, H., Robitaille, C., & Brownlee, S. (1999). Psychosocial factors in medication adherence: A model of the modeler. In D. C. Park, R. W. Morrell, & K. Shifren (Eds.), *Processing of medical information in aging patients: Cognitive and human factors perspectives* (pp. 145–165). Mahwah, NJ: Erlbaum.

Leventhal, E. A., Leventhal, H., Schaefer, P., & Easterling, D. (1993). Conservation of energy, uncertainty reduction, and swift utilization of medical care among the elderly. *Journal of Gerontology, 48*, P78–P86.

Leventhal, H., Idler, E. L., & Leventhal, E. A. (1999). The impact of chronic illness on the self system. In R. J. Contrada & R. D. Ashmore (Eds.), *Rutgers Series on Self and Social Identity: Vol. 2. Self, social identity and physical health* (pp. 185–208). New York: Oxford University Press.

Leventhal, H., Leventhal, E. A., & Cameron, L. (2001). Representations, procedures, and affect in illness self-regulation: A perceptual–cognitive model. In A. Baum, T. A. Revenson, & J. E. Singer (Eds.), *Handbook of health psychology* (pp. 19–47). Mahwah, NJ: Erlbaum.

Leventhal, H., & Nerenz, D. R. (1985). The assessment of illness cognition. In P. Karoly (Ed.), *Measurement strategies in health psychology* (pp. 517–554). New York: Wiley.

Leventhal, H., Safer, M. A., & Panagis, D. (1983). The impact of communications on the self-regulation of health beliefs, decisions, and behavior. *Health Education Quarterly, 10*, 3–29.

Ley, P. (1988). *Communicating with patients: Improving communication, satisfaction and compliance.* London: Croom Helm.

Markus, H., & Wurf, E. (1987). The dynamic self-concept: A social psychological perspective. *Annual Review of Psychology, 38*, 299–337.

Meyer, D., Leventhal, H., & Gutmann, M. (1985). Common-sense models of illness: The example of hypertension. *Health Psychology, 4*, 115–135.

Park, D. C., & Jones, T. R. (1997). Medication adherence and aging. In A. D. Fisk & W. A. Rogers (Eds.), *Handbook of human factors and the older adult* (pp. 257–287). San Diego, CA: Academic Press.

Pendleton, D., & Hasler, J. (Eds.). (1983). *Doctor–patient communication.* London: Academic Press.

Persson, L. O., Berglund, K., & Sahlberg, D. (1996). A structure of self-conceptions and illness conceptions in rheumatoid arthritis (RA). *Journal of Psychosomatic Research, 40,* 535–549.

Prohaska, T. R., Leventhal, E. A., Leventhal, H., & Keller, M. L. (1985). Health practices and illness cognition in young, middle, and elderly adults. *Journal of Gerontology, 40,* 569–578.

Rodin, J., & Timko, C. (1992). Sense of control, aging, and health. In M. G. Ory, R. P. Ables, & P. D. Lipman (Eds.), *Aging, health, and behavior* (pp. 174–206). Newbury Park, CA: Sage.

Ryff, C. D. (1991). Possible selves in adulthood and old age: A tale of shifting horizons. *Psychology and Aging, 6,* 286–295.

Scharloo, M., Kaptein, A. A., Weinman, J., Hazes, J. M., Willems, L. N. A., Bergman, W., & Rooijmans, H. G. M. (1998). Illness perceptions, coping and functioning in patients with rheumatoid arthritis, chronic obstructive pulmonary disease and psoriasis. *Journal of Psychosomatic Research, 44,* 573–585.

Showers, C. J. (2001). Self-organization in emotional contexts. In J. P. Forgas (Ed.), *Feeling and thinking: The role of affect in social cognition* (pp. 283–307). New York: Cambridge University Press.

Showers, C. J., Abramson, L. Y., & Hogan, M. E. (1998). The dynamic self: How the content and structure of the self-concept change with mood. *Journal of Personality and Social Psychology, 75,* 478–493.

Shumaker, S. A., Schron, E. B., Ockene, J. K., & McBee, W. L. (1998). *The handbook of health behavior change* (2nd ed.). New York: Springer Publishing Company.

Siegler, I. C., Bastian, L. A., & Bosworth, H. B. (2001). Health, behavior, and aging. In A. Baum, T. A. Revenson, & J. E. Singer (Eds.), *Handbook of health psychology* (pp. 469–476). Mahwah, NJ: Erlbaum.

Skinner, T. C., John, M., & Hampson, S. E. (2000). Social support and personal models of diabetes as predictors of self-care and well-being: A longitudinal study of adolescents with diabetes. *Journal of Pediatric Psychology, 25,* 257–267.

Smith, J., & Freund, A. M. (2002). The dynamics of possible selves in old age. *Journals of Gerontology Series B: Psychological Sciences and Social Sciences, 57,* P492–P500.

Taylor, S. E. (1983). Adjusting to threatening events: A theory of cognitive adaptation. *American Psychologist, 38,* 1116–1173.

Taylor, S. E., Lichtman, R. R., & Wood, J. V. (1984). Attributions, beliefs about control, and adjustment to breast cancer. *Journal of Personality and Social Psychology, 46,* 489–502.

U.S. Department of Health and Human Services. (2000). *Healthy people 2010: Understanding and improving health.* Hyattsville, MD: Author.

Wiebe, D. J., Berg, C. A., Palmer, D., Korbel, C., Beveridge, R., Lindsay, R., et al. (2002, April). *Illness and the self: Examining adjustment among adolescents with diabetes.* Paper presented at the annual meetings of the Society of Behavioral Medicine, Washington, DC.

Wyer, R. S., & Srull, T. K. (Eds.). (1994). *Handbook of social cognition.* Hillsdale, NJ: Erlbaum.

Zwahr, M. D. (1999). Cognitive processes and medical decisions. In D. C. Park, R. W. Morrell, & K. Shifren (Eds.), *Processing of medical information in aging patients: Cognitive and human factors perspectives* (pp. 55–68). Mahwah, NJ: Erlbaum.

7

TRUSTING MEDICAL AUTHORITIES: EFFECTS OF COGNITIVE AGING AND SOCIAL VIGILANCE

EMILY CHAN, OSCAR YBARRA, DENISE C. PARK, JOEL RODRIGUEZ, AND JULIE A. GARCIA

When we consider how aging affects people's relationships with medical professionals, an important question to ask is whether older adults, compared with younger adults, are more likely to take supposed medical experts at their word. This question is especially relevant in the current environment, in which much marketing of traditional and nontraditional remedies is directed at the public through the mass media by both nonprofessional and professional practitioners. The vast array of information available from the media on a particular medical issue is overwhelming and might at times contain fraudulent claims and misinformation. It has also been suggested that the elderly are more susceptible to fraud than younger adults in a variety of settings (McCabe & Gregory, 1998; McGhee, 1983). Thus, it is possible that older adults also have a greater chance of falling prey to deception when they make health care choices. It is therefore important to examine

The research reported in this chapter was supported by National Institute on Aging Grant F002048 awarded to Oscar Ybarra and Denise C. Park.

whether older adults compared with younger adults are indeed more likely to trust supposed medical experts.

Many factors contribute to whether a person is persuaded by medical treatment recommendations given to him or her by professional or nonprofessional sources. Of particular interest in this chapter is the finding showing that people are more persuaded by others who are identified as experts than those identified as laypersons (Hass, 1981). People's trust in experts is often so strong that they accept their recommendations without much scrutiny, even if a recommendation is ambiguous (Chaiken & Maheswaran, 1994; Maddux & Rogers, 1980). Research on medical adherence has also shown that patients' impressions of a health care provider can affect persuasion from medical recommendations. People who have more trust in their health care provider report greater adherence to medication regiments and other treatment recommendations than those who report less trust (DiMatteo & Lepper, 1998; Thom, Ribisl, Stewart, & Luke, 1999). In general, the more positive people perceive their relationship with their physician or health care provider, the greater is the level of medical adherence (Garrity & Lawson, 1989).

Thus, when an older adult is given medical advice from a legitimate source who is competent, his or her trust in the professional's expertise can be a positive factor in promoting adherence. However, if the medical information comes from a fraudulent source who claims to be a medical expert, being trusting can have detrimental consequences. The question to ask then is, how do people determine whether others are trustworthy and competent?

It is reasonable to expect that people should be inclined to take the advice of a person they think is honest and competent but less inclined to be persuaded by either an untrustworthy or incompetent person. In this chapter we describe research that has examined how younger and older adults process information that has to do with others' moral and competence characteristics and how cognitive functioning differences between the age groups may affect the manner in which older and younger adults generate inferences about others' personalities.

THEMES OF MORALITY AND COMPETENCE IN SOCIAL INFORMATION PROCESSING

When people perceive and think about others and try to determine their intentions, emotions, and dispositions, numerous things can come to mind. How is it that people, for the most part, have little trouble in solving this potentially overwhelming cognitive task? One possibility is that people rely on recurring themes or schemas to organize and simplify their social world. Two potential themes that people appear to use to structure and make sense of their lives are morality and competence. *Morality* refers to characteristics relevant to ethics and a sense of right and wrong in interpersonal relationships, as exemplified by traits related to honesty, helpfulness, and sincerity, or the lack thereof. *Competence* refers to characteristics relevant to achievement and the accomplishment of tasks and goals, as exemplified by traits such as intelligence, being knowledgeable, and diligence.

The dimensions of morality and competence have been labeled differently by other researchers. For example, they have been termed *socially good–bad* and *intellectually good–bad* (Rosenberg & Sedlak, 1972), *social attraction* and *intellectual attraction* (Singh & Teoh, 1999), and *liking* and *respect* (Fiske, Xu, Cuddy, & Glick, 1999; Hamilton & Zanna, 1972). Regardless of how they are labeled, the underlying features point to common definitions of the two domains, as just described.

Research on a variety of topics suggests that much of the social information people process about others is related to moral- or competence-related characteristics. When forming impressions of others, morality- and competence-related traits account for most of the variance in multidimensional analyses (Rosenberg, Nelson, & Vivekananthan, 1968). This is consistent with Anderson's (1968) finding that among the 555 traits he studied, the traits that people most desired in others were related to morality and competence. Wojciszke (1994), in an analysis of open-ended descriptions of others, also found that impressions are mostly based on morality or competence considerations. Even at the level of mate selection, men and women across 37 cultures selected kindness and understanding (morality) and intelligence as the most important characteristics in a mate (Buss, 1998).

The distinction between morality and competence is also found beyond the research domain of person perception. Leadership styles can be characterized as social-oriented leadership or task-oriented leadership (Bales, 1953; Fiedler & Chemers, 1974), with the first being concerned with the interpersonal and moral aspects of the group interaction and the latter being related to goal achievement and ability. Similarly, some groups that emerge in organizations are informal and arise to fulfill the socioemotional needs of the members, whereas other groups are more formal in nature and arise to fulfill task-oriented needs (Hammer & Organ, 1978). In another area of research, it has been shown that normative social influence (Asch, 1955) is fueled by people's interpersonal need to be accepted, whereas informational influence (Sherif, 1936) is motivated by a competence-related concern to be accurate (Cialdini & Trost, 1991).

Given how pervasive the categories of morality and competence are in social information processing, it is likely that when people interact with health care professionals in a medical context they will form impressions of the health care providers in terms of morality and competence as well. Information about the health care providers' morality and competence should influence whether or not clients will subscribe to the providers' recommendations. For example, if you heard that your doctor was able to diagnose another patient's rare condition successfully, which had been misdiagnosed by many other doctors, such displays of competence should affect your impression of the doctor and increase the likelihood that you will adhere to his or her suggestions. But if you learned that your doctor was accepting kickbacks for prescribing drugs from a particular pharmaceutical company, knowing this should influence how you evaluate the doctor and the medical information he or she gives you, making you less likely to take your doctor at his or her word.

ARE PEOPLE MORE CHRONICALLY CONCERNED ABOUT MORALITY OR COMPETENCE?

Because morality and competence information are both important and potentially informative dimensions to consider about people, under ideal circumstances it would seem that people would weight and process such information about others equally with few biases. However, as will be described presently, an individual's social cognitive repertoire of person perception skills may lead them to be biased and to favor information from one dimension over another. Therefore, a question we must consider and that served as the motivation for the first study to be described is whether the morality or competence category dominates in information processing. One way to approach this question is by examining the evolutionary context in which the human capacity for processing social information developed.

Indirect Reciprocity

As human groups became larger than groups of close kin, there were increased opportunities to interact with nonkin. People probably became more dependent on receiving help from nonkin members in such large congregates, and *indirect reciprocity*, which occurs when help offered by one individual is returned from someone other than the recipient of the assistance (Alexander, 1987), had probably become a crucial component of such complex societies. Consequently, monitoring others' morality should have become more important than monitoring their competence because morality-related information reflects whether others generally have the intention to be reciprocating members of the social exchange network. Competence-related information, although still an important component in social perception, would not be as informative about others' potential contribution to the community because it does not reflect others' intention to help. Therefore, in such systems, which are still with us today, every individual's moral reputation is constantly assessed by other group members to prevent "selfish" individuals from receiving help without ever helping others (McAndrew, 2002; Wedekind & Milinski, 2000; also see Cosmides & Tooby, 1992). Thus, being sensitive to and interested in information related to others' morality, especially their immorality, seems to provide an essential adaptation for the efficient operation of indirect reciprocity. This sensitivity might lead to morality being the primary domain of interest for perceivers in social information processing.

Morality and Social Costs

A related reason concerning why people should be more interested in morality-related than competence-related information when processing information about others is that the morality domain allows people to easily assess whether others pose potential costs and threats. As suggested by models of social inference, people hold the lay theory that *immoral* behavior is more informative regarding a person's dispositions than is *moral* behavior (Reeder & Brewer, 1979; Skowronski & Carlston, 1987; Ybarra & Stephan, 1996, 1999). This is the case because moral people tend not to do immoral things, whereas immoral people can do both moral and immoral things. Thus, the morality domain is where perceivers can readily glean information regarding potential threats and costs that stem from others' negative dispositional qualities.

The reverse tends to be the case in the competence domain. For this domain, people hold the lay theory that it is unlikely that an *incompetent* person will, all of a sudden, produce a competent performance. But it is likely that a *competent* person will on occasion, for a variety of possible reasons, do incompetent things (Reeder & Brewer, 1979; Skowronski & Carlston, 1987). Therefore, the most informative cue in the competence domain is positive person information, which should be less useful for signaling potential costs and threats in social exchange.

If the morality domain is primary in social information processing, it is likely that specific areas of the brain may be associated with the rapid and automatic processing of morality-related information. Recent research in neuropsychology suggests that this is the case. Using functional magnetic resonance imaging, Moll et al. (2002) found that people who were examining morality-related stimuli showed increased neuroactivity at the orbital and medial prefrontal cortex and the superior temporal sulcus, which were not activated when examining nonsocial stimuli or other stimuli unrelated to morality.

In another study, people who had sustained damage to the orbitofrontal cortex were shown to have an impaired ability to automatically process moral emotions (e.g., guilt, shame), although other social cognitive abilities were preserved (Eslinger & Damasio, 1985; Saver & Damasio, 1991). Together with findings from other researchers (e.g., Damasio, 1994; Farrow et al., 2001), such evidence suggests that there are specific areas of the brain that are used in the processing of morality-related information. Such specialization in the brain could possibly contribute to efficiency in the detection and processing of information that signals whether or not others are rule-abiding members of the social exchange network.

The presumed sensitivity to morality-related information may be a general adaptation that at times, though, may be modified depending on specific situational factors. For example, people are most likely to be sensitive to morality-related information when they are forming impressions of others, but because people in social interactions can have goals other than forming general impressions (Jones & Thibaut, 1958), their cognitive strategies should be flexible and sensitive to different demands.

As discussed by Hilton and Darley (1991), some goals will lead people to engage in a broad survey of others' personalities, some goals will lead people to focus on specific domains, and some goals will lead people away from seeking additional information. Certain goals might actually lead people to become more sensitive to competence-related than morality-related information or make people equally sensitive to both domains. For example, people who anticipate competition with others are more interested in seeking competence-related information than morality-related information. This is so because those who anticipate competition need such information to size up their opponents (Chan & Ybarra, 2002). However, given that social exchange is a ubiquitous feature of human life, and because forming impressions of others is a common if not obligatory goal in social interaction, it is likely that on a general level people should be more sensitive to morality- than competence-related information in others.

THE CHRONIC CONCERNS OF YOUNGER AND OLDER ADULTS

A noncontroversial premise of the present research is that there are cognitive declines as a person grows older. As people grow older, their general ability to process information is reduced (Craik & Byrd, 1982), and they experience declines in speed of processing and working memory (for a review, see Park, 2000). *Speed of processing* refers to how rapidly people perform mental operations (Salthouse, 1991, 1996), whereas working memory is the online processing capacity available to store, retrieve, and manipulate information. There is evidence that age-related decreases in speed of processing and working memory account for age differences in a broad range of behaviors, including long-term memory tasks (Park et al., 2000; Park et al., 1996); the assembly of three-dimensional figures from blocks (Morrell & Park, 1993); memory for television, radio, and print news (Frieske & Park, 1999); and reasoning about medical decisions (Zwahr, Park, & Shifren, 1999).

Despite these general age-related declines in cognition, people's chronic concern with others' morality (as opposed to their competence) is likely to be present regardless of a person's age. This should be the case because all people tend to remain embedded in a web of social relations (Antonucci & Akiyama, 1987; Charles & Carstensen, 1999), and the use of morality-related information plays a crucial role in monitoring others' status in complex social exchange. Thus, it might be expected that morality-related concepts should be more accessible in memory than competence-related concepts. In particular, it was expected that people would be fastest in reacting to concepts related to immorality. This was anticipated because such information processing supports the posited social exchange mechanism, whereby immorality signals potential costs and threats more effectively than the other types of information (e.g., positive morality- and competence-related information). In addition, it was expected that older adults would also be most sensitive to morality-related information despite being generally slower than the younger adults.

To examine these hypotheses, we conducted an experiment to compare younger and older adults' sensitivity to person information from the morality and competence domains (Ybarra, Chan, & Park, 2001). A lexical decision task (LDT) was used to examine the accessibility of morality- and competence-related concepts in memory. In an LDT, participants are asked to identify whether letter strings that are presented to them are words or nonwords as quickly and accurately as possible. Words related to concepts about which people are chronically concerned should be more accessible in memory and hence should be recognized as words faster than words related to concepts that are less accessible in memory (see Bruner, 1957). For example, people high in religiosity have been shown to be faster at identifying religion-related than religion-unrelated words (Blaine & Nguyen, 2002), and people who hold egalitarian goals have been shown to pronounce words related to egalitarianism faster than words irrelevant to egalitarianism (Moskowitz, Salomon, & Taylor, 2000).

In Ybarra et al. (2001), participants were presented with 24 words that were related to morality (e.g., *honest, unhelpful*) or competence (e.g., *intelligent, unskilled*). Half of the person cues from each trait domain were positive and half were negative in valence. An equal number of nonwords (e.g., *ostroly*) was also presented to the participants. Participants were asked to indicate if the cue that they saw was a word or nonword as quickly as

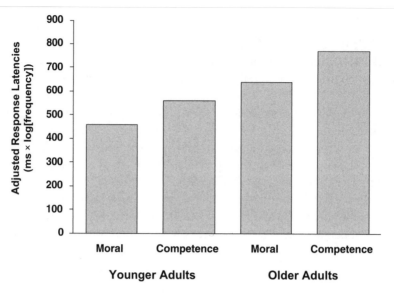

Figure 7.1. Younger and older adults' adjusted response latencies to morality- and competence-related word cues. The adjusted response latency was computed by multiplying the reaction time (ms) by log (word frequency). This was done to control for the influence of the frequency of occurrence of the words (see Balota & Chumbley, 1984). We conducted another study (Ybarra, Chan, & Park, 2001, Study 1) in which we controlled for word frequency experimentally and obtained the same results.

they could by pressing a key on the keyboard. The dependent measure of interest was how long it took participants to respond to the different person cues (traits).

Before the results were analyzed, the response time for each trait cue was corrected for frequency of occurrence (reaction time × log [word frequency]; see Balota & Chumbley, 1984). The results of the study indicated that older adults were overall slower than the younger adults in identifying the cues. This finding is consistent with much research in cognitive aging that has demonstrated age-related declines, such as in speed of processing (for a review, see Park, 2000). When the younger and older adults' reaction times to the different types of person cues were examined separately (Figure 7.1), it was apparent that both the younger and the older adults were more sensitive and faster to respond to information from the morality than the competence trait domain. This finding is consistent with the hypothesis that the processing of morality-related person information should remain a central concern for people across the life span.

A closer examination of the reaction times to the morality- and competence-related person cues as a function of cue valence revealed that both younger and older participants were fastest to respond to immoral cues than the other three types of cues (Figure 7.2). Although the analysis

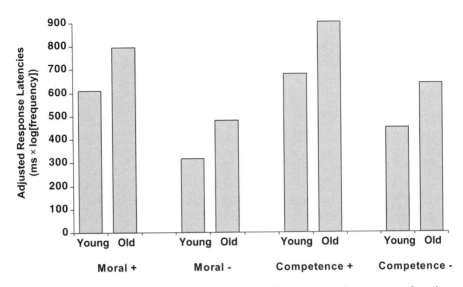

Figure 7.2. Adjusted response latencies to the positive and negative cues as a function of trait domain and participants' age.

revealed no age interactions, there was a trend that suggested that responses to the immorality cues produced the smallest difference between the younger and older adults: difference for moral negative = 160, compared with the differences for the other three types of traits: moral positive = 190, competence positive = 220, and competence negative = 190.

The findings of the first study thus indicated that people's sensitivity to morality-related information appears to be conserved across the life span. Such a pattern of responses may help people remain vigilant about others' contribution to the social exchange network and allow them to determine who is likely to default in social contracts.

FORMING MORALITY- AND COMPETENCE-RELATED PERSON IMPRESSIONS

The research reviewed in the first part of the chapter dealt with people's sensitivity to different types of person information. The findings showing that people are most sensitive to morality-related information have important implications for the manner in which people may actually form impressions and generate inferences about others' personalities. Forming impressions of others' personalities is affected by various factors, but one general factor that is bound to influence people's inferences about others is the accessibility of different types of information in memory.

The accessibility of information in memory reflects in part the frequency with which that information has been activated and used in the past. It is reasonable to expect that the more chronically accessible an information category is in memory, the more efficient its use in inference generation, such as in making judgments about others' personalities and intentions. By comparison, an information category that is less accessible in memory should result in more inefficient information processing and inference generation. Therefore, given the greater accessibility of morality-related compared with competence-related information, it would be expected that social cognitive processes that rely on or operate on morality-related information should be more efficient than those that rely on or operate on competence-related information.

The aforementioned reasoning has important implications when we consider age-related cognitive declines. Compared with less efficient processes, more efficient processes should result in social cognitive outcomes that are less likely to be disrupted by cognitive strain, such as the strain produced by age-related cognitive declines. Therefore, given that the processing of morality-related information should be efficient, impression formation that relies on morality-related information may be less affected by a person's age and the person's associated level of cognitive functioning. In contrast, the processing of competence-related information should be less efficient than the processing of morality-related information. Given age-related cognitive declines, it would thus be expected that compared with younger adults, older adults would be less able to generate appropriate inferences regarding a person's level of competence.

Older Adults and Morality Impressions: No Jumping to Conclusions

In Chan, Ybarra, and Park (2006), older and younger adults were asked to form an impression of a person whom they did not know. Inefficiency in impression formation was assessed by the extent to which participants relied on "cognitive shortcuts" to generate inferences about the person. Participants' reliance on these shortcuts was indexed by the degree to which they showed a primacy effect in impression formation, that is, a bias to base their judgments of the person using the first pieces of information they were presented compared with the last pieces of information.

Primacy reflects people's willingness to jump to conclusions without reviewing all of the available information, and the use of primacy information indicates a person's inability to devote the cognitive energy or motivation to the judgment at hand (Kruglanski & Webster, 1996). For example, the favoring of primacy cues is more likely to occur when people's cognitive resources are reduced by aversive working environments, fatigue, or when the task is tedious (Kruglanski, 1975). An absence of primacy in judgment or the presence of a recency effect (weighting the last pieces of information to a greater extent in judgment) indicates that people suspended judgment until all of the available information was evaluated. This requires the availability of cognitive resources or the execution of efficient cognitive processes (see Kruglanski & Webster, 1996).

With regard to the present conceptualization, it was thus expected that when it came to forming morality-related impressions, both the younger and older adults would fail to show a primacy effect in their impressions. This was expected because processes that use or operate on morality-related information should be efficiently executed by all people, which precludes any disruption by age-related cognitive declines. By contrast, processes that use or operate on competence-related information, because of their inefficiency, should be amenable to disruption by age-related cognitive declines. Thus, it was expected that older adults would show primacy effects when they formed competence-related person impressions, whereas the younger adults would not. We tested these hypotheses in the experiment we describe next.

Empirical Evidence: Older Adults Remain Fluent in Morality Impressions

In this experiment (Chan et al., 2006), younger and older adults were presented with either morality-related or competence-related behavioral information, and half of this information was positive and half was negative in valence. Participants formed only one impression that was based on either morality-related or competence-related information. Depending on the experimental condition, each participant read five honest and five dishonest acts (morality condition) or five intelligent and five unintelligent acts (competence condition). In addition, for both the morality and competence conditions, the presentation order of the positive and negative information was varied, so that half of the participants scrolled through all of the positive information first then the negative information, and vice versa for participants in the other condition.

After the participants read the behavior statements and formed an impression of the person, they were asked to render their judgments. Participants who formed morality-related impressions were asked to judge the target's honesty, whereas participants who formed competence-related impressions were asked to judge the target's intelligence. The dependent measure consisted of a single trait judgment that was made on a 7-point scale, with higher scores indicating more positive ratings (greater honesty or greater intelligence). From the pattern of trait judgments, we were in a position to infer whether or not participants favored the primacy cues in their impressions.

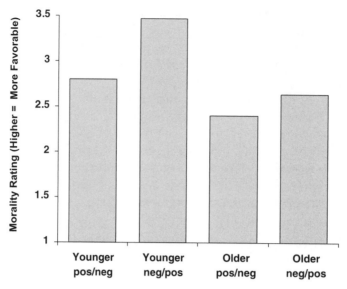

Figure 7.3. Younger and older adults' morality trait judgments as a function of trait domain and presentation orders.

Overall, the findings indicated that morality impressions received lower ratings (i.e., more negative) than competence impressions, despite the fact that both positive and negative information was processed in both conditions. This finding is consistent with the earlier discussion regarding people's greater sensitivity to immorality-related information because such information signals potential costs and threats.

To determine whether participants favored primacy cues in the different conditions, we examined the effect of presentation order (positive-negative or negative-positive) on participants' trait judgments (Chan et al., 2006). A primacy effect was defined as a more positive judgment when the first pieces of the presented information were positive and a more negative judgment when the first pieces of presented information were negative.

With regard to the participants who formed morality-related impressions (honesty, dishonesty), the results indicated that both younger and older adults showed no tendency toward using the primacy information in their judgments (see Figure 7.3). In fact, consistent with expectations, the presentation order effect was significant, indicating that a recency effect was obtained. The trait judgments were more positive if the last pieces of information were positive and more negative if the last pieces of information were negative. Such a pattern of findings indicates that all of the participants suspended their judgments until all of the morality-related information was processed.

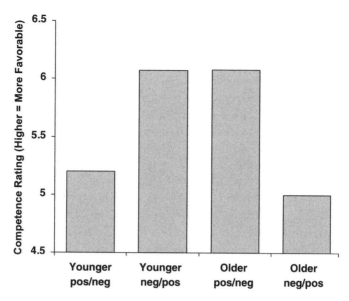

Figure 7.4. Younger and older adults competence trait judgments as a function of trait domain and presentation orders.

For the participants who formed impression judgments related to competence (intelligent, unintelligent), the results indicated that the older adults favored using the primacy cues whereas the younger adults did not (Figure 7.4). The trait judgments made by the older participants were more positive when the first pieces of information were positive but more negative when the first pieces of information were negative. In contrast, the younger adults did not favor the primacy cues but appeared to have suspended judgments until they reviewed all of the available information, resulting in a recency effect. Thus, the older adults appeared to have jumped to conclusions regarding the person's level of competence.

CONCLUSIONS AND IMPLICATIONS

The results from the first study (Ybarra et al., 2001) indicated that people are poised to process and recognize information that has to do with a person's morality, especially any indication of immorality. These findings were obtained for both younger and older adults, suggesting that the morality category is more accessible in memory than the competence category, and this sensitivity to morality-related information is conserved across the life span. On the basis of these results, we suggested that the accessibility of person information in memory should affect the efficiency with which perceivers form impressions and generate inferences that are based on either morality- or competence-related information. This issue was taken up in the second reported study.

In the second study (Chan et al., 2006), the findings showed that in forming morality-related impressions, participants' impressions were not based on the first pieces of presented information, which suggests a suspension of judgment until all of the information was processed. These results were not affected by participants' age. In contrast, participants who formed competence-related impressions showed differences in their inferences as a function of their age. The younger adults once again appeared able to suspend their judgments, as they did not show a primacy effect. However, the older adults showed strong primacy effects in forming competence-based impressions, consistent with the idea that they were unable to suspend judgment until they evaluated all of the competence-related information.

Taken together, the results described in this chapter indicate that certain domains of person information are more efficiently processed than others. Social cognitive processes that rely on or operate on morality-related information tend to be more efficient, which makes them more likely to preclude disruption by cognitive strain such as that created by age-related cognitive declines. In contrast, the processes that use or operate on competence-related information seem less efficient, which appears to leave them open to disruption by age-related cognitive declines.

People's sensitivity to morality-related information and their seeming efficiency in processing such information make sense in that it provides a social cognitive medium through which indirect reciprocity in social systems can operate. In all social systems, each person's moral reputation is constantly assessed by other group members to prevent cheaters from receiving help without ever helping others (McAndrew, 2002; Wedekind & Milinski, 2000; see also Cosmides & Tooby, 1992). This is a constant concern for people, which may help explain people's sensitivity to these aspects of others across the life span. In contrast, although competence-related information is an important component in social perception, it is not as informative about others' potential contribution to the community because it does not reflect others' intention to help or inclination to cheat. Thus, compared with the processing of morality-related information, it makes sense that the use of and processing of competence-related information would be less efficient.

When we consider medical situations, the general implication of the present research is that older adults may be apt to jump to conclusions when evaluating the competence of the source giving the medical recommendation. This tendency may be exacerbated by the fact that medical situations are often surrounded by a sense of crisis and urgency, which should further increase older adults' propensity to rely on primacy cues. This should be the case because the presence of stress, fatigue, and the pressure to learn new medical information may further reduce their cognitive capacity. If the first bits of information they receive about the source of the medical advice are positive, older adults may develop more positive impressions than if the first pieces of information are negative. In terms of the former possibility, this could put older adults in the position of prematurely favoring a promising miracle treatment suggested by a con artist who presents himself or herself as an expert, even though subsequent information may clearly indicate incompetence. With regard to jumping to the conclusion that the health care provider possesses negative dispositions, this inference could sway the older adults to terminate their relations with the health care provider or to not abide by his or her recommendations, even though later it is discovered that this individual is indeed quite competent and highly regarded.

Some research indicates that older adults generally believe their own physicians are very competent but that physicians and health care providers in general are not highly competent in making judgments regarding older adults (Gould & McDonald-Miszczak, 1996). Thus, another implication of the present research is that older adults are likely to maintain beliefs regarding their health care provider's competence even if they encounter subsequent information that would disconfirm these initial expectations. As a result, an older patient may be less likely to question and be more likely to adhere to medical advice that he or she receives from a practitioner with whom he or she has an established relationship. This should not be a concern in cases in which the practitioner is truly competent. However, in rare cases in which the practitioner is not qualified to provide medical advice and treatment or when the practitioner actually has deceptive intentions, it might be difficult for the older patient to recognize the incompetence of the current practitioner. In addition, the belief that health care providers in general are not highly competent may serve as a barrier to older adults who need to switch to a new practitioner.

Finally, it is of interest to consider research with younger adults in which researchers have provided a mix of morality- and competence-related information to be used in impression formation. The findings from these studies have shown that under such circumstances, impressions of others tend to be swayed more by the morality- than the competence-related information (e.g., De Bruin & Van Lange, 1999; Martijn, Spears, Van der Pligt, & Jakobs, 1992). Thus, one implication of these findings is that to induce a healthy skepticism in older adults when evaluating medical personnel and other sources of medical information, it may be useful to have them focus on determining not only the person's competence but, more important, the person's morality, for example, whether or not the person is honest and helpful. Such a focus may have the unintended effect of allowing older adults to consider more of the available information before making important medical decisions.

REFERENCES

Alexander, R. D. (1987). *The biology of moral systems*. New York: Aldine de Gruyter.

Anderson, N. H. (1968). Likableness ratings of 555 personality-trait words. *Journal of Personality and Social Psychology, 9*, 272–279.

Antonucci, T. C., & Akiyama, H. (1987). An examination of sex differences in social support in mid and late life. *Sex Roles, 17*, 737–749.

Asch, S. E. (1955). Opinions and social pressure. *Scientific American, 19*, 31–35.

Bales, R. F. (1953). The equilibrium problem in small groups. In T. Parsons, R. F. Bales, & E. A. Shils (Eds.), *Working papers in the theory of action* (pp. 111–161). Glencoe, IL: Free Press.

Balota, D. A., & Chumbley, J. I. (1984). Are lexical decisions a good measure of lexical access? The role of word frequency in the neglected decision stage. *Journal of Experimental Psychology: Human Perception and Performance, 10*, 340–357.

Blaine, B. E., & Nguyen, D. B. (2002). Believing is seeing: Religiousness and perceptual expertise. *International Journal for the Psychology of Religion, 12*, 93–107.

Bruner, J. S. (1957). On perceptual readiness. *Psychological Review, 64*, 123–152.

Buss, D. M. (1998). The psychology of human mate selection: Exploring the complexity of the strategic repertoire. In C. Crawford & D. L. Krebs (Eds.), *Handbook of evolutionary psychology: Ideas, issues, and applications* (pp. 405–430). Mahwah, NJ: Erlbaum.

Chaiken, S., & Maheswaran, D. (1994). Heuristic processing can bias systematic processing: Effects of source credibility, argument ambiguity, and task importance on attitude judgment. *Journal of Personality and Social Psychology, 66*, 460–473.

Chan, E., & Ybarra, O. (2002). Interaction goals and social information processing: Underestimating one's partners but overestimating one's opponents. *Social Cognition, 20*, 409–439.

Chan, E., Ybarra, O., & Park, D. C. (2006). *Primacy versus recency in impression formation: The role of trait domains*. Manuscript in preparation.

Charles, S. T., & Carstensen, L. L. (1999). The role of time in the setting of social goals across the lifespan. In T. M. Hess & F. Blanchard-Fields (Eds.), *Social cognition and aging* (pp. 319–342). San Diego, CA: Academic Press.

Cialdini, R. B., & Trost, M. R. (1991). Social influence: Social norms, conformity, and compliance. In D. T. Gilbert, S. T. Fiske, & G. Lindzey (Eds.), *Handbook of social psychology* (Vol. 2, pp. 151–192). Boston: McGraw-Hill.

Cosmides, L., & Tooby, J. (1992). Cognitive adaptations for social exchange. In J. Barkow (Ed.), *The adapted mind* (pp. 163–228). New York: Oxford University Press.

Craik, F. I. M., & Byrd, M. (1982). Aging and cognitive deficits: The role of attentional resources. In F. I. M. Craik & S. Trehub (Eds.), *Aging and cognitive processes* (pp. 191–211). New York: Plenum Press.

Damasio, A. R. (1994). *Descartes' error: Emotion, reason, and the human brain.* New York: Putnam.

De Bruin, E. N. M., & Van Lange, P. A. M. (1999). Impression formation and cooperative behavior. *European Journal of Social Psychology, 29,* 305–328.

DiMatteo, M. R., & Lepper, H. S. (1998). Promoting adherence to courses of treatment: Mutual collaboration in the physician–patient relationship. In L. D. Jackson & B. K. Duffy (Eds.), *Health communication research: A guide to developments and directions* (pp. 75–86). Westport, CT: Greenwood Press.

Eslinger, P. J., & Damasio, A. R. (1985). Severe disturbance of higher cognition after bilateral frontal lobe ablation: Patient EVR. *Neurology, 35,* 1731–1741.

Farrow, T. F. D., Zheng, Y., Wilkinson, I. D., Spence, S. A., Deakin, J. F., Tarrier, N., et al. (2001). Investigating the functional anatomy of empathy and forgiveness. *NeuroReport, 12,* 2433–2438.

Fiedler, F. E., & Chemers, M. M. (1974). *Leadership and effective management.* Glenview, IL: Scott Foresman.

Fiske, S. T., Xu, J., Cuddy, A. C., & Glick, P. (1999). (Dis)respecting versus (dis)liking: Status and interdependence predict ambivalent stereotypes of competence and warmth *Journal of Social Issues, 55,* 473–489.

Frieske, D. A., & Park, D. C. (1999). Memory for news in young and old adults. *Psychology and Aging, 14,* 90–98.

Garrity, T. F., & Lawson, E. J. (1989). Patient–physician communication as a determinant of medication misuse in older, minority women. *Journal of Drug Issues, 19,* 245–259.

Gould, O. N., & McDonald-Miszczak, L. (1996, May). *Perceptions of ageism in health care workers.* Poster session presented at the Third International Conference on Communication, Aging, and Health, Kansas City, MO.

Hamilton, D. L., & Zanna, M. P. (1972). Differential weighting of favourable and unfavourable attributes in impressions of personality. *Journal of Experimental Research: Personality, 6,* 204–212.

Hammer, W. C., & Organ, D. W. (1978). *Organizational behavior: An applied psychological approach.* Dallas, TX: Business Publications.

Hass, R. G. (1981). Effects of source characteristics on the cognitive processing of persuasive messages and attitude change. In R. Petty, T. Ostrom, & T. Brock (Eds.), *Cognitive responses in persuasion* (pp. 141–172). Hillsdale, NJ: Erlbaum.

Hilton, J. L., & Darley, J. M. (1991). The effects of interaction goals on person perception. In M. P. Zanna (Ed.), *Advances in experimental social psychology* (Vol. 24, pp. 236–262). New York: Academic Press.

Jones, E. E., & Thibaut, J. W. (1958). Interaction goals as bases of inference in interpersonal perception. In R. Tagiuri & L. Petrillo (Eds.), *Person perception* and *interpersonal behavior* (pp. 151–178). Stanford, CA: Stanford University Press.

Kruglanski, A. W. (1975). The endogenous–exogenous partition in attribution theory. *Psychological Review, 82,* 387–406.

Kruglanski, A. W., & Webster, D. M. (1996). Motivated closing of the mind: "Seizing" and "freezing." *Psychological Review, 103,* 263–283.

Maddux, J. E., & Rogers, R. W. (1980). Effects of source expertness, physical attractiveness, and supporting arguments on persuasion: A case of brains over beauty. *Journal of Personality and Social Psychology, 39,* 235–244.

Martijn, C., Spears, R., Van der Pligt, J., & Jakobs, E. (1992). Negativity and positivity effects in person perception and inference: Ability versus morality. *European Journal of Social Psychology, 22,* 453–463.

McAndrew, F. T. (2002). New evolutionary perspectives on altruism: Multilevel-selection and costly signaling theories. *Current Directions in Psychological Science, 11,* 79–82.

McCabe, K. A., & Gregory, S. S. (1998). Elderly victimization: An examination beyond the FBI's index crimes. *Research on Aging, 20,* 363–372.

McGhee, J. L. (1983). The vulnerability of elderly consumers. *International Journal of Aging and Human Development, 17,* 223–246.

Moll, J., de Oliveira-Souza, R., Eslinger, P. J., Bramati, I. E., Mourão-Miranda, J., Amdreiuolo, P. A., & Pessoa, L. (2002). The neural correlates of moral sensitivity: A functional magnetic resonance imaging investigation of basic and moral emotions. *Journal of Neuroscience, 22,* 2730–2736.

Morrell, R., & Park, D. C. (1993). Effects of age, illustrations and task variables on the performance of procedural assembly tasks. *Psychology and Aging, 8,* 389–399.

Moskowitz, G. B., Salomon, A. R., & Taylor, C. M. (2000). Preconsciously controlling stereotyping: Implicitly activated egalitarian goals prevent the activation of stereotypes. *Social Cognition, 18,* 151–177.

Park, D. C. (2000). The basic mechanisms accounting for age-related decline in cognitive function. In D. C. Park & N. Schwarz (Eds.), *Cognitive aging: A primer* (pp. 3–21). Philadelphia: Psychology Press.

Park, D. C., Davidson, N., Lautenschlager, G., Smith, A. D., Smith, P., & Hedden, T. (2000). Models of visuospatial and verbal memory across the adult life span. *Psychology and Aging, 17,* 299–320.

Park, D. C., Smith, A. D., Lautenschlager, G., Earles, J., Frieske, D., Zwahr, M., & Gaines, C. (1996). Mediators of long-term memory performance across the life span. *Psychology and Aging, 11,* 621–637.

Reeder, G. D., & Brewer, M. B. (1979). A schematic model of dispositional attribution in interpersonal perception. *Psychological Review, 86,* 61–79.

Rosenberg, S., Nelson, C., & Vivekananthan, P. S. (1968). A multidimensional approach to the structure of personality impressions. *Journal of Personality and Social Psychology, 9,* 283–294.

Rosenberg, S., & Sedlak, A. (1972). Structural representations of implicit personality theory. In L. Berkowitz (Ed.), *Advances in experimental social psychology* (Vol. 6, pp. 235–297). New York: Academic Press.

Salthouse, T. A. (1991). *Theoretical perspectives on cognitive aging.* Hillsdale, NJ: Erlbaum.

Salthouse, T. A. (1996). The processing-speed theory of adult age differences in cognition. *Psychological Review, 103,* 403–428.

Saver, J. L., & Damasio, A. R. (1991). Preserved access and processing of social knowledge in a patient with acquired sociopathy due to ventromedial frontal damage. *Neuropsychologia, 29,* 1241–1249.

Sherif, M. (1936). *The psychology of social norms.* New York: HarperCollins.

Singh, R., & Teoh, J. B. P. (1999). Attitudes and attraction: A test of two hypotheses for the similarity–dissimilarity asymmetry. *British Journal of Social Psychology, 38,* 427–443.

Skowronski, J. J., & Carlston, D. E. (1987). Social judgment and social memory: The role of cue diagnosticity in negativity, positivity, and extremity biases. *Journal of Personality and Social Psychology, 52,* 689–699.

Thom, D. H., Ribisl, K. M., Stewart, A. L., & Luke, D. A. (1999). Further validation and reliability testing of the Trust in Physician Scale. *Medical Care, 37,* 510–517.

Wedekind, K., & Milinski, M. (2000, May 5). Cooperation through image scoring in humans. *Science, 288,* 561–574.

Wojciszke, B. (1994). Multiple meanings of behavior: Construing actions in terms of competence and morality. *Journal of Personality and Social Psychology, 67,* 222–232.

Ybarra, O., Chan, E., & Park, D. (2001). Young and old adults' concerns with morality and competence. *Motivation and Emotion, 25,* 85–100.

Ybarra, O., & Stephan W. G. (1996). Misanthropic person memory. *Journal of Personality and Social Psychology, 70,* 691–700.

Ybarra, O., & Stephan, W. G. (1999). Attributional orientations and the prediction of behavior: The attribution-prediction bias. *Journal of Personality and Social Psychology, 76,* 718–727.

Zwahr, M. D., Park, D. C., & Shifren, K. (1999). Judgments about estrogen replacement therapy: The role of age, cognitive abilities and beliefs. *Psychology and Aging, 14,* 179–191.

III

ADHERENCE TO TREATMENT

8

MOTIVATIONAL MODELS AND VOLITIONAL PROCESSES IN THE PROMOTION OF HEALTH BEHAVIORS

SHEINA ORBELL

Concerns about health in aging have prompted attention to preventive behavior change and to medical, surgical, and self-management strategies for improving mobility and independence in later years (Orbell, 1996). Technical and epidemiological knowledge will have little or no impact on health, however, unless people adopt recommended procedures or make changes to their behavior. I begin this chapter by considering the role of several important social cognitive models in explaining health-related behavior. A conceptual distinction is drawn between those theoretical models that emphasize the deliberative processes regarding the *nature* of a health threat (e.g., the commonsense model of illness representations; Leventhal, Meyer, & Nerenz, 1980) and those models that emphasize the deliberation of the costs and benefits of performing a recommended health protective *behavior* (e.g., protection-motivation theory, Rogers, 1975, 1983; theory of reasoned action, Fishbein & Ajzen, 1975; theory of planned behavior, Ajzen, 1985). I review empirical evidence for these various approaches to understanding motivation for health behaviors. In the next part of the chapter I turn to examination of the sufficiency of these motivational theories and review evidence concerning the strength of the relationship between intentions to act and actual behavior (see Orbell, 2004). Next, an analysis of the nature of inconsistency between intention and behavior is presented. It is argued that there are good empirical and theoretical grounds for supposing that positive intentions do not always translate into intended actions. One important approach to this difficulty is to identify the role of volitional self-regulatory processes in explaining how and under what circumstances people may shift from a state of willingness to adopt recommended health-related behaviors to actual enactment and maintenance of those recommendations. I turn to this issue in the final section of the chapter.

MOTIVATION FOR HEALTH PROTECTIVE BEHAVIORS

It is useful to draw a distinction between behaviors that are recommended for the purposes of maintaining a state of good health and those that are recommended for the purposes of correcting a state of ill health or minimizing its adverse consequences. Behaviors recommended for maintaining health may be performed by people who are in good health and do not believe themselves to be ill. Behavioral motivation in this domain has often been examined within social psychological frameworks that focus on evaluations of the behavior itself. For example, the theory of planned behavior (Ajzen, 1985) specifies the variables attitude, subjective norm, and perceived behavioral control over performing the behavior. Frameworks for performing illness-specific behaviors, such as injecting insulin or practicing physical therapy exercises, tend to emphasize variables that address cognitions about the nature of illness itself. For example, the commonsense model of illness representations (Leventhal et al., 1980) specifies the variables identity, timeline, cause, consequences, and cure–control as determinants of whether an individual copes with illness by adopting a recommended behavioral response. In principle, it is possible to view both preventive behaviors and corrective behaviors as coping responses to illness threat. Indeed protection-motivation theory (Rogers, 1983) incorporates variables concerned with illness threat (perceived severity, perceived susceptibility) as well as variables concerned with behavioral evaluation and performance (response efficacy, response costs, and self-efficacy). Nonetheless, it is important to acknowledge in reviewing and in comparing these theoretical approaches that they have tended to focus on different classes of behavior and used different types of population. From a theoretical point of view, the relative importance of social cognitive beliefs about illness versus beliefs about behavior is an important issue for the study of motivation in the health domain (Orbell, Hagger, Brown, & Tidy, in press).

The Commonsense Model of Illness Representations

People's cognitions regarding illness are thought to be schematically organized along five dimensions: *identity* (symptoms, illness label), *causes* (attributions for the cause of illness), *timeline* (Is the illness going to be acute or chronic?), *consequences* (Will the illness have serious physical or psychosocial consequences?), *and cure–control* (Can the illness be effectively controlled by one's behavior or by treatment? see Linz, Penrod, & Leventhal, 1982; Meyer, Leventhal, & Gutmann, 1985). These illness cognitions are proposed to determine whether an individual will adopt a recommended personal coping behavior or treatment regime (for a review, see Hagger & Orbell, 2003).

Illness representations have been studied in a range of contexts, including diabetes self-management (Hampson, Glasgow, & Stryker, 2000; Hampson, Glasgow, & Toobert, 1990), chronic fatigue syndrome (Heijmans, 1998), common cold (Lau, Bernard, & Hartman, 1989), myocardial infarction (Petrie, Weinman, Sharpe, & Buckley, 1996), rheumatoid arthritis (Schiaffino, Shawaryn, & Blum, 1998), osteoarthritis (Orbell, Johnston, Rowley, Espley, & Davey, 1998), and atrial fibrillation (Steed, Newman, & Hardman, 1999), with many studies using samples of older adults. One difficulty in examining consistency of associations of illness representations with coping outcomes in research to date arises from the heterogeneity of measurement approaches, both to illness representations and to coping behaviors. To address this difficulty, Hagger and Orbell (2003) conducted a content analysis of measures prior to a meta-analytic synthesis of results and obtained an average weighted correlation of .28 between the control–cure dimension of illness representations and the use of problem-focused coping behaviors (defined as any active attempt to directly address the illness). By using Cohen's (1992) criteria for interpreting effect size, a correlation of .28 might be interpreted as approaching a medium effect. This finding suggests that adoption of recommended behaviors for dealing with illness is primarily a function of beliefs that the illness may be controlled by those behaviors. Identity, consequences, and timeline were not significantly associated with problem-focused coping in either a positive or negative direction but were associated with avoidance or denial of illness.

Protection-Motivation Theory

The origins of protection-motivation theory have been attributed to earlier research on fear appeals. Protection-motivation theory provides an account of cognitive processes that explain how a threatening or fear-arousing communication is translated into a state of "protection motivation," or readiness to act to address the threat (Rogers, 1975, 1983). The theory proposes two forms of cognitive process accounting for the development of protection motivation: threat appraisal and coping appraisal. *Threat appraisal* concerns appraisals of personal vulnerability to illness, perceived severity of that illness to the individual, and fear arousal. *Coping appraisal* summarizes the person's assessment of the recommended coping response to the appraised threat and comprises response efficacy (perceived efficacy of the recommended response), self-efficacy (perceived ability to perform the recommended response; see Bandura, 1977), and response costs (perceived psychological costs of performing the recommended response). Where an individual feels vulnerable to a serious illness and perceives that the recommended coping response is effective, relatively easy to perform, and not too costly, he or she is proposed to develop protection motivation or an intention to perform the recommended coping response.

Protection-motivation theory has been used in a range of contexts, including condom use (Abraham, Sheeran, Abrams, & Spears, 1994), breast cancer screening (Boer & Seydel, 1996), cervical cancer screening (Orbell & Sheeran, 1998), parents' compliance with child's physical therapy (Flynn, Lyman, & Prentice-Dunn, 1995), breast self-examination (Hodgkins & Orbell, 1998), smoking cessation (Maddux & Rogers, 1983), tooth flossing (Sheeran & Orbell, 1996), testicular self-examination (Steffen, 1990), and dietary supplement use (Wurtele, 1988). Components of protection-motivation theory (like the commonsense model) may be used to predict not only the enactment of recommended responses but also the use of maladaptive strategies such as avoidance or denial. In a meta-analytic review, Milne, Sheeran, and Orbell (2000) obtained weighted average correlations of .16, .10, and .20 between intention and vulnerability, severity, and fear, respectively. Response efficacy, self-efficacy, and response costs obtained correlations with intention of .29, .33, and −.34, respectively. Thus, threat appraisals might be considered to have small associations with protection motivation, whereas coping appraisals obtain moderate associations. The apparent superiority of coping appraisal in explaining protection motivation was further supported by findings from a vote count, implying that evaluation of coping behavior is a primary source of motivation for adopting recommended health protective behaviors.

The Theories of Reasoned Action and Planned Behavior

The theory of reasoned action (Fishbein, 1980; Fishbein & Ajzen, 1975) evolved from research concerning the relationship of attitude to behavior. The theory proposes that to understand the effects of attitude on behavior, it is necessary to consider first the relation of attitude to the development of behavior-specific motivation, that is, the development of a behavioral intention. The theory of reasoned action proposes that intentions are proximally determined by a person's attitude toward behavior and his or her subjective norm for the behavior. *Attitude* refers to a person's overall favorable or unfavorable evaluation of performing the behavior, whereas *subjective norm* summarizes a person's belief that important others believe he or she should perform the behavior. Thus, unlike the common-sense model or protection-motivation theory, the theory of reasoned action explicitly acknowledges the role of social influence in governing people's motivation to act.

To account for behaviors that require resources, opportunity, or cooperation of others, Ajzen (1985) developed the theory of planned behavior. The theory of planned behavior postulates an additional predictor of intentions and behavior—perceived behavioral control. *Perceived behavioral control* refers to people's appraisals of their ability to perform the behavior and comprises Bandura's (1977) concept of self-efficacy, together with perceptions of control over behavior. A positive intention to act is therefore said to arise when an individual possesses a positive attitude toward the behavior, perceives that important others would support the behavior, and perceives that he or she has control over performing the behavior.

The theories of reasoned action and planned behavior have been examined in relation to a wide range of health-related behaviors, including motivation to provide care to elderly parents (Rapaport & Orbell, 2000), cervical screening uptake (Sheeran & Orbell, 2000b), physical activity (Hagger, Chatzisarantis, Biddle, & Orbell, 2001), uptake of breast screening (Rutter, 2000), recovery of physical activity after joint replacement surgery (Orbell & Sheeran, 2000), illicit drug use (e.g., Conner, Sherlock, & Orbell, 1998; Orbell, Blair, Sherlock, & Conner, 2001), vehicle driver behavior (e.g., Parker, 1997), and blood donation (e.g., Warshaw, Calantone, & Joyce, 1986). A number of reviews are also available (e.g., Ajzen, 1991; Armitage & Conner, 2001; Sheppard, Hartwick, & Warshaw, 1988), of which the most pertinent to the present chapter might be the meta-analysis by Godin and Kok (1996), which focused on the performance of health-related behaviors. Godin and Kok obtained a weighted average correlation of .46 between attitude and intention, .34 between subjective norm and intention, and .46 between perceived behavioral control and intention. Effect sizes for attitude and perceived behavioral control thus approached large effect sizes, whereas the effect size for subjective norm was moderate, lending considerable support to the role of attitude, subjective norm, and perceived behavioral control in predicting intention to perform health protective behaviors.

EVALUATION OF DETERMINANTS OF MOTIVATION

Meta-analytic evidence to date suggests that motivation for health behaviors is a proximal function of people's expectancies regarding a recommended behavior. Moderate associations with intentions and behavior have been reliably obtained for treatment control from the commonsense model and for response efficacy from protection-motivation theory. Each of these constructs concerns beliefs about the expectancy that performing a recommended behavior (including uptake of a treatment) will be effective in reducing illness threat. Similarly, response costs from protection-motivation theory and attitude from the theory of planned behavior relate to an individual's evaluation of the desirability of the behavior, whereas self-efficacy from protection-motivation theory and perceived behavioral control from the theory of planned behavior relate to a person's confidence in his or her ability to carry out the recommended action. Research using the theory of planned behavior also obtains evidence for the role of social influence in the form of social normative beliefs in governing the development of motivation. Thus a parsimonious account of motivation for health behavior might focus on these social cognitive beliefs.

A number of factors might account for the relatively less impressive performance of illness-related beliefs in the models considered here. On the face of it, a moderate degree of perceived health-related threat ought to be a prerequisite for preventive or corrective behavior. It is possible that relatively small correlations between perceived severity and health-related motivation occur in part because the populations studied tend to be well informed and the diseases studied tend to have high salience and be very serious conditions. These considerations may lead to relatively low variance in measures of severity and consequently small correlations with intentions and behavior. One solution to this difficulty is to use measures of severity that emphasize psychosocial as opposed to simply physical or epidemiological notions of disease severity. A further difficulty may arise if the population studied already has an illness, as in most research concerning the commonsense model, and consequently, perceptions of severity may be a function of current and past coping behaviors. Although it is arguable that the role of perceived illness threat might be more clearly illuminated if it were examined among a naïve population and in relation to a novel disease threat, it is also possible that small correlations between threat appraisal and intentions and behavior can be accounted for by the principle of correspondence (Ajzen & Fishbein, 1973, 1974). Measures of attitude, self-efficacy, treatment control, response costs, and so on are measures of specific beliefs about performing a specific behavior and therefore show correspondence in terms of action, target, time, and context. Measures of consequences, severity, and susceptibility, however, do not possess these qualities of correspondence to specific behavioral acts.

Global assessments of disease threat might be expected to predict global assessments of health-related behavior but do less well in explaining a specific intention to perform a specific behavior.

The success of models such as the commonsense model, protection-motivation theory, and the theory of planned behavior in explaining cognitive prerequisites of health-related motivation has led to their use in the development of interventions at a community and individual level (for reviews, see Hardeman et al., 2002; Milne et al., 2000; Rutter & Quine, 2002). Particularly useful has been the development of tailored interventions (see chap. 10, this volume) in which social cognitive variables specified by these models are selectively manipulated to address person-specific motivational deficits. Individual differences may also affect the success of interventions. For example, Orbell, Perugini, and Rakow (2004) showed that people may differ in terms of the extent to which they are influenced by potential immediate versus distant outcomes when considering how to act now. In an experimental study, this individual difference (the Consideration of Future Consequences [CFC] scale; Strathman, Gleicher, Boninger & Edwards, 1994) moderated the processing of a message in which the same consequences of taking up screening for colorectal cancer were presented as occurring in either the short or long term. People low on CFC were more likely to view screening as beneficial when positive consequences of participation were communicated as occurring in the short term, whereas the opposite was true for those high on CFC. These processing differences were shown to have substantive impacts on the development of positive attitudes, perceived behavioral control, and intentions to participate (see also Orbell & Hagger, 2006). An important additional finding is that CFC appears to decrease with age, implying that health communications aimed at older age groups might be more likely to lead to positive intentions to act if they emphasize the positive consequences of acting as occurring in the shorter term.

THE RELATIONSHIP OF MOTIVATION TO BEHAVIORAL ENACTMENT

The theoretical perspectives considered thus far may be characterized as motivational or deliberative models of behavioral decision making. Each model proposes that behavior, be it the performance of self-care activity, taking medication, changing one's diet or physical activity regime, or taking up a preventive health service, follows from a process of deliberation. Several of these accounts, including the theory of reasoned action (Fishbein, 1980), the theory of planned behavior (Ajzen, 1985, 2001), protection-motivation theory (Rogers, 1983), and recent developments such as the model of goal-directed behavior (Perugini & Bagozzi, 2001), propose that the process of deliberation culminates in the formation of an intention to act. Behavioral intention, according to each of these models, mediates the impact of prior variables on subsequent behavior. Both the model of goal-directed behavior and the theory of planned behavior also allow for the possibility that in some circumstances a person may not have complete control over behavior and therefore may be unable to act on his or her intention. Thus, behavior in these models may be predicted from intention and perceived behavioral control. An intention may be either positive ("I intend to do Z") or negative ("I do not intend to do Z") and is assumed to capture the motivational import of prior variables so as to determine the tenacity with which an individual intends to pursue a given behavior or goal. An intention that is strongly held is supposed to be pursued with more vigor and be more likely to lead to enactment. A fundamental issue for the sufficiency of each of these theories and for the prediction of health-related behavior must therefore be to consider how satisfactory *is* the theoretically causal relationship between intention and behavior.

How Strong Is the Relationship Between Intention and Behavior?

Many studies concerned with a wide range of behaviors have considered the relationship of intentions to behavior. It is important to note that many tests of the intention–behavior relation are available with respect to ecologically valid behaviors occurring in natural contexts, and many studies have used nonstudent samples (see Sears, 1986). If we as researchers are to evaluate (and improve on) the ability of intentions to determine behavior, it is important that we do so in social contexts in which possible obstacles to translating an intention into behavior are permitted to occur naturally, as they do in everyday life. Several meta-analytic reviews are available to assist in evaluating the size of the association between intention and behavior, some derived from literatures relating to specific behaviors, such as physical activity (Hagger, Chatzisarantis, & Biddle, 2002), condom use (Sheeran & Orbell, 1998), and health behaviors (Godin & Kok, 1996), or specific theories such as the theory of reasoned action (Sheppard et el., 1988), the theory of planned behavior (Armitage & Conner, 2001), or the protection-motivation theory (Milne et al., 2000). Sheeran (2002) provided an overview of meta-analytic evidence from studies relating to these different theories and behavior by performing a meta-analysis of 10 previously published meta-analyses, giving a total sample size of 82,107, and 422 hypothesis tests. His analysis shows that although correlations between intentions and behavior obtained in individual meta-analyses ranged from .40 to .82, the overall sample weighted average correlation was .53, a large effect according to Cohen's (1992) criteria. In regression terms, this implies that intentions account for 28% of the variance in behavior, on average, in longitudinal studies. This is particularly impressive given that the size of the relation is likely to be attenuated by the compatibility of scales used to measure intentions and behavior and by the reliability with which both intentions and behavior are assessed (Ajzen, 1991, 2002; Orbell, 2004; Sutton, 1998). In sum, evidence from longitudinal studies implies that the ability of the intention construct to predict behavior is good, and interventions to modify intention and its proximal determinants are highly likely to lead to behavior change.

Decomposition of the Relationship Between Intentions and Behavior

Notwithstanding the power of behavioral intentions to account for substantial variance in subsequent behavior, there are both theoretical and empirical grounds for supposing that not all people who intend to perform a given behavior will actually do so. In fact, the high positive correlations obtained between intention and behavior can tell us only that those who intend to act are more likely to act than those who do not intend to act. Although this is clearly reassuring for all motivational accounts of health-related behavior, in fact there are two possible sources of consistency and two possible sources of inconsistency between intention and behavior that cannot be readily discerned from correlational data (or from regression analyses; see McBroom & Reid, 1992; Orbell & Sheeran, 1998). If intention and behavior are cross-tabulated (see Table 8.1), it can be shown that consistency between intention and behavior will arise when those with positive intentions act or when those with negative intentions do not act. Conversely, inconsistency between intention and behavior will arise when those with positive intentions do not act or those with negative intentions do act. It is useful to recognize that this analysis applies to the direction of an intention, irrespective of whether the focal behavior is an *approach* behavior (e.g., "I intend to take my insulin" [positive] vs. "I do not intend to take my insulin" [negative]) or an *avoidance* behavior (e.g., "I intend to try not to eat snacks" [positive] vs. "I do not intend to try not to eat snacks" [negative]). In this latter instance, an individual who intends to avoid snacking and does so is classified as an *inclined actor* and an individual who does not intend to avoid snacking and does not do so is classified as a *disinclined abstainer*.

Orbell and Sheeran (1998) examined data from a study in which women's uptake of a cervical screening test, an objectively verifiable behavior, was predicted from their intentions 1 year previously (see the partition into the four discrete patterns of intention–behavior relationship illustrated in bold in Table 8.1: inclined actor, inclined abstainer, disinclined actor, and disinclined abstainer). By examining the data in this manner, it was

TABLE 8.1

Decomposition of Sources of Consistency Between Intentions and Behavior

Previous behavior	Subsequent behavior	Approach		Avoid	
		Positive intention	Negative intention	Positive intention	Negative intention
		I intend to exercise	*I do not intend to exercise*	*I intend not to smoke*	*I do not intend not to smoke*
Acts	Acts	Inclined actor *Continues to exercise*	Disinclined actor *Continues to exercise*	Inclined actor *Continues not to smoke*	Disinclined actor *Continues not to smoke*
Does not act	Acts	**Inclined actor** *Starts to exercise*	**Disinclined actor** *Starts to exercise*	Inclined actor *Stops smoking*	Disinclined actor *Stops smoking*
Acts	Does not act	Inclined abstainer *Stops exercising*	Disinclined abstainer *Stops exercising*	Inclined abstainer *Starts smoking*	Disinclined abstainer *Starts smoking*
Does not act	Does not act	**Inclined abstainer** *Continues not to exercise*	**Disinclined abstainer** *Continues not to exercise*	Inclined abstainer *Continues to smoke*	Disinclined abstainer *Continues to smoke*

Note. The four discrete patterns of intention–behavior relationship are illustrated in bold.

possible to reveal that the main source of consistency in intention–behavior relations is derived from the perhaps unremarkable ability of nonintenders not to act. People are, it would appear, very good at not doing what they do not intend to do. Some 88% of the disinclined acted consistently with their intention and were classified as disinclined abstainers, compared with only 12% classified as inconsistent disinclined actors. Intenders, however, were much less likely to carry out their intention to act. Just 43% of this group were screened during the year and were classified as inclined actors, whereas some 57% behaved in a way that was inconsistent with their intention and were classified as inclined abstainers.

Orbell and Sheeran's (1998) finding can be corroborated by evidence from other studies and data concerning different types of behavior. Table 8.2 illustrates the decomposition of inclined actors, disinclined abstainers, inclined abstainers, and disinclined actors for studies concerned with three classes of health-related behavior. Approach behaviors that are discrete acts require that an intender perform a focal behavior once, such as in the case of a single attendance at cancer screening (Sheeran & Orbell, 2000b; Sutton, Bickler, Sancho-Aldridge, & Saidi, 1994). Approach behaviors that involve repeated behaviors, such as regular physical activity (Orbell, 2000a) or consistent condom use (Gallois et al., 1992; Orbell, 2001; Stanton et al., 1996), require that intenders consistently perform the focal behavior over a period of time. The third class of behaviors is avoidance behaviors in which an intender must successfully resist performing a focal behavior consistently over a period of time (e.g., Orbell, 2000b). For each class of intention–behavior relationship, intenders were more likely to fail to act on their intentions (median number of inclined abstainers = 46%) than were nonintenders (median number of disinclined actors = 9.5%).

Although these observations do not represent a comprehensive review of all available evidence, findings to date provide reasonable evidence that the main source of inconsistency between intention and behavior and that which leaves most variance in behavior unaccounted for is derived from the tendency of people with positive intentions not to act on those intentions. Moreover, this relationship obtains whether one considers intentions to approach or avoid a focal behavior, whether one considers single behaviors or repeated behaviors, and whether one uses objectively verifiable or self-report measures of behavior.

Explanations for Inconsistency Between Intention and Behavior

Given the emphasis in models of health-related behavior on intention and its various determinants as predictors of behavior, an important issue for understanding intention–behavior inconsistency is to consider whether the variables contained in those models might be able to discriminate

TABLE 8.2
Percentages of Samples From Different Studies Behaving Consistently and Inconsistently With Their Intentions by Type of Behavioral Intention

Behavior type	Consistent		Inconsistent	
	Inclined actors	Disinclined abstainers	Inclined abstainers	Disinclined actors
Approach: Discrete				
Screening uptake (Orbell & Sheeran, 1998)	43	88	57	12
Screening uptake[a] (Sheeran & Orbell, 2000b)	70	97	30	3
Screening uptake[a] (Sutton et al., 1994)	74	65	26	35
Approach: Repeated				
Condom use (Orbell, 2001)	33	98	67	2
Condom use[a] (Gallois et al., 1992)	43	90	57	10
Condom use[a] (Stanton et al., 1994)	61	100	39	0
Exercise[a] (Sheeran & Orbell, 2001)	46	97	54	3
Sports club attendance (Orbell, 2000)	63	83	37	17
Avoidance: Repeated				
Not eating late night junk food (Orbell & Sheeran, 2002)	38	91	62	9

[a]Figures based on secondary analysis of data presented in Sheeran (2002).

between inclined actors and inclined abstainers. Orbell and Sheeran (1998) conducted just such a discriminant analysis using variables from protection-motivation theory. Although these variables were able to provide reasonable prediction of behavior for the sample as a whole and to discriminate the inclined from the disinclined, it was not possible to derive a significant discriminant function capable of distinguishing between inclined actors and inclined abstainers. Thus, it would appear that people with statistically equivalent motivation might nonetheless differ in their likelihood of performing a behavior.

The intention–behavior relationship has been the subject of previous conceptual analyses (e.g., Ajzen, 1991, 2001, 2002; Greve, 2001; Orbell, 2004; Sheeran, 2002), pointing in particular to the need to address properties of intentions that might affect their stability or the tenacity with which they are held. According to this perspective, equivalent intentions, assessed in terms of direction and intensity, may differ in other properties, and it is these properties that affect their relationship to behavior.

One obvious reason why people may not appear to enact their positive intentions is that they might modify their intentions in the time interval between assessing intention and behavior (Ajzen, 1985, 1991; Fishbein, 1980; Fishbein & Ajzen, 1975). There is both indirect and direct evidence for the stability hypothesis. Indirect tests based on comparisons of the strength of the intention–behavior correlation in which there is a short time interval between the two measures versus a long time interval show evidence of moderation for within-behavior comparisons (Sheeran & Orbell, 1998) but not for across-behavior comparisons (Randall & Wolff, 1994). Sheeran, Orbell, and Trafimow (1999) conducted a direct test in which intention stability was measured by computing within-participants' correlations between intention scores at two time points, prior to assessing behavior. Their findings showed that stable intentions were indeed better predictors of subsequent behavior than unstable intentions (cf. Ajzen, 2002; Conner & Norman, 2002; Conner, Sheeran, Norman, & Armitage, 2000). These findings, together with evidence for a moderating role of other variables (e.g., degree of intention formation, Bagozzi & Yi, 1989; Sheeran, Norman, & Orbell, 1999; anticipated regret, Parker, Manstead, & Stradling, 1995; Sheeran & Orbell, 1999a; self-schemas, Sheeran & Orbell, 2000a), which may themselves influence intention–behavior relations by their influence on temporal stability (Sheeran & Abraham, 2003), are persuasive. One might consider, however, whether instability ought, in practice, to be equally likely to occur among people with initially positive or negative intentions. If this were the case, we might generally expect to observe equivalent inconsistency between intention and behavior among people holding either positive or negative intentions, which we do not (Table 8.2).

Alternatively, it might even be suggested that the failure of people to turn their intentions into action be taken as indicative of the need to turn to alternative, nondeliberative, and nonconscious explanations of human action (e.g., Wegner & Wheatley, 1999). Perugini and Bagozzi (2004) estimated the size of effect that might be attributed to automatic processes (such as primes outside of conscious awareness) in classic experiments by Bargh, Chen, and Burrows (1996) and by Chen and Bargh (1999). On the basis of 11 manipulations, Perugini and Bagozzi estimated that automaticity might account for 12% of variance in behavior, clearly leaving substantial variance unaccounted for. Such automatic processes can certainly be demonstrated, even outside of the laboratory and with general population samples. For example, Orbell and Guinote (2005) showed that healthy older people attending two day centers (where they receive social contact, lunch, and recreation) could be induced to speed or slow their walking pace after being primed with a youthful or positive elderly prime, respectively. It is not clear, however, how enduring such effects might be.

Within a self-regulatory perspective, two lines of argument lead to the conclusion that further exploration of the intention–behavior relationship is worthwhile. As will be seen in the following sections of this chapter, there are reasons to believe that behaviors may originate as intentional acts and become automatic after satisfactory repetition (cf. Ajzen, 2002; Brandstätter, Lengfelder, & Gollwitzer, 2001). The ability of past behavior to predict behavior over and above behavioral intention has also been seen as indicative of a role for automatic, usually referred to as habitual, processes in predicting future actions. Although this issue remains open to further research (see Ajzen, 2002), it might be argued that even if past behavior effects were attributed to habit, this raises the important self-regulatory question of how people might overcome past behavioral tendencies and act according to their intentions (see Table 8.1; see also Orbell, Hodgkins, & Sheeran, 1997).

VOLITIONAL PROCESSES AND THE PROMOTION OF HEALTH BEHAVIORS

Having formed a behavioral intention, the actor may encounter a host of problems in actually translating the intention into action. For example, people may possess intentions that cannot be enacted immediately but have to await a suitable opportunity, they may procrastinate about getting started, they may possess other competing intentions that gain priority or exhaust their self-regulatory resources, or they may have difficulty sticking to a behavior that requires repeated performance or sustained effort and avoiding getting distracted by other goals en route (Kuhl, 1985). The identification of self-regulatory solutions to these difficulties represents an important step forward in explaining the intention–behavior relation.

An important contribution to understanding the intention–behavior relation in recent years is Gollwitzer's concept of an implementation intention (see Gollwitzer, 1993, 1999; Gollwitzer & Brandstätter, 1997; see also chap. 2, this volume). An *implementation intention* is a powerful self-regulatory strategy that takes the form "If I encounter situation X, then I will perform behavior Y." Implementation intentions should be distinguished from intentions to achieve certain outcomes or perform certain behaviors, which have been the focus of the chapter up to now. Whereas a goal intention of this sort simply reflects an individual's positive orientation toward the behavior or outcome and the intensity of that intention, an implementation intention is proposed to commit the individual to action initiation. This is because when an implementation intention is formed, a mental link is created between a future specific situation and the intended response. As a consequence of this mental link, suitable opportunities for initiating action are not missed or forgotten or overlooked because attention is directed elsewhere.

There is now considerable evidence from a number of behavioral domains that supplementing a positive intention with an implementation intention specifying where and when to initiate behavior can increase the likelihood that the intention will be translated into action (see Table 8.3). Evidence shows not only that behaviors are more likely to be performed but that they are likely to be performed sooner (e.g., Dholakia & Bagozzi, 2003), suggesting that behavior will be initiated at the first available opportunity or as soon as the contextual cue for action is encountered. Behaviors that may be perceived as costly or unpleasant to perform are also promoted by forming implementation intentions. For example, Orbell et al. (1997) showed that women were 4 times as likely to perform a breast self-examination if they supplemented their intention with an implementation intention. The powerful effects of implementation intentions are not restricted to discrete behavioral acts. Behaviors that have to be repeated, where frequent performance (e.g., dental hygiene; Orbell & Verplanken, 2003a) or not forgetting (e.g., taking a daily vitamin pill; Sheeran & Orbell, 1999b) is crucial, can also be established by forming an implementation intention. Forming an implementation intention to assist in the performance of a task can also protect self-control resources (Baumeister, Heatherton, & Tice, 1994), as evidenced by improved performance on a subsequent task while in a state of "ego depletion" (Webb & Sheeran, 2003). Implementation intentions have also been shown to facilitate action initiation among older adult samples, in which prospective memory (e.g., Guynn, McDaniel, & Einstein, 2001) may be particularly poor (Chasteen, Park, & Schwarz, 2001; Orbell & Sheeran, 2000), and among patients going through opiate withdrawal (Brandstätter et al., 2001). The effects of implementation intentions are dramatic, generalizable to a wide range of behaviors and populations, and have been well established using both self-report and objectively verifiable behaviors.

Given the success of implementation intentions, one might wonder if people actually possess the tendency to spontaneously self-regulate their behavior in this way. There is some evidence to suggest that they may. Orbell and Sheeran (2000) gave participants booklets in which they had to form their own implementation intentions on a weekly basis over a 12-week period. Rise, Thompson, and Verplanken (2003) developed a multi-item method for measuring implementation intentions in correlational

TABLE 8.3
Behavioral Impact of Forming an Implementation (IMP) Intention

Behavior type	Behavioral outcome among those forming IMP intentions	Behavioral outcome among those not forming IMP intentions
Discrete		
Write a report at Christmas (Gollwitzer & Brandstätter, 1997, Study 2)	70% completion	30% completion
Complete an assignment (Koole & Spijker, 2000)	Completed after 1.02 days	Completed after 2.90 days
Collect an assignment (Dholakia & Bagozzi, 2003, Study 1)	72% (low difficulty) 10% (high difficulty)	9.5% 0%
Check a Web site (Dholakia & Bagozzi, 2003, Study 2)	70% completion	33% completion
Collect a coupon (Aarts et al., 1999)	80% completion	50% completion
Perform breast self-exam (Orbell et al., 1997)	64% completion	14% completion
Resume functional activity after surgery (older adults) (Orbell & Sheeran, 2000)	18 out of 32 activities resumed faster than those without IMPs	—
Uptake cervical screening test (Sheeran & Orbell, 2000b)	92% uptake	69% uptake
Exercise (Milne et al., 2002)	91% completion	29% completion
Attend worksite fire training (Sheeran & Silverman, 2003)	39% attendance	12% attendance
Write a cv (opiate withdrawal patients) (Brandstätter et al., 2001, Study 1)	80% completion	0% completion
Write a cv (postwithdrawal patients) (Brandstätter et al., 2001, Study 1)	40% completion	0% completion
Exercise (Orbell & Verplanken, 2003a)	79% completion	54% completion

(continued)

TABLE 8.3 *(Continued)*

Behavior type	Behavioral outcome among those forming IMP intentions	Behavioral outcome among those not forming IMP intentions
Repeated		
Recycling drinking cartons (Rise et al., 2003)	IMPs r = .58 with behavior	—
Exercise (Rise et al., 2003)	IMPs r = .67 with behavior	—
Dental flossing daily Orbell & Verplanken, 2003b)	M = flossed 10 out of 14 days	M = flossed 4 out of 14 days
Take a daily vitamin pill (Sheeran & Orbell, 1999b, Study 1)	1.57 out of 21 days missed	3.53 out of 21 days missed
Take a daily vitamin pill (Sheeran & Orbell, 1999b, Study 2)	.90/21 days missed 26% missed a pill	2.50 out of 21 days missed 61% missed a pill
Writing date on 6 test material sheets of paper (older adults) (Chasteen et al., 2001)	M = .57 out of 6.0 sheets dated	M = .22 out of 6.0 sheets dated

research and showed that the measure predicted significant variance in behavior independent of goal intention. Webb and Sheeran (2003) conducted a retrospective questionnaire study in which self-reported implementation intentions were shown to discriminate between those who completed versus did not complete their goals. People appear to be most likely to form an implementation intention when they expect that completion of the task will be difficult (Bargh & Gollwitzer, 1994), thus forming an implementation intention may be viewed as a willful step to urge oneself on.

Implementation intentions are proposed to supplement the effects of goal intentions on behavioral performance. Important for the analysis of inclined abstainers, most studies have sought to demonstrate that participants possess positive intentions before being asked to form an implementation intention (e.g., Brandstätter et al., 2001). These studies show that among people *equally motivated to act*, in terms of their goal intention, forming an implementation intention regarding when and where to initiate action significantly increases goal completion (e.g., Orbell et al., 1997; Sheeran & Orbell, 1999b). Three studies that investigated the combined effects of a motivational intervention based on protection-motivation theory with an implementation intention intervention (Dholakia & Bagozzi, 2003; Milne, Orbell, & Sheeran, 2002; Milne & Sheeran, 2001) each showed that motivation was necessary but not sufficient for action initiation. Orbell et al. (1997) and Sheeran and Orbell (1999b) additionally examined the possibility that implementation intentions might alter or specifically increase commitment to goal intentions. In both studies, intention was unaltered by the formation of an implementation intention, indicating that the process by which implementation intentions led to behavioral enactment can be attributed to postdeliberative processes affecting the translation of an intention into action.

Given that implementation intentions do not operate by modifying traditional motivational or deliberative variables (e.g., by modifying intentions), how do they exert their effects? Gollwitzer (1993, 1999; Gollwitzer & Sheeran, 2006) proposed that the critical feature of implementation intentions is the linking of action to a specified context in memory. When the context is encountered, action is proposed to follow (a) immediately; (b) efficiently, that is, without requiring much cognitive processing capacity; and (c) without conscious intent. Put another way, implementation intentions delegate control of behavior to the environment. Various forms of evidence speak to these proposed mechanisms. Orbell et al. (1997), for example, showed that all but one person in their study reported enacting breast self-examination in the time and place specified in their implementation intentions 1 month previously. Although these findings suggest that people are able to detect situations specified in their implementation intentions, they do not speak directly to speed in detecting those contexts, or to speed of action initiation, once those contexts are detected. Gollwitzer and Brandstätter (1997, Study 3) demonstrated that participants who formed implementation intentions regarding suitable opportunities to present counterarguments in a debate were faster to seize opportunities to express themselves when those opportunities arose than were participants who only identified suitable opportunities. Webb and Sheeran (2004) also demonstrated that enhanced cue detection did not occur at the expense of distraction from other nonrelevant or ambiguous stimuli. Similarly, Aarts and Dijksterhuis (2000) showed that people who formed implementation intentions regarding travel mode choices were faster to respond with choices specified in their implementation intentions when presented with computer-generated cues regarding journeys they might make. Aarts, Dijksterhuis, and Midden (1999) further showed that the heightened accessibility of environmental cues specified in an implementation intention to collect a coupon on the way to the cafeteria mediated the likelihood of actually collecting that coupon. Thus, supplementing an intention with an implementation intention ensures that situations for enactment are rapidly detected and acted on, even in the chaos of everyday life, as in students heading for the cafeteria or participants in Orbell et al.'s (1997) study going about their daily routines.

In fact, many of the experiments previously described have been conducted in ecologically valid environments where goal intentions under investigation might be considered to be competing with other cognitive activities (e.g., Milne et al., 2002; Sheeran & Orbell, 1999b, 2000b). This does not, however, constitute hard evidence that implementation intentions operate efficiently and require limited processing capacity. Brandstätter et al. (2001) provided just such evidence by examining the effects of forming implementation intentions under conditions of high cognitive load. Two studies showed that patients with schizophrenia (Study 2) and students under cognitive load generated by a dual task (Studies 3 and 4) were faster to respond in a go/no-go computerized task than those who had not formed implementation intentions. Thus, implementation intentions produced behavior in an efficient manner. In fact, it is intriguing to note from Brandstätter et al.'s findings that the effects appeared to be enhanced by higher cognitive load, suggesting that the willful act of forming an implementation intention can ensure action initiation especially when a person has a great many competing intentions. Bayer, Moskowitz, and Gollwitzer (2002) have extended this finding to show that a behavior specified in an implementation intention was enacted faster in response to a subliminal cue. This recent evidence suggests that having formed a goal intention and supplemented it by an implementation intention, the initiation of behavior does not require further conscious intent.

Evidence to date provides strong support for the notion that implementation intentions operate by delegating control to the environment (Gollwitzer, 1993, 1999). Evidence that the situational context specified in an implementation intention is capable of producing responses (a) immediately, (b) efficiently, and (c) outside of conscious awareness constitute three critical features of automatic responding (e.g., Bargh, 1994, 1996, 1997). This is an intriguing possibility, indicating that the deliberative processes, which might lead to development of a goal intention, can, by virtue of being supplemented by the willful act of forming an implementation intention, ultimately produce responses that may be characterized as automatic. In terms of understanding the establishment of novel behaviors, this implies that implementation intentions are a simple and willful means of creating habits. Habits also possess the characteristics of automaticity (Aarts & Dijksterhuis, 2000; Wood, Quinn, & Kashy, 2002) but, crucially, are developed as a result of repeated behavioral responses to a particular environmental cue rather than as a result of a conscious mental act of forming an implementation intention (Verplanken & Aarts, 1999). In practical terms, this analysis implies that "good" habits might be created rather quickly if implementation intentions were used in intervention studies.

Verplanken and Orbell (2003) developed a self-report habit index (SRHI), which provides a measure of metasubjective awareness of automaticity in behavioral responding (see Verplanken, Myrbakk, & Rudi, 2005). The measure is not intended to capture automaticity as it occurs but captures people's awareness that they do something, or have done something, automatically, perhaps without realizing they were doing it. Because this measure provides an assessment of *quality* of behavioral responses, it may have particular value in research in which memory for *frequency* of behavior is unreliable, but people are able to characterize their behavior, using this measure, as occurring automatically. Orbell and Verplanken (2003a, 2003b) showed that an implementation intention manipulation produces rapid increases in scores on the SRHI in two health behavioral domains: exercise and dental flossing. Moreover, Orbell and Verplanken (2003b) demonstrated that forming an implementation intention was capable of attenuating the impact of premanipulation (previous) habit on subsequent behavior in regression analyses. These findings point to the validity of the measure in that it is sensitive to a manipulation (i.e., formation of an implementation intention), which has been independently demonstrated to create automatic responses. Further work with this measure might contribute to research seeking to make or break habits in health behavior and to distinguish between those with past behavioral experience who enact an intention to change their behavior and those who do not (see Table 8.1).

SELF-REGULATION AND PURSUIT OF COMPLEX GOALS

Thus far, we have been primarily concerned with the pursuit of relatively simple goal intentions referring to specific behavioral responses (e.g., "I intend to perform breast self-examination" or "I intend to floss my teeth"). However, in considering the tasks of self-regulation, it is useful to distinguish other forms of goal intention (cf. Bagozzi, 1992; Bagozzi & Dholakia, 1999). The general conceptualization ("I intend to do Z") may also apply to the achievement of more complex behavioral goals in which a number of behavioral steps are required to reach the intended behavior (e.g., "I intend to control my blood sugar," "I intend to stop snacking," or "I intend to give up smoking") or to the outcomes of behaviors (e.g., "I intend to get fit" or "I intend to lose weight"). These more complex goal intentions require attention to (a) the identification of instrumental acts that might lead to goal achievement and (b) the self-regulatory skills that might contribute to those acts being successfully initiated and maintained. The formation of a goal intention to achieve a complex goal or to achieve an outcome may initiate a search for means (i.e., implemental mindsets; Gollwitzer, Heckhausen, & Steller 1990; Taylor & Gollwitzer, 1995) or the formation of plans as to what instrumental acts are needed to pursue a goal. The extent to which these activities lead to goal attainment will depend, however, on the selection of appropriate (effective) instrumental acts and the successful execution of those acts.

In an investigation of the role of implementation intentions in pursuit of a complex behavioral goal, Sheeran and Orbell (2000b) theorized that the goal intention to get a cervical screening test would be achieved by performing the instrumental act of telephoning to make an appointment ("I intend to do Y in order to achieve behavioral goal Z"). Participants in that study were asked to form implementation intentions regarding when and where they would make an appointment to have a screening test ("If I encounter situation X, I will do Y, in order to achieve behavioral goal Z"). In that study, implementation intentions were highly successful in both ensuring that the instrumental act was performed and, consequently, that participants underwent a cervical screening test. Although appropriate means to an end may be readily apparent in some instances, the identification of instrumental acts and the execution of those acts may be less clear. The plethora of pamphlets and publications relating to how to give up smoking or how to lose weight attests to this possibility. Orbell and Sheeran (2002; cf. Schaal & Gollwitzer, 1999, cited in Gollwitzer, 1999) investigated people's knowledge of possible instrumental acts that might contribute to avoiding eating snacks. Although people were able to suggest three distinct strategies that they might use to achieve this goal, subsequent studies showed that only one type of strategy concerned with maintaining attentional focus away from snacking was actually effective in reducing snack consumption. When people formed an implementation intention to enact this strategy, they not only were more likely to use the strategy, and presumably did so in an automatic manner, but also were more likely to achieve the goal of reducing snack consumption.

Some goal intentions may be difficult to achieve, not only because of the difficulty in initiating a behavioral intention or an intention to pursue an instrumental act but also because it may be difficult to stick with a behavior requiring concentration, deal with setbacks, or resume activity following an interruption. These capacities are the focus of Kuhl's (1996, 2000; Kuhl & Kazen, 1994) personality systems interactions theory. Kuhl suggested that an individual may possess positive intentions to enact a goal but lack the necessary volitional abilities to actually perform that behavior. Personality systems interactions theory describes the complex interplay of conscious and nonconscious processes (e.g., emotions, attention, arousal, cognitive processing), which comprise two distinct types of volitional efficiency: *goal maintenance*, which is achieved by mechanisms of self-control, and *self-maintenance*, which is achieved by mechanisms of self-regulation.

Self-control was originally referred to as *action control* in the theory of action control (Kuhl, 1981, 1984, 1985, 1992) and functionally supports the maintenance and enactment of conscious goals and intentions in an explicit memory structure. Self-control is akin to common notions of will-power and essentially refers to conscious processes such as planning that inhibit other cognitive and emotional processes to protect an ongoing intention from competing alternatives. Because processes related to the self are suppressed when operating in this mode (self-control: "control of self"), self-control can permit an individual to pursue goals that may not be self-chosen or that have been assigned by others.

Unlike action-control theory, personality systems interactions theory postulates a second mode of volition referred to as self-regulation. Self-regulation (self as agent) maintains actions in line with the needs, values, and beliefs of the self. When operating in this volitional mode, self-generated actions and goals are protected and maintained by means of largely unconscious processes that integrate as many cognitive and emotional subsystems as possible for the support of a chosen action. Because the self-regulation mode relies on access to the self-system, an individual operating in this mode will have access to self-motivational and cognitive resources for finding new solutions and will be able to identify and reject self-alien unwanted thoughts or social demands set by others that might otherwise interfere with goal-directed activity. Whereas self-control is facilitated by negative mood, self-regulation is facilitated by positive mood.

An exciting development in recent years has been the availability of scales to assess the various functional volitional components proposed by personality systems interactions theory (Kuhl & Fuhrmann, 1998). The Volitional Competence Inventory (VCI) assesses subjective concomitants of the various functions of self-control and self-regulation under conditions that require the person to overcome difficulties of enactment, such as competing motivations, strong habitual tendencies, and over- or underarousal. Scales assessing self-regulation include attention control, implicit attention control, motivation control, emotion control, self-determination, and decision control, whereas self-control competencies include intention control, planning, initiating, impulse control, and failure control.

Orbell (2003) examined the ability of volitional competence as assessed by the VCI to enhance prediction of a challenging behavior after taking account of intensity of intention and prior variables. When faced with a challenging task such as studying, a person who can activate the self-system by using self-regulation is hypothesized to experience positive mood, which in turn enhances access to memory and causes an increase in motivational energy for strengthening commitment to self-compatible goals, so that he or she can stay focused on the self-chosen activity and avoid unwanted self-alien thoughts (Kuhl, 2000). Consistent with theory, participants with high scores on scales assessing these competencies—conscious attention control, implicit attention control, and self-determination—were more likely to translate their intentions into action. Moreover, participants with low subjective norms (which might be interpreted as low social encouragement for studying or self-alien demands) were able to perform at least as well as those with high subjective norm if they used self-regulation. This study suggests that social influences may play a part in the postintentional phase of persisting at a behavioral goal, rather than simply in the formation of a behavioral intention. Moreover, the study demonstrates that the activation of important self-regulatory competencies may overcome deficits in social normative support in a given goal pursuit situation. Future research might usefully examine other effects of volitional competence posed by this intriguing theory on the successful completion of health-related behavioral goals.

CONCLUDING COMMENTS

A good deal of progress has been made in understanding motivational and volitional determinants of health-related actions. Although behavioral and outcome goals may be prescribed by medical and epidemiological evidence, the task of turning those goals into behavioral reality is an important one for psychology. There have been relatively few attempts to integrate or compare different accounts of self-regulation or motivation (e.g., Bagozzi & Kimmel, 1995; Orbell et al., in press; Weinstein, 1993), and evidence presented in this chapter suggests that there may be scope for further parsimony in a model integrating some of the important determinants of health-related intentions. Moreover, self-regulatory mechanisms that address some of the fundamental obstacles to achieving behavioral goals require further attention. Evidence presented here suggests that intentions and their determinants, implementation intentions, methods of focusing attention on the goal or away from distractions, social influences, and self-regulatory volitional competencies may all be important in achieving health behavioral goals.

REFERENCES

Aarts, H., & Dijksterhuis, A. (2000). Habits as knowledge structures: Automaticity in goal-directed behaviors. *Journal of Personality and Social Psychology, 78,* 53–63.

Aarts, H., Dijksterhuis, A., & Midden, C. (1999). To plan or not to plan? Goal achievement or interrupting the performance of mundane behaviors. *European Journal of Social Psychology, 29,* 971–979.

Abraham, C. S., Sheeran, P., Abrams, D., & Spears, R. (1994). Exploring teenagers' adaptive and maladaptive thinking in relation to the threat of HIV infection. *Psychology and Health, 9,* 253–272.

Ajzen, I. (1985). From intentions to actions: A theory of planned behavior. In J. Kuhl & J. Beckmann (Eds.), *Action control: From cognition to behavior* (pp. 11–39). Berlin: Springer-Verlag.

Ajzen, I. (1991). The theory of planned behavior. *Organizational Behavior and Human Decision Processes, 50,* 179–211.

Ajzen, I. (2001). Nature and operation of attitudes. *Annual Review of Psychology, 52,* 27–58.

Ajzen, I. (2002). Residual effects of past on later behavior: Habituation and reasoned action perspectives. *Personality and Social Psychology Review, 6,* 107–122.

Ajzen, I., & Fishbein, M. (1973). Attitudinal and normative variables as predictors of specific behaviors. *Journal of Personality and Social Psychology, 27,* 41–57.

Ajzen, I., & Fishbein, M. (1974). Factors influencing intentions and the intention–behavior relation. *Human Relations, 27,* 1–15.

Armitage, C. J., & Conner, M. (2001). Efficacy of the theory of planned behavior: A meta-analytic review. *British Journal of Social Psychology, 40,* 471–499.

Bagozzi, R. P. (1992). The self-regulation of attitudes, intentions and behavior. *Social Psychology Quarterly, 55,* 178–204.

Bagozzi, R. P., & Dholakia, U. (1999). Goal setting and goal striving in consumer behavior. *Journal of Marketing, 63,* 19–32.

Bagozzi, R. P., & Kimmel, S. K. (1995). A comparison of leading theories for the prediction of goal-directed behaviours. *British Journal of Social Psychology, 34,* 437–461.

Bagozzi, R. P., & Yi, Y. (1989). The degree of intention formation as a moderator of the attitude–behavior relationship. *Social Psychology Quarterly, 52,* 266–279.

Bandura, A. (1977). Self-efficacy: Toward a unifying theory of behavioral change. *Psychological Review, 84,* 191–215.

Bargh, J. A. (1994). The four horsemen of automaticity: Awareness, intention, efficiency and control in social cognition. In R. S. Wyer Jr. & T. K. Srull (Eds.), *Handbook of social cognition* (2nd ed., pp. 1–40). Hillsdale, NJ: Erlbaum.

Bargh, J. A. (1996). Principles of automaticity. In E. T. Higgins & A. Kruglanski (Eds.), *Social psychology: Handbook of basic principles* (pp. 169–183). New York: Guilford Press.

Bargh, J. A. (1997). The automaticity of everyday life. In R. S. Wyer Jr. (Ed.), *The automaticity of everyday life: Advances in social cognition* (Vol. 10, pp. 1–61). Mahwah, NJ: Erlbaum.

Bargh, J. A., Chen, M., & Burrows, L. (1996). Automaticity of social behavior: Direct effects of trait construct and stereotype activation on action. *Journal of Personality and Social Psychology, 71,* 230–244.

Bargh, J. A., & Gollwitzer, P. M. (1994). Environmental control of goal-directed action: Automatic and strategic contingencies between situations and behavior. In J. A. Bargh & P. M. Gollwitzer (Eds.), *Nebraska symposium on motivation: Integrative views of motivation, cognition and emotion* (pp. 71–124). Lincoln: University of Nebraska Press.

Baumeister, R. F., Heatherton, T. F., & Tice, D. M. (1994). *Losing control: How and why people fail at self-regulation.* London: Academic Press.

Bayer, U. C., Moskowitz, G. B., & Gollwitzer, P. M. (2002). *Implementation intentions and action initiation without conscious intent.* Unpublished manuscript.

Boer, H., & Seydel, E. R. (1996). Protection motivation theory. In M. Conner & P. Norman (Eds.), *Predicting health behaviour: Research and practice with social cognition models* (pp. 95–120). Buckingham, England: Open University Press.

Brandstätter, V., Lengfelder, A., & Gollwitzer, P. M. (2001). Implementation intentions and efficient action initiation. *Journal of Personality and Social Psychology, 81,* 946–960.

Chasteen, A. L., Park, D. C., & Schwarz, N. (2001). Implementation intentions and facilitation of prospective memory. *Psychological Science, 12,* 457–461.

Chen, M., & Bargh, J. A. (1999). Consequences of automatic evaluation: Immediate behavioral predispositions to approach or avoid the stimulus. *Personality and Social Psychology Bulletin, 25,* 215–224.

Cohen, J. (1992). A power primer. *Psychological Bulletin, 112,* 155–159.

Conner, M., & Norman, P. (2002). The theory of planned behaviour and dietary change. *Health Psychology, 21,* 194–201.

Conner, M., Sheeran, P., Norman, P., & Armitage, C. J. (2000). Temporal stability as a moderator of relationships in the theory of planned behavior. *British Journal of Social Psychology, 39,* 469–494.

Conner, M., Sherlock, K., & Orbell, S. (1998). Psychosocial determinants of ecstasy use in young people in the UK. *British Journal of Health Psychology, 3,* 295–317.

Dholakia, U. M., & Bagozzi, R. P. (2003). As time goes by: How implementation intentions influence enactment of short-fuse behaviors. *Journal of Applied Social Psychology, 33,* 889–922.

Fishbein, M. (1980). A theory of reasoned action: Some applications and implications. In H. Howe & M. Page (Eds.), *Nebraska symposium on motivation* (Vol. 27, pp. 65–116). Lincoln: University of Nebraska Press.

Fishbein, M., & Ajzen, I. (1975). *Belief, attitude, intention and behavior: An introduction to theory and research.* Reading, MA: Addison-Wesley.

Flynn, M. F., Lyman, R. D., & Prentice-Dunn, S. (1995). Protection motivation theory and adherence to medical treatment regimens for muscular dystrophy. *Journal of Social and Clinical Psychology, 14,* 61–75.

Gallois, C., Kashima, Y., Terry, D., McCamish, M., Timmins, P., & Chauvin, A. (1992). Safe and unsafe sexual intentions and behavior: The effects of norms and attitudes. *Journal of Applied Social Psychology, 22,* 1521–1545.

Godin, G., & Kok, G. (1996). The theory of planned behavior: A review of its applications to health-related behaviors. *American Journal of Health Promotion, 11,* 97–98.

Gollwitzer, P. M. (1993). Goal achievement: The role of intentions. *European Review of Social Psychology, 4,* 141–185.

Gollwitzer, P. M. (1999). Implementation intentions: Strong effects of simple plans. *American Psychologist, 54,* 493–503.

Gollwitzer, P. M., & Brandstätter, V. (1997). Implementation intentions and effective goal pursuit. *Journal of Personality and Social Psychology, 73,* 186–199.

Gollwitzer, P. M., Heckhausen, H., & Steller, B. (1990). Deliberative and implemental mindsets: Cognitive tuning toward congruous thoughts and information. *Journal of Personality and Social Psychology, 59,* 1119–1127.

Gollwitzer, P. M., & Sheeran, P. (2006). Implementation intentions and goal achievement: A meta-analysis of effects and processes. *Advances in Experimental Social Psychology, 38,* 69–119.

Greve, W. (2001). Traps and gaps in action explanation: Theoretical problems of a psychology of human action. *Psychological Review, 108,* 435–451.

Guynn, M. J., McDaniel, M., & Einstein, G. O. (2001). Remembering to perform actions: A different type of memory? In H. Zimmer & R. Cohen (Eds.), *Memory for action: A distinct form of episodic memory?* (pp. 25–48). Oxford, England: Oxford University Press.

Hagger, M. S., Chatzisarantis, N. L. D., & Biddle, S. J. H. (2002). A meta-analytic review of the theories of reasoned action and planned behavior in physical activity: Predictive validity and the contribution of additional variables. *Journal of Sport and Exercise Psychology, 24,* 3–32.

Hagger, M. S., Chatzisarantis, N. L. D., Biddle, S. J. H., & Orbell, S. (2001). Antecedents of children's physical activity intentions and behavior: Predictive validity and longitudinal effects. *Psychology and Health, 16,* 391–407.

Hagger, M. S., & Orbell, S. (2003). A meta-analytic review of the common-sense model of illness representations. *Psychology and Health 18,* 141–184.

Hampson, S., Glasgow, R. E., & Stryker, L. A. (2000). Beliefs versus feelings: A comparison of personal models and depression for predicting multiple outcomes in diabetes. *British Journal of Health Psychology, 5,* 27–40.

Hampson, S., Glasgow, R. E., & Toobert, D. J. (1990). Personal models of diabetes and their relations to self-care activities. *Health Psychology, 9,* 632–646.

Hardeman, W., Johnston, M., Johnston, D., Bonetti, D., Wareham, N. J., & Kinmonth, A. L. (2002). Application of the theory of planned behaviour in behaviour change interventions: A systematic review. *Psychology and Health, 17,* 123–158.

Heijmans, M. (1998). Coping and adaptive outcome in chronic fatigue syndrome: Importance of illness cognitions. *Journal of Psychosomatic Research, 45,* 39–51.

Hodgkins, S., & Orbell, S. (1998). Does protection-motivation theory predict behavior? A longitudinal test and exploration of the role of previous behavior. *Psychology and Health, 13,* 237–250.

Koole, S., & Spijker, M. (2000). Overcoming the planning fallacy through willpower: Effects of implementation intentions on actual and predicted task-completion times. *European Journal of Social Psychology, 30,* 873–888.

Kuhl, J. (1981). Motivational and functional helplessness: The moderating effect of state versus action orientation. *Journal of Personality and Social Psychology, 40,* 155–170.

Kuhl, J. (1984). Volitional aspects of achievement motivation and learned helplessness: Toward a comprehensive theory of action control. In B. A. Maher (Ed.), *Progress in experimental personality research* (Vol. 13, pp. 99–171). New York: Academic Press.

Kuhl, J. (1985). Volitional mediators of cognition–behavior consistency: Self-regulatory processes and action control. In J. Kuhl & J. Beckmann (Eds.), *Action control: From cognition to behavior* (pp. 101–128). Berlin: Springer-Verlag.

Kuhl, J. (1992). A theory of self-regulation: Action versus state orientation, self-discrimination and some applications. *Applied Psychology: An International Review, 41,* 97–129.

Kuhl, J. (1996). Who controls whom when "I control myself"? *Psychological Inquiry, 7,* 61–68.

Kuhl, J. (2000). A functional-design approach to motivation and self-regulation: The dynamics of personality systems interactions. In M. Boekaerts, P. R. Pintrich, & M. Zeidner (Eds.), *Self-regulation: Directions and challenges for future research* (pp. 111–169). San Diego, CA: Academic Press.

Kuhl, J., & Fuhrmann, A. (1998). Decomposing self-regulation and self-control: The volitional components checklist. In J. Heckhausen & C. Dweck (Eds.), *Life span perspectives on motivation and control* (pp. 15–49). Mahwah, NJ: Erlbaum.

Kuhl, J., & Kazen, M. (1994). Self-discrimination and memory: State orientation and false self-ascription of assigned activities. *Journal of Personality and Social Psychology, 66,* 1103–1115.

Lau, R. R., Bernard, T. M., & Hartman, K. A. (1989). Further explorations of common-sense representations of common illnesses. *Health Psychology, 8,* 195–219.

Leventhal, H., Meyer, D., & Nerenz, D. (1980). The common sense model of illness danger. In S. Rachman (Ed.), *Medical psychology* (Vol. 2, pp. 7–30). New York: Pergamon Press.

Linz, D., Penrod, S., & Leventhal, H. (1982, July). *Cognitive organisation of disease among laypersons.* Paper presented at the 20th International Congress of Applied Psychology, Edinburgh, Scotland.

Maddux, J. E., & Rogers, R. W. (1983). Protection motivation theory and self-efficacy: A revised theory of fear appeals and attitude change. *Journal of Experimental Social Psychology, 19,* 242–253.

McBroom, W. H., & Reid, F. W. (1992). Towards a reconceptualization of attitude–behavior consistency. *Social Psychology Quarterly, 55,* 205–216.

Meyer, D., Leventhal, H., & Gutmann, M. (1985). Common-sense models of illness: The example of hypertension. *Health Psychology, 4,* 115–135.

Milne, S. E., Orbell, S., & Sheeran, P. (2002). Combining motivational and volitional interventions to promote exercise participation: Protection-motivation theory and implementation intentions. *British Journal of Health Psychology, 7,* 163–184.

Milne, S. E., & Sheeran, P. (2001, September). *Testing interaction effects in implementation intentions.* Paper presented at the annual conference of the Division of Health Psychology of the British Psychological Society, St Andrews, Scotland.

Milne, S., Sheeran, P., & Orbell, S. (2000). Prediction and intervention in health-related behavior: A meta-analytic review of protection-motivation theory. *Journal of Applied Social Psychology, 30,* 106–143.

Orbell, S. (1996). Informal care in social context: A social psychological analysis of participation, impact and intervention in care of the elderly. *Psychology and Health, 11,* 155–178.

Orbell, S. (2000a). [Acquiring a novel behavior: Development of attitudes and intentions during the establishment of a regular behavior]. Unpublished raw data.

Orbell, S. (2000b). [The theory of planned behavior and behavior change]. Unpublished raw data.

Orbell, S. (2001). [Attitudes, intentions and consideration of future consequences as determinants of consistent condom use]. Unpublished raw data, University of Essex, England.

Orbell, S. (2003). Personality systems interactions theory and the theory of planned behavior: Evidence that self-regulatory volitional components enhance enactment of studying behavior. *British Journal of Social Psychology, 42,* 95–112.

Orbell, S. (2004). Intention–behavior relations: A self-regulation perspective. In G. Haddock & G. R. Maio (Eds.), *Contemporary perspectives on the psychology of attitudes* (pp. 145–168). London: Psychology Press.

Orbell, S., Blair, C., Sherlock, K., & Conner, M. (2001). The theory of planned behavior and ecstasy use: Roles for habit and perceived control over taking versus obtaining substances. *Journal of Applied Social Psychology, 31,* 31–47.

Orbell, S., & Guinote, A. (2005). *Priming activity in older people.* Manuscript submitted for publication.

Orbell, S., & Hagger, M. (2006). Temporal framing and the decision to take part in Type 2 diabetes screening: Effects of individual differences in consideration of future consequences. *Health Psychology, 25,* 537–548.

Orbell, S., Hagger, M., Brown, V., & Tidy, J. (in press). Comparing two theories of health behaviour: A prospective study of non-follow-up after abnormal cervical screening results. *Health Psychology.*

Orbell, S., Hodgkins, S., & Sheeran, P. (1997). Implementation intentions and the theory of planned behavior. *Personality and Social Psychology Bulletin, 23,* 953–962.

Orbell, S., Johnston, M., Rowley, D., Espley, A., & Davey, P. (1998). Cognitive representations of illness and functional and affective adjustment following surgery for osteoarthritis. *Social Science and Medicine, 47,* 93–102.

Orbell, S., Perugini, M., & Rakow, T. (2004). Individual differences in sensitivity to health communications: Consideration of future consequences. *Health Psychology, 23,* 388–396.

Orbell, S., & Sheeran, P. (1998). "Inclined abstainers": A problem for predicting health behavior. *British Journal of Social Psychology, 37,* 151–166.

Orbell, S., & Sheeran, P. (2000). Motivational and volitional processes in action initiation: A field study of implementation intentions. *Journal of Applied Social Psychology, 30,* 780–797.

Orbell, S., & Sheeran, P. (2002). *Implementation intentions and complex goals.* Manuscript in preparation.

Orbell, S., & Verplanken, B. (2003a). *Implementation intentions and the creation of a healthy habit.* Manuscript in preparation.

Orbell, S., & Verplanken, B. (2003b). *Implementation intentions and the SRHI.* Manuscript in preparation.

Parker, D. (1997, April). *The relationship between speeding attitudes and speeding behavior.* Paper presented to the Department of Transport at the Behavioural Studies Seminar, Esher, England.

Parker, D., Manstead, A. S. R., & Stradling, S. G. (1995). Extending the theory of planned behavior: The role of personal norm. *British Journal of Social Psychology, 34,* 127–137.

Perugini, M., & Bagozzi, R. P. (2001). The role of desires and anticipated emotions in goal-directed behaviors: Broadening and deepening the theory of planned behavior. *British Journal of Social Psychology, 40,* 79–98.

Perugini, M., & Bagozzi, R. P. (2004). An alternative view of pre-volitional processes in decision-making: Conceptual issues and empirical evidence. In G. R. Maio & G. Haddock (Eds.), *Contemporary perspectives on the psychology of attitudes* (pp. 169–201). Hove, England: Psychology Press.

Petrie, K. J., Weinman, J., Sharpe, N., & Buckley, J. (1996). Role of patients' view of their illness in predicting return to work and functioning after myocardial infarction: Longitudinal study. *British Medical Journal, 312,* 1191–1194.

Randall, D. M., & Wolff, J. A. (1994). The time interval in the intention–behavior relationship: Meta-analysis. *British Journal of Social Psychology, 33,* 405–418.

Rapaport, P., & Orbell, S. (2000). Augmenting the theory of planned behaviour: Motivation to provide practical assistance and emotional support to parents. *Psychology and Health, 15,* 309–324.

Rise, J., Thompson, M., & Verplanken, B. (2003). Measuring implementation intentions in the context of the theory of planned behavior. *Scandinavian Journal of Psychology, 44,* 87–95.

Rogers, R. W. (1975). A protection motivation theory of fear appeals and attitude change. *Journal of Psychology, 91,* 93–114.

Rogers, R. W. (1983). Cognitive and physiological processes in fear appeals and attitude change: A revised theory of protection motivation. In B. L. Cacioppo

& L. L. Petty (Eds.), *Social psychophysiology: A source book* (pp. 153–176). London: Guilford Press.

Rutter, D. R. (2000). Attendance and reattendance for breast cancer screening: A prospective 3-year test of the theory of planned behaviour. *British Journal of Health Psychology, 5,* 1–13.

Rutter, D. R., & Quine, L. (2002). *Changing health behaviour.* Buckingham: Open University Press.

Sears, D. O. (1986). College sophomores in the laboratory: Influences of a narrow data base on social psychology's view of human nature. *Journal of Personality and Social Psychology, 51,* 515–530.

Schiaffino, K. M., Shawaryn, M. A., & Blum, D. (1998). Examining the impact of illness representations on psychological adjustment to chronic illness. *Health Psychology, 17,* 262–268.

Sheeran, P. (2002). Intention–behavior relations: A conceptual and empirical review. In M. Hewstone & W. Stroebe (Eds.), *European review of social psychology* (Vol. 12, pp. 1–36). Chichester, England: Wiley.

Sheeran, P., & Abraham, C. (2003). Mediator of moderators: Temporal stability of intention and the intention–behavior relation. *Personality and Social Psychology Bulletin, 29,* 205–215.

Sheeran, P., Norman, P., & Orbell, S. (1999). Evidence that intentions based on attitudes better predict behavior than intentions based on subjective norms. *European Journal of Social Psychology, 29,* 403–406.

Sheeran, P., & Orbell, S. (1996). How confidently can we infer health beliefs from questionnaire responses? *Psychology and Health, 11,* 273–290.

Sheeran, P., & Orbell, S. (1998). Does intention predict condom use? A meta analysis and test of four moderators. *British Journal of Social Psychology 37,* 231–250.

Sheeran, P., & Orbell, S. (1999a). Augmenting the theory of planned behavior: Roles for anticipated regret and descriptive norms. *Journal of Applied Social Psychology, 29,* 2107–2142.

Sheeran, P., & Orbell, S. (1999b). Implementation intentions and repeated behaviors: Enhancing the predictive validity of the theory of planned behavior. *European Journal of Social Psychology, 29,* 349–369.

Sheeran, P., & Orbell, S. (2000a). Self-schemas and the theory of planned behavior. *European Journal of Social Psychology, 30,* 533–550.

Sheeran, P., & Orbell, S. (2000b). Using implementation intentions to increase attendance for cervical cancer screening. *Health Psychology, 19,* 283–289.

Sheeran, P., Orbell, S., & Trafimow, D. (1999). Does the temporal stability of behavioral intentions moderate intention–behavior and past behavior–future behavior relations? *Personality and Social Psychology Bulletin, 25,* 721–730.

Sheeran, P., & Silverman, M. (2003). Evaluation of three interventions to promote workplace health and safety: Evidence for the utility of implementation intentions. *Social Science and Medicine, 56,* 2153–2163.

Sheppard, B. H., Hartwick, J., & Warshaw, P. R. (1988). The theory of reasoned action: A meta-analysis of past research with recommendations for modifications and future research. *Journal of Consumer Research, 15*, 325–342.

Stanton, B. F., Li, X., Black, M. M., Ricardo, I., Galbraith, J., Feigelman, S., & Kaljee, L. (1996). Longitudinal stability and predictability of sexual perceptions, intentions and behaviors among early adolescent African-Americans. *Journal of Adolescent Health, 18*, 10–19.

Stanton, B., Li, X., Black, M., Ricardo, I., Galbraith, J., Kaljee, L., & Feigelman, S. (1994). Sexual practices and intentions among preadolescent and early adolescent low-income urban African-Americans. *Pediatrics, 93*, 966–973.

Steed, L., Newman, S. P., & Hardman, S. M. C. (1999). An examination of the self-regulation model in atrial fibrillation. *British Journal of Health Psychology, 4*, 337–347.

Steffen, V. J. (1990). Men's motivation to perform the testicle self-exam: Effects of prior knowledge and an educational brochure. *Journal of Applied Social Psychology, 20*, 681–702.

Strathman, A., Gleicher, F., Boninger, D. S., & Edwards, C. S. (1994). The consideration of future consequences: Weighing immediate and distant outcomes of behavior. *Journal of Personality and Social Psychology, 66*, 742–752.

Sutton, S. (1998). Predicting and explaining intentions and behavior: How well are we doing? *Journal of Applied Social Psychology, 28*, 1317–1338.

Sutton, S., Bickler, G., Sancho-Aldridge, J., & Saidi, G. (1994). Prospective study of predictors of attendance for breast screening in inner London. *Journal of Epidemiology and Community Health, 48*, 65–73.

Taylor, S., & Gollwitzer, P. M. (1995). Effects of mindset on positive illusions. *Journal of Personality and Social Psychology, 69*, 213–226.

Verplanken, B., & Aarts, H. (1999). Habit, attitude and planned behavior: Is habit an empty construct or an interesting case of goal-directed automaticity? *European Review of Social Psychology, 10*, 101–134.

Verplanken, B., & Faes, S. (1999). Good intentions, bad habits and effects of forming implementation intentions on healthy eating. *European Journal of Social Psychology, 29*, 591–604.

Verplanken, B., Myrbakk, V., & Rudi, E. (2005). The measurement of habit. In T. Betsch & S. Haberstroh (Eds.), *The routines of decision making* (pp. 231–247). Mahwah, NJ: Erlbaum.

Verplanken, B., & Orbell, S. (2003). Reflections on past behavior: A self-report index of habit strength. *Journal of Applied Social Psychology, 33*, 1313–1330.

Warshaw, P. R., Calantone, R., & Joyce, M. (1986). A field application of the Fishbein and Ajzen intention model. *Journal of Social Psychology, 126*, 135–136.

Webb, T. L., & Sheeran, P. (2003). Can implementation intentions help to overcome ego-depletion? *Journal of Experimental Social Psychology, 39*, 279–286.

Webb, T. L., & Sheeran, P. (2004). Identifying good opportunities to act: Implementation intentions and cue detection. *European Journal of Social Psychology, 34*, 407–419.

Wegner, D. M., & Wheatley, T. (1999). Apparent mental causation: Sources of the experience of will. *American Psychologist, 54*, 480–492.

Weinstein, N. D. (1993). Testing four competing theories of health-protective behavior. *Health Psychology, 12*, 324–333.

Wood, W., Quinn, J. M., & Kashy, D. A. (2002). Habits in everyday life: Thought, emotion and action. *Journal of Personality and Social Psychology, 83*, 1281–1297.

Wurtele, S. K. (1988). Increasing women's calcium intake: The role of health beliefs, intentions and health value. *Journal of Applied Social Psychology, 18*, 627–639.

9

JUDGMENT AND DECISION PROCESSES IN OLDER ADULTS' COMPLIANCE WITH MEDICAL REGIMENS

LINDA L. LIU AND RICHARD GONZALEZ

A recent trend in health care is characterized by increases in patient autonomy and shared medical decision making between patients and their doctors or health care providers. Medical decisions are no longer made solely by physicians, because patients are increasingly encouraged to play an active role in researching their own illnesses and deciding which treatment options they will pursue. This shift in medical decisions from doctor to patient has the potential to affect the health care of older adults negatively. Substantial research in cognitive aging indicates that older adults frequently have more difficulty comprehending and remembering medical information compared with younger adults (e.g., Brown & Park, 2002; Halter, 1999; Morrell, Park, & Poon, 1989; Park & Kidder, 1996). These deficits in information processing may translate into suboptimal decision making as older adults are increasingly expected to play a more active role in researching their illnesses, choosing between multiple treatment options, and planning how they will implement new medical behaviors.

Although considerable research on aging and decision making has focused on studying the effects of aging on patients' ability to make competent decisions regarding consent to treatment (see Appelbaum & Grisso, 1998), it is also increasingly important to investigate older patients' normative decision-making skills—how they make decisions that maximize utility (Kahneman & Tversky, 2000)—and to assess the processes and outcomes of their decisions. Important skills include weighing the risks and benefits in selecting and eliminating medications and treatments from consideration (Deyo, 2001) and accurately estimating the likelihood of future outcomes (Yates & Patalano, 1999). The burgeoning availability of medical information on the Internet has increased patients' ability to access medical information and advice from a variety of sources, including other physicians and other patients, with obtaining health information being cited as one of the most common uses for the Internet (Morrell, Mayhorn, & Bennett, 2000). For all of these reasons, how older adults evaluate and integrate medical information from different sources in making medical decisions has become a vital topic for investigation.

In this chapter, we discuss the impact of aging on older adults' ability to make medical decisions that are relevant to following doctors' instructions. Within the scope of this discussion, we use the term *medical judgment* to describe the cognitive processes involved in estimations of likelihood, ranking the relative likelihood of different outcomes, and assessments of severity. A *medical decision*, in turn, represents a choice that is made after alternatives with different attributes are weighed and compared. The ability to make sound medical judgments and decisions is determined by a complex interaction of factors, including age-related changes in information-processing ability and cognitive biases that are automatically elicited by the use of well-known cognitive heuristics. Consequently, older adults' success on decision-making tasks can be measured by examining both measures of process and outcome. We first present a brief survey of changes in information-processing abilities that accompany aging (for a detailed discussion, see chap. 5, this volume) and that provide the backdrop for older adults' performance of medical judgments and decisions. We continue with a discussion of how these age-related changes fit into a well-articulated theoretical framework of judgment and decision making. Then we present evidence for how age-related changes in cognition induce differences in strategy use among older adults and discuss how these age differences in cognitive function and strategy translate into decision-making outcomes. Finally, we propose some directives on how the interplay of aging and information processing can be taken into consideration when presenting medical decisions to older adults.

AGE-RELATED CHANGE IN
COGNITIVE FUNCTION

Although judgments and decisions are considered to be distinct processes, judgments often form the backdrop for future decisions. Judgments encompass a wide range of behaviors that include the ability to weigh multiple pieces of information, rank the likelihood of various outcomes, and assess the severity of outcomes; decisions also encompass the choice among multiple options and the selection of options that represent solutions to a problem or a scenario (Yates & Patalano, 1999). Consider, for example, an older adult woman who begins to experience a collection of symptoms, including a sore throat, sneezing, coughing, and runny nose. Between the time of symptom onset to the time she receives treatment, she will make a number of judgments regarding the severity of her symptoms and estimate their frequency of occurrence; she will make decisions about how to react on the basis of the outcomes of these judgments. She may attempt to determine whether these symptoms are indicative of a cold or a seasonal allergy by judging the overall similarity of the collection of symptoms to her cognitive representation of colds and allergies. If she regards the symptoms as severe enough to treat and estimates that their occurrence will be infrequent, she may decide to purchase an over-the-counter remedy. On the other hand, if the symptoms occur with high frequency, she may decide to make a doctor's appointment and request a prescription medication. There are, of course, judgments of severity of the symptoms, but in this section we focus on the judgments of likelihood.

Once the decision is made to seek treatment, the patient is faced with the task of selecting a medication from several that are available. Table 9.1 is a hypothetical tabular summary of a possible array of choices with key accompanying features. Although this organization of options as an Alternative × Attribute matrix (Payne, 1976) is useful for the purposes of presentation in an academic chapter, an older adult who is collecting information about each drug in a naturalistic setting (e.g., a drug store or a doctor's office) is unlikely to receive this type of summary. Instead, the patient will likely face the task of learning the features of each medication individually. Consequently, the patient in this case must make multiple evaluations and judgments on her own, such as choosing the method of drug administration (e.g., oral or nasal), determining which side effects are acceptable and which are not, and establishing how much she is willing to pay. If she is making these decisions within a doctor's office or a drugstore, there is additional time pressure as well. Finally, she must also select a treatment that she is relatively confident she can remember to carry out at home. If she is not

TABLE 9.1
Alternative × Attribute Matrix

Drug option	Price (30-day supply)	Administration	Availability	Most common side effects
Drug A	Excellent	Oral (swallow)	OTC	Excitability, drowsiness, sleep disturbance
Drug B	Poor	Oral (swallow)	Prescription	Coughing, upper respiratory tract infection, back pain
Drug C	Excellent	Oral (swallow)	OTC	Drowsiness, excitability, dry mouth
Drug D	Very good	Oral (swallow)	OTC	Headache, drowsiness, fatigue
Drug E	Excellent	Nasal spray	OTC	Burning, stinging, sneezing
Drug F	Fair	Nasal spray	Prescription	Sneezing, stuffy nose, unpleasant taste/smell
Drug G	Fair	Nasal spray	Prescription	Headache, dry nose, throat irritation
Drug H	Poor	Inhaler	Prescription	Headache, nosebleed, sore throat
Drug I	Very good	Inhaler	OTC	Nervousness, rapid heart beat, heart problems
Drug J	Fair	Nasal spray	Prescription	Nosebleed, nasal/throat irritation, cough
Drug K	Poor	Oral (chew)	Prescription	Diarrhea, stomach upset, cough
Drug L	Very good	Oral (swallow)	OTC	Nervousness, dizziness, sleeplessness
Drug M	Good	Inhaler	Prescription	Nasal dryness/irritation, burning, stinging
Drug N	Good	Oral (swallow)	Prescription	Drowsiness, dry mouth

Note. A matrix depicting popular brands of allergy medication. OTC = over the counter.

confident of her ability to do so, she may opt to visit the doctor regularly to receive allergy shots instead.

Thus, the decision to seek treatment for an ailment comprises a number of cognitively demanding tasks in which options previously seen must be remembered while new options are being considered. In the above example, the decision of whether to purchase one drug versus another will be guided by a set of judgments, such as those involved in ranking the drugs according to personal preferences for how they are administered and the severity of accompanying side effects. Consequently, the decision outcome will be based on these judgments and the relative importance of these dimensions to the decision maker. The molar task of making a medical judgment or decision regarding an ailment thus consists of a number of subprocesses, including remembering previously seen options, ranking them by relative importance, and executing a decision outcome that is consistent with this evaluation. Each of these subprocesses taps a number of cognitive functions, all of which change with age.

Effects of Age-Related Declines in Memory and Processing

Because judgments and decisions frequently depend on balancing a constellation of information including personal preferences, risks, and benefits, the performance of optimal judgment and decision making requires a great deal of online processing. Considerable work in cognitive aging has shown that online-processing components of cognition, such as working memory and processing speed, show marked declines in older individuals (Park, 2000; Salthouse & Babcock, 1991), and age-related changes in cognition have the potential to affect older adults' performance of nearly all of the processes that underlie judgment and decision making.

Decreases in working memory capacity are characterized by declines in the ability to store and manipulate multiple pieces of information simultaneously in conscious awareness. *Slowing in processing speed* refers to declines in the ability to complete a task accurately but quickly under time constraints, and the effects of slowing in processing speed are often most evident when older adults are faced with novel situations or must make decisions within a time limit (Park, 2000). Under time constraints, older adults may require more time to make an optimal decision compared with younger adults.

Given the multiple cognitive declines that occur with age, aging is frequently hypothesized to have a generally negative impact on judgment and decision processes (Peters, Finucane, MacGregor, & Slovic, 2000), representing a combination of changes in physiological function. Both decreases in frontal lobe volume (Raz, 2000; Scheibel, 1996) and increases in bilateral recruitment of brain regions (Reuter-Lorenz, Stanczak, & Miller,

1999) appear to accompany advanced age, and research is beginning to shed light on how these physiological changes might lead to a host of psychological changes, such as an increased reliance on the limbic system and increased attention to emotional information (Blanchard-Fields, 1998). Substantial evidence suggests that older and younger adults make decisions differently and that they arrive at these decisions using not only different strategies but through different physiological pathways.

Furthermore, physiological differences may underlie some of the more general characteristics of decision-making styles. Older adults are generally believed to reason in a more top-down fashion compared with younger adults' bottom-up, data-driven style of thinking (Sinnott, 1989). This has been characterized by others as an age-related increase in affective styles of processing (Blanchard-Fields, 1998), theory-driven or heuristic processing (Mutter & Pliske, 1994), or risk aversion in the sense of avoiding decision making altogether when given the option to do so (Calhoun & Hutchison, 1981). Others have proposed that older adults engage in simplification processes to conserve emotional as well as cognitive processing resources. Leventhal, Leventhal, Schaefer, and Easterling (1993) found that older adults seeking medical care do so more immediately yet request less information when doing so. They proposed that older adults "conserve energy" by seeking medical attention quickly, thus allowing physicians to assume more of the burden of decision making and reducing their own anxiety. Thus, older adults also may reduce the amount of information they seek in order to reduce their emotional investment. Meyer, Russo, and Talbot (1995) also found that older women were more likely to make an immediate decision after hearing one surgeon's recommendation than were younger women, who were willing to risk delaying treatment to hear additional opinions. Taken together, these findings suggest that older adults may choose to conserve energy by avoiding the task of making difficult decisions on their own.

Age-related declines in long-term memory function may also lead older adults to have increased difficulty with retrieving information learned in the past and to have difficulty with *prospective remembering*—retrieving a relevant behavior that one intends to perform at a specific time in the future (see chap. 3, this volume). Recent work has also shown that over time older adults' long-term memory is subject to distortions, such that even when they are able to recall the basic content of information, they may lose details regarding its valence (Skurnik, Yoon, Park, & Schwarz, 2005) or the trustworthiness of its source (Ybarra & Park, 2002). Individuals who are presented with a great amount of information may lose details of information they receive, leading to systematic distortions in the information they recall and leaving them with only a general positive or negative affective impression.

Schwarz and Clore (1996) found that in situations in which older individuals must make complex or speeded decisions, information is often encoded in terms of its emotional value to the individual rather than its actual content. The tendency to base judgments on a positive or negative feeling that one associates with particular options is referred to as an *affect heuristic* (Finucane, Alhakami, Slovic, & Johnson, 2000). Bargh (1996) argued that affective processing occurs automatically. Blanchard-Fields (1998) proposed that this occurs in part because one's emotional state becomes integrated with cognitive representation of events in memory, and she argued that the affective information is available but not necessarily used unless task demands are heightened because of increases in task complexity or time pressure. In some cases, the efficiency of an affective response can be advantageous, as when individuals display heightened sensitivity to information conveyed about risk (Loewenstein, Weber, Hsee, & Welch, 2001), and increases in the ability to use emotional as well as cognitive information observed with age (Labovie-Vief, 1992) can sometimes be important for good decision making (Bechara, Tranel, & Damasio, 2000; Wilson & Schooler, 1991). However, when an affective or emotional assessment of a situation conflicts with one's cognitive assessment of the situation, this might result in older adults' remembering only a negative impression of a treatment—for example, that it was very painful to a friend or relative—and ruling out this treatment despite there being many other factors to recommend it. As another example, the older adult searching for an allergy medication who finds it difficult to keep track of her different options might make her decision on the basis of the relative affective reaction to different side effects or on the memorability of the different options (e.g., resulting from their frequency of appearance in commercials) rather than on their utility to treating her illness. Older adults who have difficulty recalling to-be-remembered information may resort to choosing an alternative that looks familiar (Jacoby, Jennings, & Hay, 1996), elicits positive feelings (Klaczynski & Robinson, 2000), or is consistent with their prior beliefs about quality (Mutter & Pliske, 1994).

Other basic changes in cognitive functions such as working memory also serve as a fundamental component of many higher order cognitive processes, such as reading and comprehension. Specifically, declines in working memory may result in older adults' having difficulty with understanding information that is lengthy or complex (Light & Capps, 1986). In particular, older adults have difficulty revising recently read information, particularly if it is inconsistent with the beliefs they have formed about what they have read (Hamm & Hasher, 1992). Difficulty in revising beliefs that have been formed can be attributed to the increased role that automatic processes play in older adults' thinking (Peters et al., 2000) as well as declines in older adults' ability to inhibit irrelevant information (Hamm & Hasher, 1992).

The addition of time pressure seems to increase difficulty with revising automatically generated inferences; Blanchard-Fields (1998) noted that older adults are capable of revising conclusions automatically drawn from reading a passage of information but only did so when given sufficient time.

Chasseigne, Mullet, and Stewart (1997) demonstrated that this decrease in the ability to perform cognitive "revisions" in older adults also leads to a decreased sensitivity to cue–criterion relationships. The ability to identify a cue–criterion relationship is medically important because it allows individuals to detect a correlation between a situation and an illness or symptom (e.g., being near freshly cut grass and having an allergy attack). Although they found no age differences in older and younger adults' ability to detect simple cue–criterion relationships (i.e., the cue shared a direct relationship with the criterion), the inclusion of an inverse relationship resulted in older adults having significantly more difficulty in accommodating this change. Explicitly stating that the change helped a younger subset of the older group but not the oldest old revised their theories about the relationships. Thus, it is not simply the case that declines in cognitive abilities reduce older adults' sensitivity to probability cues; instead, these declines may make some of the component processes more difficult to execute and may be clearly evident in only the most cognitively demanding situations.

Older adults' difficulty in revising previously held beliefs can also increase their susceptibility to being deceived. A series of studies by Ybarra, Chan, and Park (2001) found that age-related change in cognition may make older adults less capable of being skeptical and socially vigilant when dealing with individuals they have just met. Furthermore, Ybarra and Park (2002) found that older adults were less able to be socially vigilant and to undertake the processes of revising their impressions of people once they were formed. They demonstrated that under cognitively taxing conditions, older adults tended to retain a more positive impression of the individuals who had been discredited since their initial meeting, indicating that they were less able to be cognitively skeptical. These results suggest that older adults may be particularly susceptible to first impressions about drugs and doctors and that they will find it difficult to revise their initial beliefs about a medication they have just learned about if, for example, the medication is recalled or proven to be ineffective.

Summary

Because age declines in cognition may have a negative impact on older adults' ability to engage in cognitive processes that require effort (Craik & Byrd, 1982), fast responding (Schwarz & Clore, 1996), or filtering out irrelevant and focusing on relevant information (Hasher & Zacks, 1988), cognitive aging may lead to the suboptimal execution of some or many of the constituent processes of judgment and decision making. This suboptimal execution includes increased reliance on initial affective reactions to a situation, preference for avoiding a decision (or delegating the decision to a physician), decreased ability to remember the original valence of information, deficits in the ability to revise initial inferences generated about information read, and increased susceptibility to being deceived. Furthermore, within distracting contexts such as a noisy drugstore or a busy doctor's office, older adults may be less able to filter out unhelpful or uninformative information, particularly if it is attractive or salient, because of age-related decreases in inhibitory processes (Hasher & Zacks, 1988).

What do laboratory declines on tests of cognition tell us about how older adults make decisions in real life? One possible consequence of aging is that age-related declines in effortful cognition among older adults may lead to their increased reliance on heuristics or cognitive shortcuts to simplify and reduce the cognitive effort of executing decisions (Klaczynski & Robinson, 2000; Mutter & Pliske, 1994). Another is that older adults may adopt alternative information-processing strategies to circumvent these cognitive changes. In this next section, we review some of the research on normative decision making and suggest what this body of research might tell us about how older adults perform on standard decision-making tasks.

AGING AND NORMATIVE DECISION MAKING

Age-related declines in cognition may affect how and whether normative responses are given on standard tasks of judgment and decision making. Because heuristic use is often conceptualized as a cognitive shortcut that results from the inability to process information exhaustively, older adults, given their cognitive deficits, should be even more likely to use heuristics and, consequently, be more likely to display the biases reported for younger adults (Peters et al., 2000). For example, older adults given the task of choosing between different medications in Table 9.1 may find it difficult to compare two medications that vary on a number of features. Determining how to weigh different traits and how to combine the weights into a composite score representing the utility to the decision maker may be taxing and difficult for older adults. Reductions in working memory capacity might also limit older adults' ability to multitask so that they can consider a new item of information while assessing how it compares with the ones seen previously. Given that a large amount of information will require a number of judgments and comparisons, it is often necessary to simplify these judgments and decisions.

Automatic processing components of cognition, in part, support older adults' decision-making ability, and older adults can use these intact resources to counteract the effects of aging and support declining cognitive functions. Automatic processes underlie many fundamental aspects of cognition such as heuristic use, stereotype activation, and affective reactions to stimuli (Bargh, 1996). Thus, the use of heuristics is governed by processes that are insensitive to the effects of aging (Peters et al., 2000). Because older adults do not experience the same declines in automatic processes as in effortful processes like working memory and processing speed (Park, 2000), reliance on heuristics that depend on automatic processing should remain stable with age.

The use and overuse of heuristics in simplifying these types of tasks have guided much of the research on normative judgment and decision making. When faced with situations in which people must make a decision in which many conditions are uncertain or unknown, individuals may use heuristics in forming their judgments and decisions. These heuristics can be adaptive (Gigerenzer 1991a, 1991b) and are an important cognitive tool that allow individuals to simplify a complex judgment. For example, doctors often use a similarity heuristic when diagnosing a patient who is exhibiting a host of symptoms. Rather than matching individual symptoms to a mental list of illnesses, physicians may simply assess the similarity of the patient's case to different illness prototypes to make a diagnosis (Elstein, 1999).

However, in some cases, the use of heuristics can lead to errors in reasoning, and the predictable use of a given heuristic in relation to a given type of problem is frequently referred to as a *cognitive bias* (Kahneman & Tversky, 1982). For example, an older adult choosing an allergy medication may be faced with the task of estimating the likelihood of encountering the different side effects associated with each drug. If the older adult is evaluating Drug H versus Drug J, he or she might consider whether it is more likely that he or she will experience headache or nosebleed. Although the package notes might report that nosebleeds have a higher incidence of occurrence (3%) than headaches (1%), the older adult might be unduly influenced by the fact that he or she can imagine having a headache more easily than a nosebleed. In this case, heavier reliance on his or her heuristic might lead the older adult to a suboptimal decision outcome: choosing Drug J. Because the vast majority of research on decision making in younger adults has focused on the inappropriate use of heuristics and the cognitive biases that result, younger adults' decision making provides an excellent framework within which to compare younger and older adults' judgments and decisions (see Kahneman, Slovic, & Tversky, 1982).

Forming Judgments on the Basis of Mental Availability

A typical result observed with young adults is that the judgments of quantity or likelihood tend to be larger for sets that come to mind easily than they are for less mentally available sets. For example, individuals who are asked to judge whether there are more seven-letter words ending in -*ing* or whose sixth letter is an *n* are typically biased to say that words in the first category are more numerous because it is easier to generate these words mentally. Tversky and Kahneman (1983) theorized that the judgment of set size initiates a mentally effortful task of generating exemplars for the set described and during which the amount of effort expended is used as a metric for estimating the size of the set. By this view, the set of items that comes to mind easily (-*ing* words) is generally estimated (incorrectly) to be larger than the set of items that is more difficult to generate (sixth-letter-*n* words). The underestimation of the size of the logically larger set is evidence that younger adults use an availability heuristic to perform set size judgments.

Within a medical domain, the use of the availability heuristic might lead to older adults' tendency to over- or underestimate their likelihood of becoming ill or of suffering side effects, depending on the relative salience of the illness in question (Peters et al., 2000; Tversky & Kahneman, 1974). Older adults might be disproportionately influenced by the popular discussion of a particular illness's symptoms (e.g., severe acute respiratory illness, or SARS) and overestimate their risk for becoming infected with the disease. If this question were posed in 2003, with the increased media attention given to SARS and the relative reduction in salience of influenza, this might lead older adults to (incorrectly) respond that they are at greater risk of catching SARS than the flu. In this case, the vividness of the SARS symptoms and their resulting heightened mental availability would likely inflate estimates of likelihood for being affected by the disease despite its low incidence in the population relative to a more immediate concern for elderly adults such as the flu (Centers for Disease Control and Prevention, 2003).

Order Effects on Memory

A perfect model of normative decision making would predict that individuals presented with the same pieces of information should produce the same judgment or decision regardless of the order in which the information is given. However, Chapman, Bergus, and Elstein (1996) found that the order in which multiple pieces of information was presented affected the eventual decision that was made. Both novice and experienced physicians read three pieces of information sequentially from a patient file indicating the following:

1. The patient had a history of lung cancer.
2. The patient exhibited a neurological disturbance.
3. The patient's computed tomography (CT) scan was normal.

Physicians were asked to estimate the probabilities of the following two diagnoses: (a) that the patient had had a transient ischemic attack (a stroke) and (b) that the patient had a brain tumor. In the absence of all other information, a past diagnosis of lung cancer would be suggestive of a brain tumor. A normal CT scan would be evidence against the presence of a brain tumor. Half of the physicians in the study read the patient information in the order described above (i.e., 1-2-3), and the other half read it in the reverse order (i.e., 3-2-1). Chapman et al. found a significant asymmetry in decisions made as a function of presentation order. Specifically, they found a recency effect in which physicians who received information about the previous diagnosis of lung cancer last (in the third position in the series) were significantly more likely to give a diagnosis of a brain tumor compared with physicians who received this information first in the series. This effect of recency was found regardless of physicians' level of experience. Among older patients, recency effects might lead them to choose later presented treatments disproportionately often, especially in cases in which options are presented orally rather than in a written format, as is common in a doctor's office. Indeed, in a study of older adults' choices of response options in telephone surveys, Schwarz and Knäuper (2000) found that the tendency to endorse the last response option presented orally in a series tended to occur with greater frequency among older interviewees.

What can be done to remedy recency effects? Chapman et al. (1996) suggested that one way to "debias" physicians would be to encourage physicians to consider clinical evidence in different orders and to review the most relevant information immediately before making a diagnosis to increase its weight. Older patients might be provided with a summary at the end of their appointment in which the treatment options are presented in a different order than was presented verbally by the physician, and additional care could be exercised to present lists of treatment options in both an auditory and a written format. Recent follow-up work supports the efficacy of these strategies, suggesting that recency effect can be remedied by initiating a process of self-review in which the decision maker completes an ongoing comparison between his or her decision and the original goal (Ashton & Kennedy, 2002). Thus, individuals can be encouraged to "stay on track" and not be disproportionately influenced by the last piece of information encountered. Although the research on order effects has largely focused on younger adults, age-related changes that are typically observed in information-processing behavior suggest that susceptibility to order effects may be magnified with age. Webster, Richter, and Kruglanski (1996) demonstrated that mental fatigue induces inefficiencies in processing and increases primacy effects in information use in decision making. To the extent that particularly demanding tasks in which there are multiple options and multiple features to be compared are particularly taxing for older adults, this may induce similar levels of fatigue and increase older adults' susceptibility to these types of order effect.

Judgments Based on Representativeness or Similarity

When individuals are asked to judge the probability of an event, such as the likelihood that they have breast cancer, they tend to use a shortcut in which they evaluate the similarity between the event and some prototypical event and use similarity to estimate the probability that the event will occur. In this situation, if the individual in question is very similar to the stereotype they hold for a typical breast cancer patient, they will produce higher estimates of likelihood than if there is a low level of similarity. This use of the representativeness heuristic (Tversky & Kahneman, 1983) allows individuals who are uncertain about how to judge the probability of populations to make this judgment on the basis of an easier judgment of similarity. Thus, the use of this heuristic would produce a predictable pattern of results in which a female would judge herself to have a high probability of having breast cancer, whereas a male would be less likely to produce a self-diagnosis of having the disease. Although in this situation the heuristic produces an estimate that is consistent with the relative risk for the disease, when more salient or memorable options exert greater influence in the judgment than less salient, but perhaps more important, information, this can lead to inappropriate probability judgments. For example, an individual who is short of breath may perceive high similarity between the present symptom and a heart attack, inflating the perceived probability judgment that he or she is experiencing a heart attack and leading, perhaps, to an unnecessary trip to the emergency room. Because older adults are more prone to rely on stereotypes in situations with greater degrees of uncertainty (Mather, Johnson, & DeLeonardis, 1999), this would lead to increases in using representativeness as a metric for probability and an accompanying increase in these kinds of medical errors.

Fortunately, whether individuals display a representativeness bias depends to a great extent on the salience or strength of the stereotype. For example, if the individual feels strongly that being female is a critical feature of the typical breast cancer patient, then a male patient will perceive his risk for this disease as being very small. However, if a patient vignette is worded in neutral language, to avoid eliciting stereotypes that can be embraced or discounted, this may decrease individuals' display of the representativeness bias. On the other hand, if the objective is to warn a patient that his or her risky behavior is likely to lead to an illness, highlighting the high degree of similarity between their own case and a patient vignette may be desirable. Tymchuk, Ouslander, Rahbar, and Fitten (1988) found that the use of storybook vignettes was effective in improving patients' comprehension of medical procedures, possibly because the introduction of a character highlighted the similarities between the individual receiving the procedure in the story and the individual about to undergo the procedure. Thus, the perceived distance between the patient and a prototypical patient may be an important metric for how the patient assesses risks associated with illness or various medical procedures.

Violation of the Conjunction Rule

Patients embarking on medical treatments may also be asked to estimate and compare the relative magnitude of two probabilities. For example, in making a decision about his or her chance of having a heart attack, a patient may be asked whether there are more individuals who have had one or more heart attacks or individuals who are over the age of 55 and have had one or more heart attacks (Kahneman et al., 1982). Younger adults typically estimate the latter to be greater, with the explanation being that having multiple heart attacks is consistent with many people's stereotypes of elderly adults. Thus, for an individual to be both over the age of 55 and prone to heart attacks is especially consistent with their stereotype and, invoking the representativeness heuristic (Kahneman & Tversky, 1982), college-age participants wrongly estimate that the size of the group representing the conjunction of the two events would be larger than the size of the group defined by the single criterion. It follows from the literature on age-related cognitive declines that older adults might have difficulty overriding the automatically generated response that is consistent with their stereotype of older adults.

Anchoring and Adjustment

In judgments requiring an estimation of quantity or likelihood, a typical heuristic is to generate an initial estimate based on subjective evidence and then revise that estimate on the basis of incoming information. This heuristic is adaptive if the initial estimate is accurate, but frequently it results in inaccurate judgments when the estimate is not revised sufficiently to reflect new evidence (i.e., a primary effect). This may be problematic for older adults, who experience decreases in cognitive flexibility and may have particular difficulty revising their theories or estimates once they have made them mentally. Taken with evidence suggesting that older adults in some cases display more risk-averse tendencies compared with younger adults (Dror,

Katona, & Mungur, 1998), it may be the case that older adults allow their predispositions (low-risk seeking) to guide their initial estimates or decisions and that any revisions of these estimates that occur subsequently will be insufficiently small or will not occur at all.

Summary

Older adults typically experience a variety of cognitive declines such that making decisions may force them to rely more heavily on heuristics that allow them to simplify decisions at hand and reduce cognitive effort. Like young adults, older adults may find it difficult to judge the relative likelihood of occurrence of two outcomes (e.g., likelihood of two different side effects) and use the relative mental ease or availability of the two side effects to judge which is more likely to occur. Decreases in working memory capacity and processing speed might also hinder older adults' ability to process multiple alternatives when making a decision and lead them to place disproportionate weight on the first or last options they hear. Finally, older adults may find it especially difficult to revise inferences that they have already generated about an illness or a diagnosis. These stereotypic patterns of cognitive bias are found reliably when younger adults are presented with these decision-making scenarios, and age-related changes in cognitive function may lead older adults to make similar or even more biased judgments and decisions. However, increases in cognitive bias may not present a complete picture of older adults' performance of decision making in everyday contexts. In the next section, we present evidence that although this standard framework for evaluating decision-making outcomes on the basis of their normative value captures judgment and decision making within specific tasks, it does not provide a way to assess the constituent processes of decision making in which older adults demonstrate an ability to compensate for these changes in age-related cognitive function.

STRATEGY USE AND EVERYDAY DECISION MAKING

A recent surge of interest in everyday decision-making processes has led to a shift in focus away from regarding decision making as a purely probabilistic task in which there is a clear, normatively defined correct response. Classic research on decision making (Kahneman et al., 1982) is characterized by two central issues: (a) the establishment of a normative yardstick against which judgment and decision behavior are measured and (b) a focus on the product of judgment and decision processes as typically measured by college-aged adults' responses to a standard set of tasks. Defined in this way, normative responding on classic judgment and decision-making tasks (Kahneman & Tversky, 2000; Tversky & Kahneman, 1974) entails responding in a way that is consistent with Bayesian probabilities and that adheres to axioms of rationality such as expected utility theory (Sen, 1971; Von Neumann & Morgenstern, 1947). Normative responding might include making judgments and estimations of magnitude or quantity that reflect base-rate probabilities, choosing consistently (as opposed to inconsistently) among a set of alternatives (Simonson & Tversky, 1992), accurately weighing multiple pieces of information based on informative value, and ranking the likelihood of various outcomes in a way that is consistent with background information (Yates & Patalano, 1999).

However, recent work suggests that a normative yardstick may not provide a complete means for evaluating the quality of everyday decision-making behaviors. Huber, Wider, and Huber (1997) found that individuals presented with naturalistic decision-making tasks, in which they actively collected information to reach a decision, rarely sought or used exact probability information to assess the relative risk presented by different alternatives and to choose a course of action. They suggested that naturalistic decision making in a context that involves risk may not induce the same pattern of heuristic use and cognitive biases traditionally exhibited when a decision is presented as a gamble, possibly because gambles involve the presentation of relevant information up front, whereas naturalistic decisions require the decision maker to search and acquire information and determine its relevance before making the decision. Among the types of naturalistic decisions included here are the types of behavior that are required when evaluating options in medical, financial, and legal settings as well as more traditional settings that involve the purchasing of goods and services.

Ruling-Out Strategy

M. M. S. Johnson (1990) presented older adults with a car-purchasing task in which the participants were asked to choose which of six cars they would purchase. Each car's description consisted of its performance on nine different criteria, such as fuel economy, riding comfort, and maintenance cost. At any given time, participants could press a key allowing them to view a single piece of information about a single car, and participants guided their own information searches by selecting which cars they wished to evaluate and what types of information they chose to view. Participants were under no time constraints and were allowed to view as many pieces of information about as many cars as they wished.

M. M. S. Johnson (1990) found that older adults making a decision to buy a car tended to seek out less information and to spend less time reviewing each option compared with younger adults. Although this processing difference would initially seem to be maladaptive, M. M. S. Johnson and Drungle (2000) provided evidence that this abbreviated search behavior may be indicative of higher quality of search behavior: They found that older adults choosing between over-the-counter medications demonstrated more organized patterns of search. Sanfey and Hastie (2000) characterized these abbreviated types of search strategies as noncompensatory strategies—using a set of minimal criteria to rule out options found to be unacceptable in order to reduce the number of options that must be considered. This strategy of ruling out eliminates decision options with certain features and does not allow them to enter the comparison process at all. It is contrasted with compensatory strategies, which require more effort and in which the pros offset the cons of an individual option but in which all options are weighed and taken into consideration to make some options seem better than others. It is also evidenced in older adults' decisions made about medical options. When making decisions in which they are choosing between multiple medical options, Meyer et al. (1995) found that older patients seek out less information, suggesting that they self-regulate the amount of information they will have to consider in making a decision, and that they require less time to reach their decisions. Zwahr, Park, and Shifren (1999) found that older women considering estrogen replacement therapy made fewer comparisons of treatment alternatives and perceived that they had fewer options.

Several factors are thought to increase noncompensatory decision making, including increased decision complexity (J. E. V. Johnson & Bruce, 1997) and reductions in time given to make a decision (Maule, Hockey, & Bdzola, 2000). To the extent that increased processing demands resemble age-related declines in cognitive function, declines in processing abilities with age may lead to an increase in older adults' engagement of noncompensatory styles of decision making. Thus, an elimination strategy reduces the amount of information that must be considered and may thus be a particularly useful strategy for older adults, and older adults appear to engage in information collection strategies that successfully compensate for their cognitive declines.

Summary

Normative decision-making tasks may not provide a complete means for evaluating the quality of everyday decision-making behaviors. Process-oriented models of decision making (M. M. S. Johnson, 1990; Payne, 1979) have demonstrated that older adults adapt their acquisition of information in ways that compensate for their declining ability to engage in the simultaneous processing of multiple pieces of information and consider fewer options because of their slower ability to process this information. Thus, an inspection of older adults' processing strategies provides insight into what might be the most effective way to support older adults' decision-making performance.

ASPECTS OF DECISION MAKING PRESERVED WITH AGE

Age-related declines in cognition notwithstanding, much of the research on aging and decision making has demonstrated that the quality or outcome of older adults' decisions is comparable to that of younger adults. For example, although older adults consider less information and make their decisions more quickly, younger and older adults typically arrive at the same decisions (Meyer et al., 1995; Zwahr et al., 1999). Meyer et al. (1995) found no age differences in final treatment selection among younger and older women presented with information about treatments for breast cancer. Using a financial decision-making task, Hershey and Wilson (1997) found no evidence to support the supposition that older adults exhibited more overconfidence or were otherwise maladaptively biased in their decisions. In the previous section, we reviewed evidence suggesting that older adults frequently use strategies to adapt tasks in ways that accommodate age-related reductions in their processing resources. In this section, we illustrate how age-related changes in cognition can also support the continued ability of older adults to make competent decisions in a variety of domains and suggest how these competencies can be developed into strategies for facilitating medical compliance in older adults.

The preservation of competent decision-making ability is demonstrated pragmatically as well as empirically through research demonstrating that the performance of molar decision-making behaviors, such as workplace and managerial behaviors (Park, 1994; Taylor, 1975), remain at high levels with age. Similarly, expertise in specific domains such as chess playing does not appear to decline with age (Charness, 1981). Thus, older adults appear to maintain high levels of decision-making ability through a combination of compensatory strategies and accommodation of tasks to fit their cognitive deficits (Salthouse, 1987). In fact, some recent work has provided evidence that older adults' greater experience in making decisions may even remediate tendencies to "irrational" decision making that have been reliably documented in younger adults. Tentori, Osherson, Hasher, and May (2001) showed that a consumer decision elicited a pattern of irregular choice making in younger adults but not in older adults. Specifically, they demonstrated that after groups of younger and older adults stated which of two options they preferred, younger adults showed a greater tendency than older adults to reverse that preference when an irrelevant, third option was presented. This preference reversal violates a standard axiom called *regularity*, because the addition of the third option is irrelevant and therefore should not influence the decision in any way. Thus, although numerous declines in cognition and processing speed occur as individuals age, these declines do not necessarily signify declines in judgment or decision-making skills.

A number of explanations have been proposed to account for stability in decision-making ability across the life span. First, the fact that older adults often remain capable of executing critical activities in their daily life despite demonstrated deficits in laboratory tests of memory suggests that laboratory testing conditions may not be comparable to demands encountered by older adults in everyday life. This may be because skills that appear superficially similar in the laboratory may not show similar patterns of age-related decline in real life. Salthouse (1984) illustrated that although both laboratory reaction time tasks and typing tasks in which individuals read and typed texts engage superficially similar motor skills, only the reaction time tasks evidenced the typical pattern of age-related slowing that is attributed to general slowing of processing speed. Thus, seemingly similar tasks may not exhibit similar age differences in performance.

Cognitive declines also can be offset or masked by compensating mechanisms such as practice or experience. Salthouse and Somberg (1982) showed that older adults improved with practice at performing a task requiring them to verify whether an item currently being presented was present in a set of items seen earlier, with the set size of items varying from one to four. The improvement, however, did not manifest itself as a reduction in the gross age difference in mean reaction time collapsed across set size. On the contrary, older adults remained on the whole slower than younger adults. However, measures of the slope of the relationship between the reaction time as the set size of items presented increased showed an important age difference. With practice, this slope measure was greatly reduced in older adults such that the initial large age difference between older and younger adults virtually disappeared after 50 sessions of practice. The reduction in slope was typically interpreted as reflecting older adults' improvement through practice in making the comparison between the probe stimulus and the previously viewed objects. With practice, the comparison with one item versus multiple comparisons with four items became easier. The explanation is that memory scanning becomes more automatic with practice; thus, the attenuation of the age difference in slope can be attributed to the fact that the automatization of the memory comparison process is developed equally easily by younger and older adults. Older adults can catch up to the performance levels of younger adults through practice.

Older adults also may compensate for age-related deficits on some processes by masking these deficits with gains in performance on other processes. Charness (1981) demonstrated that older chess players whose memory deficits were evidenced in poorer accuracy for configurations of pieces also considered fewer alternatives when selecting moves in a game. Older and younger players were equally skilled in the molar behavior of playing the game of chess, however, which suggests that the observed reductions and abbreviations in a subset of the component behaviors were offset by gains in other areas, such as possibly faster searches among available alternatives and faster identification.

Finally, older adults may also be able to support declining cognitive functions by relying on cognitive functions that are relatively resistant to the effects of aging. Park et al. (2002) noted that measures of world knowledge, such as verbal fluency, remain intact and even show slight improvements as individuals age. Similarly, Salthouse (1996) found that older adults showed little evidence for decline on measures of crystallized knowledge, such as measures of vocabulary. Meyer et al. (1995) suggested that increases in reading ability, specifically, may support older adults' ability to make faster decisions compared with younger adults, because they identify critical information more quickly and remember it later when making their decision. In addition to increases in specific cognitive abilities (e.g., verbal ability), older adults' automatic processes are also relatively spared from the effects of aging (Park et al., 2002). Thus, older adults' competencies in decision making may also receive support from abilities that remain preserved with age.

In addition to supporting older adults' performance of everyday activities, automatic processes can be trained to close gaps in performance that arise from age-related declines in cognition. The success of older adults' automatic processes in compensating for cognitive deficits is best evidenced in work on medical compliance. With regard to practical medical behaviors, older adults who have been treated for a number of years for high blood pressure are in fact more adherent to medications than are middle-aged adults (Morrell, Park, Kidder, & Martin, 1997; Park et al., 1999). This is surprising, given that medication adherence is a cognitively demanding task. However, although older adults do show declines in the ability to perform self-initiated processing, their highly routinized schedules allow them to be in familiar contexts frequently, which provides the environmental support for a regularly occurring activity such as the taking of medications. When a pattern of behavior is repeated over time, such as taking medication with breakfast, it becomes automatized and takes on features of an automatic, well-learned behavior such as driving a car with a standard transmission or riding a bicycle.

Other laboratory research supports the effectiveness of using mental rehearsal to recruit automatic processes that support medical and health behaviors. Mental rehearsal has proved effective in promoting a range of health behaviors from performing monthly breast self-exams (Orbell, Hodgkins, & Sheeran, 1997) to maintaining a healthy diet (Verplanken & Faes, 1999; for a review, see Gollwitzer, 1999). Perhaps even more surprising is that older adults are capable of extending strategies that tap into automatic processes in service of maintaining high levels of medical adherence on new medical behaviors, including those that are complex and challenging.

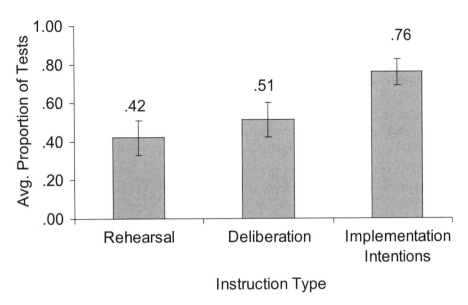

Figure 9.1. Proportion of blood glucose tests performed within 10 minutes of the target times as a function of instruction group. Error bars represent +/– standard error of the mean. Rehearsal = repeating instructions out loud; deliberation = generating pros and cons; implementation intentions = forming specific plans; avg. = average. From "Aging and Medical Adherence: The Use of Automatic Processes to Achieve Effortful Things," by L. L. Liu and D. C. Park, 2004, *Psychology and Aging, 19,* p. 321. Copyright 2004 by the American Psychological Association.

Liu and Park (2004) demonstrated that older adults taught a strategy for a prospective memory task of remembering to perform a new medical behavior—the performance of blood glucose testing four times daily for a 3-week period—were highly successful at remembering to perform their tests (Figure 9.1). These results are consistent with research that has performed direct comparisons of effortful and automatic retrieval from memory, which generally has shown large differences in performance between older and younger adults for when retrieval requires effort but small or no differences when memory retrieval is automatic.

In summary, cognitive declines can be offset or masked by compensating mechanisms such as experience or practice and if only normative behavior is examined—that is, assessing only right and wrong answers. This may present an overly pessimistic view of decision making in aging individuals. Thus, the process of aging distinguishes between tasks requiring the active engagement of processing resources (processing declines) and tasks serving a maintenance function, such as those that are well rehearsed and that do not require as many new decisions to be made (Murphy, 1989).

Older adults may use practice to remediate the effects of aging, develop alternative strategies to accommodate these deficits, or use their combined years of experience in solving other types of problems to mask these deficits. Through the use of noncompensatory decision strategies and attempts to focus their efforts on only decision options most likely to be favorable, older adults' performance of molar decision-making behaviors can remain at high levels. Age-invariant cognitive functions such as verbal and reading ability and automatic processing capabilities are also important supports for decision making in older adults. Automatic processes, in particular, are important because they can support declines in other types of processing. Thus, an understanding of the competencies in older adults' decision-making ability not only sheds light on why there are processing differences between younger and older adults' decision making (e.g., why older adults consider fewer options) but also suggests ways in which medical judgment and decision making can best be supported.

PRESCRIPTIVES FOR PRESENTING MEDICAL DECISIONS TO OLDER ADULTS

Approaches to improving older adults' judgment and decision-making skills that focus solely on compensating for age-related deficits without taking into account preserved aspects of cognitive function may overlook the fact that older adults frequently make good decisions despite approaching decision-making tasks in fundamentally different ways than younger adults. Peters et al. (2000) suggested that an overly pessimistic view of decision making in old age also may be harmful in that it may induce biased decisions about whether older adults are competent to give or refuse consent to medical care. Furthermore, it is also important to be mindful that older adults' decision-making strategies are not simply pared-down versions of younger adults' approaches. With these caveats in mind, we conclude with a discussion of ways in which judgments and decisions might be structured to take advantage of the processes that continue to function well in older adults and to improve older adults' compliance with medical instructions.

Highlight General Principles That Relate Similar Decisions

Decision-making ability does not appear simply to decline over the life span. Rather, older adults may approach decision making using strategies or general rules that they have learned by experience (Baltes & Staudinger, 1993). Thus, practitioners who design decision-making aids for older adults should not focus exclusively on compensating for age-related deficits in cognition (e.g., presenting information more slowly or reducing the number of options presented). Rather, interventions should also consider that older adults have experience in making a variety of judgments and decisions and should highlight general principles (e.g., basic rules of set theory) that may be useful in guiding decisions across multiple contexts. For example, an older adult who is considering getting a smallpox vaccine instead of a flu vaccine might be encouraged to place less emphasis on what is being reported in the media and be reminded of the relative risks presented by both illnesses. Although there may be a tendency to process the risks heuristically and to inflate the likelihood of becoming infected with the illness that is more salient at the moment, this tendency can be corrected by highlighting the parallels with past decisions in which inflated risks of contracting a more "famous" but statistically less common illness was adjusted (e.g., choosing between getting tested for anthrax and getting tested for high blood pressure or diabetes).

Highlight Differences Between Critical and Noncritical Information

Although it is logical to assume that older adults' reductions in processing capacity would suggest a preference for less information, it is more often the case that older adults prefer more rather than less information (Beisecker & Beisecker, 1990). However, differentiating more from less important information is as crucial as regulating the total amount of information given, because increasing the amount of information available is not guaranteed to produce the same effects on all patients. For example, Deyo (2001) investigated the medical decisions made among patients with back problems, comparing those who received a written booklet of treatment options and those who received both a videodisk and a booklet. Patients included those who suffered from a herniated disk and those who suffered from spinal stenosis (a compression of the spaces in the spine that leads to pressure on the spinal cord or nerves, often resulting in pain or numbness in the legs). Deyo found that although the inclusion of the videodisk resulted in a 22% lower surgery rate among the patients with herniated disk, it produced a higher rate of surgery among the patients with spinal stenosis. It is important to note, however, that among the two information groups there were no significant effects in any of the outcome measures, such as measures of pain.

On closer examination, the differential effect of the videodisk is apparent. The symptoms resulting from a herniated disk are characterized by gradual recovery without treatment. The effects of spinal stenosis, however, tend to remain constant and rarely improve without surgery. Hence, the videodisk essentially improved decision making merely by highlighting the most important information for making the decision, although this resulted in different decisions being made by both groups. The end result was favorable from a practitioner's point of view: All patients achieved equally positive outcomes, with a 22% lower surgery rate among one of the groups. This indicates that the optimal decision was made both by individuals who elected to have and by those who elected not to have the surgery (Deyo, 2001).

Counterbalance Order of Information

Although older adults are experienced at making many types of decisions, given the cognitive declines that may stand in the way of older adults' ability to consider all alternatives exhaustively, physicians and health care providers presenting older adults with multiple medical alternatives should consider whether information is consistently being presented in the same order and consequently whether one alternative is being given excessive consideration. It appears that even experienced decision makers are prone to being unduly influenced by the last piece of information presented in a series. Thus, care should be taken to present the most important information first or last rather than embedding it in the middle of other information. Furthermore, encouraging patients to engage in self-review in which they continually compare their decisions with their original goal may prevent patients from being overwhelmed by a large amount of intervening information. For example, a patient who is surveying the options in Table 9.1 may proceed through the first five drugs listed (Drugs A–D) and become focused on choosing between traditional oral medications (tablets) without allowing him- or herself to consider either the nasal sprays or the chewable or dissolving medications. Encouraging patients to prioritize their needs (e.g., ease of administration) and to continually evaluate each medication option against these needs may help patients to stay on track and consider a wider range of options rather than being unduly influenced by the first or last medications seen.

Present Valence of Information Positively

Older adults' increased gullibility and increased sensitivity to the "illusion of truth" under conditions of cognitive load suggest that older adults can be misled easily (Skurnik et al., 2005). If older adults are frequent visitors to a particular Web site and are exposed repeatedly to false information, of particular concern is that repeatedly warning older adults that a piece of information is false will "backfire" and that over time this information will gain an illusion of truth. Older adults also may experience some cognitive stress when using new technologies on the Internet or when learning about new technologies from a doctor or a salesperson. In particular, those who interact with older adults should be advised to phrase their directives in terms of positives rather than warning against negative results (e.g., "Take this medication with food" rather than "Don't take this medication on an empty stomach"). Furthermore, older adults should be warned against making quick judgments when they encounter salespeople or vendors on the Web.

Be Sensitive to Numerical Presentation

Given the research reporting that equivalent numerical representations of probabilities, such as percentages and proportions, are not regarded as equivalent by individuals, it is important for physicians to be sensitive to this difference in perception. Specifically, because frequency representations of probability (a 1 in 10 chance) elicit more of an affective reaction than percentage representations (a 10% chance), physicians and other health care providers should consider presenting statistics on long-term survival or mortality rates as percentages to minimize alarm. In contrast, they may wish to present risks associated with unhealthful behaviors such as smoking or failing to monitor blood glucose levels as frequencies (i.e., a 1 in 10 risk vs. a 10% risk) to emphasize patients' personal vulnerability to the ill effects of these behaviors.

Use a "Forced-Choice" Format When Prescribing Health Behaviors

Older adults given the opportunity to defer making a choice will often do so (Calhoun & Hutchison, 1981). Thus, if a physician or health care provider is seeking to institute a healthy behavior into a patient's schedule, he or she may be more successful by offering Option A (adding one vegetable to the diet everyday) or Option B (taking a 15-minute walk everyday) rather than suggesting one option or the other alone. In the latter case, the choice is either "choose A or do nothing" or "choose B or do nothing." Presenting the choice as "choose A or B," however, may increase the chance that at least one of the two desirable behaviors will be performed.

Increase Rehearsal and Practice in Making Decisions

With an increasing number of elderly becoming familiar with the Internet, we suggest that another means to improving medication adherence is simply to encourage older adults to practice the act of making decisions. Honing the automatic component of the process may be especially useful. For example, when older adults are presented with a new set of choices, they may form the following implementation intention to read instructions slowly and carefully: "When my doctor presents me with more than one option, I will stop and read each option out loud slowly and carefully." This may encourage older adults to engage in more deliberative processing and override initial automatic affective feelings or prejudices.

Using the Internet, older adults can also read a variety of health reports about different medical technologies and procedures so that they become accustomed to weighing different information sources and making decisions about their own care. Older adults may have considerably less experience than do younger adults in being active consumers of different types of medical information (Petrisek, Laliberte, Allen, & Mor, 1997). They may also be unaccustomed to having multiple choices and may have less practice in weighing different features to reach a decision. The widespread availability of medical information on the Internet may be an important resource in helping older adults to practice processing information and drawing conclusions from what they have read (Liu & Park, 2003). For example, rather than simply being told to take their medications, older adults can read about drug interactions to learn why some drugs must be taken on an empty stomach and others must be taken with food. In particular, information on the Internet may be especially helpful in highlighting contraindications for certain medicines. A warning sticker on a medication vial may include a brief warning to "avoid sunlight while taking this medication," but additional elaboration of these warnings on the Internet may include a more detailed explanation for why the medication increases the skin's sensitivity to sunlight and could include pictures detailing what can occur if precautions are not taken, both of which can improve an individual's memory for the warning.

CONCLUSIONS

Although the cognitive declines that accompany aging are well documented (Park et al., 1996, 2002), acknowledging that these declines are accompanied by improvements in other cognitive functions provides an important piece of the puzzle of identifying the types of judgments and decisions that are likely to be most problematic for older adults. We have argued in this chapter that decision-making ability does not simply decline over the life span. Although numerous declines in cognition and processing speed occur as individuals age, the preservation of well-practiced, automatic behaviors may explain the classic paradox of cognitive aging that older adults continue to make reasonably good decisions in many domains despite experiencing age-related decline. This perspective has important implications for designing interventions, because it suggests that practitioners who design decision-making aids for older adults should not focus exclusively on compensating for age-related cognitive deficits (e.g., presenting information more slowly or reducing the number of options presented). Rather, interventions should also consider older adults' experience with making a variety of judgments and decisions and highlight general principles that may be useful in guiding decisions across multiple contexts with problems that share a common structure. For example, older adults asked to decide between a generic or full-cost prescription drug could be unduly lured by the widespread brand recognition of the full-cost drug. However, an intervention that encourages them to resist their initial impressions and to take time to review their options could encourage them to think about the common list of active ingredients in both drugs and the similar effects each will have on their health. This decision strategy of waiting and then weighing and prioritizing the features of two different options could then be transferred to other decision contexts. Understanding how different judgments and decisions are more and less sensitive to age-related cognitive decline may help to highlight the best ways in which to present them to older adults and may suggest ways to optimize decision-making efficiency to minimize the negative effects of aging in important situations.

REFERENCES

Appelbaum, P. S., & Grisso, T. (1998). *Assessing competence to consent to treatment: A guide for physicians and other health professionals.* New York: Oxford University Press.

Ashton, R. H., & Kennedy, J. (2002). Eliminating recency with self-review: The case of auditors' "going concern" judgments. *Journal of Behavioral Decision Making, 15,* 221–231.

Baltes, P. B., & Staudinger, U. M. (1993). The search for a psychology of wisdom. *Current Directions in Psychological Science, 2,* 75–80.

Bargh, J. A. (1996). Automaticity in social psychology. In E. T. Higgins & A. W. Kruglanski (Eds.), *Social psychology: Handbook of basic principles* (pp. 169–183). New York: Guilford Press.

Bechara, A., Tranel, D., & Damasio, A. R. (2000). Poor judgment in spite of high intellect: Neurological evidence for emotional intelligence. In R. Bar-On & J. D. A. Parker (Eds.), *The handbook of emotional intelligence: Theory, development, assessment, and application at home, school, and in the workplace* (pp. 192–214). San Francisco: Jossey-Bass.

Beisecker, A. E., & Beisecker, T. D. (1990). Patient information-seeking behaviors when communicating with doctors. *Medical Care, 28,* 19–28.

Blanchard-Fields, F. (1998). The role of emotion in social cognition across the adult life span. In K. W. Schaie & M. P. Lawton (Eds.), *Annual review of gerontology and geriatrics: Vol. 17. Focus on emotion and adult development* (pp. 238–265). New York: Springer.

Brown, S. C., & Park, D. C. (2002). Roles of age and familiarity in learning of health information. *Educational Gerontology, 28,* 695–710.

Calhoun, R. E., & Hutchison, S. L. (1981). Decision-making in old age: Cautiousness and rigidity. *International Journal of Aging and Human Development, 13,* 89–98.

Centers for Disease Control and Prevention. (2003). *Flu in the United States*. Retrieved January 2, 2003, from http://www.cdc.gov/ncidod/diseases/flu/fluvirus. htm

Chapman, G. B., Bergus, G. R., & Elstein, A. S. (1996). Order of information affects clinical judgment. *Journal of Behavioral Decision Making, 9,* 201–211.

Charness, N. (1981). Aging and skilled problem solving. *Journal of Experimental Psychology: General, 110,* 21–38.

Chasseigne, G., Mullet, E., & Stewart, T. R. (1997). Aging and multiple cue probability learning: The case of inverse relationships. *Acta Psychologica, 97,* 235–252.

Craik, F. I. M., & Byrd, M. (1982). Aging and cognitive deficits: The role of attentional resources. In F. I. M. Craik & S. Trehub (Eds.), *Aging and cognitive processes* (pp. 191–211). New York: Plenum Press.

Deyo, R. A. (2001). A key medical decision maker: The patient. *British Medical Journal, 323,* 466–467.

Dror, I. E., Katona, M., & Mungur, K. (1998). Age differences in decision making: To take a risk or not? *Gerontology, 44,* 67–71.

Elstein, A. S. (1999). Heuristics and biases: Selected errors in clinical reasoning. *Academic Medicine, 74,* 791–799.

Finucane, M. L., Alhakami, A., Slovic, P., & Johnson, S. M. (2000). The affect heuristic in judgments of risks and benefits. *Journal of Behavioral Decision Making, 13,* 1–17.

Gigerenzer, G. (1991a). From tools to theories: A heuristic of discovery in cognitive psychology. *Psychological Review, 98,* 254–267.

Gigerenzer, G. (1991b). How to make cognitive illusions disappear: Beyond heuristics and biases. *European Review of Social Psychology, 2,* 83–115.

Gollwitzer, P. M. (1999). Implementation intentions: Strong effects of simple plans. *American Psychologist, 54,* 493–503.

Halter, J. B. (1999). The challenge of communicating health information to elderly patients: A view from geriatric medicine. In D. C. Park, R. W. Morrell, & K. Shifrin (Eds.), *Processing of medical information in aging patients: Cognitive and human factors perspectives* (pp. 23–28). Mahwah, NJ: Erlbaum.

Hamm, V. P., & Hasher, L. (1992). Age and the availability of inferences. *Psychology and Aging, 7,* 56–64.

Hasher, L., & Zacks, R. T. (1988). Working memory, comprehension, and aging: A review and a new view. In G. H. Bower (Ed.), *The psychology of learning and motivation: Advances in research and theory* (Vol. 22, pp. 193–225). San Diego, CA: Academic Press.

Hershey, D. A., & Wilson, J. A. (1997). Age differences in performance awareness on a complex financial decision-making task. *Experimental Aging Research, 23,* 257–273.

Huber, O., Wider, R., & Huber, O. W. (1997). Active information search and complete information presentation in naturalistic risky decision tasks. *Acta Psychologica, 95,* 15–29.

Jacoby, L. L., Jennings, J. M., & Hay, J. F. (1996). Dissociating automatic and consciously controlled processes: Implications for diagnosis and rehabilitation of memory deficits. In D. J. Herrmann, C. L. McEvoy, C. Hertzog, P. Hertel, & M. K. Johnson (Eds.), *Basic and applied memory research: Vol. 1. Theory in context* (pp. 161–193). Mahwah, NJ: Erlbaum.

Johnson, J. E. V., & Bruce, A. C. (1997). A probit model for estimating the effect of complexity on risk taking. *Psychological Reports, 80,* 763–772.

Johnson, M. M. S. (1990). Age differences in decision making: A process methodology for examining strategic information processing. *Journal of Gerontology, 45,* P75–P78.

Johnson, M. M. S., & Drungle, S. C. (2000). Purchasing over-the-counter medications: The influence of age and familiarity. *Experimental Aging Research, 26,* 245–261.

Kahneman, D., Slovic, P., & Tversky, A. (1982). *Judgment under uncertainty: Heuristics and biases.* Cambridge, England: Cambridge University Press.

Kahneman, D., & Tversky, A. (1982). The psychology of preferences. *Scientific American, 246,* 160–173.

Kahneman, D., & Tversky, A. (2000). *Choices, values and frames.* Cambridge, England: Cambridge University Press.

Klaczynski, P. A., & Robinson, B. (2000). Personal theories, intellectual ability, and epistemological beliefs: Adult age differences in everyday reasoning biases. *Psychology and Aging, 15,* 400–416.

Labouvie-Vief, G. (1992). A neo-Piagetian perspective on adult cognitive development. In R. J. Sternberg & C. A. Berg (Eds.), *Intellectual development* (pp. 52–86). New York: Cambridge University Press.

Leventhal, E. A., Leventhal, H., Schaefer, H., & Easterling, D. (1993). Conservation of energy, uncertainty reduction, and swift utilization of medical care among the elderly. *Journal of Gerontology, 48,* P78–P86.

Light, L. L., & Capps, J. L. (1986). Comprehension of pronouns in young and older adults. *Developmental Psychology, 22,* 580–585.

Liu, L. L., & Park, D. C. (2003). Technology and the promise of independent living for older adults: A cognitive perspective. In K. W. Schaie & N. Charness (Eds.), *Impact of technology on successful aging* (pp. 262–289). New York: Springer Publishing Company.

Liu, L. L., & Park, D. C. (2004). Aging and medical adherence: The use of automatic processes to achieve effortful things. *Psychology and Aging, 19,* 318–325.

Loewenstein, G. F., Weber, E. U., Hsee, C. K., & Welch, N. (2001). Risk as feelings. *Psychological Bulletin, 127,* 267–286.

Mather, M., Johnson, M. K., & DeLeonardis, D. M. (1999). Stereotype reliance in source monitoring: Age differences and neuropsychological test correlates. *Cognitive Neuropsychology, 16,* 437–458.

Maule, A. J., Hockey, G. R., & Bdzola, L. (2000). Effects of time-pressure on decision-making under uncertainty: Changes in affective state and information processing strategy. *Acta Psychologica, 104,* 283–301.

Meyer, B. J. F., Russo, C., & Talbot, A. (1995). Discourse comprehension and problem solving: Decisions about the treatment of breast cancer by women across the life span. *Psychology and Aging, 10,* 84–103.

Morrell, R. W., Mayhorn, C. B., & Bennett, J. (2000). A survey of World Wide Web use in middle-aged and older adults. *Human Factors, 42,* 175–182.

Morrell, R. W., Park, D. C., Kidder, D. P., & Martin, M. (1997). Adherence to antihypertensive medications across the lifespan. *The Gerontologist, 37,* 609–617.

Morrell, R. W., Park, D. C., & Poon, L. W. (1989). Quality of instructions on prescription drug labels: Effects on memory and comprehension in young and old adults. *The Gerontologist, 29,* 345–354.

Murphy, K. R. (1989). Is the relationship between cognitive ability and job performance stable over time? *Human Performance, 2,* 183–200.

Mutter, S. A., & Pliske, R. M. (1994). Aging and illusory correlation in judgments of co-occurrence. *Psychology and Aging, 9,* 53–63.

Orbell, S., Hodgkins, S., & Sheeran, P. (1997). Implementation intentions and the theory of planned behavior. *Personality and Social Psychology Bulletin, 23,* 945–954.

Park, D. C. (1994). Aging, cognition, and work. *Human Performance, 7,* 181–205.

Park, D. C. (2000). The basic mechanisms accounting for age-related decline in cognitive function. In D. C. Park & N. Schwarz (Eds.), *Cognitive aging: A primer* (pp. 3–21). Philadelphia: Psychology Press.

Park, D. C., Hertzog, C., Leventhal, H., Morrell, R. W., Leventhal, E., Birchmore, D., et al. (1999). Medication adherence in rheumatoid arthritis patients: Older is wiser. *Journal of the American Geriatrics Society, 47,* 172–183.

Park, D. C., & Kidder, D. P. (1996). Prospective memory and medication adherence. In M. Brandimonte, G. O. Einstein, & M. A. McDaniel (Eds.), *Prospective memory: Theory and applications* (pp. 369–390). Hillsdale, NJ: Erlbaum.

Park, D. C., Lautenschlager, G., Hedden, T., Davidson, N., Smith, A. D., & Smith, P. (2002). Models of visuospatial and verbal memory across the adult life span. *Psychology and Aging, 17,* 299–320.

Park, D. C., Smith, A. D., Lautenschlager, G., Earles, J., Frieske, D., Zwahr, M., & Gaines, C. (1996). Mediators of long-term memory performance across the lifespan. *Psychology and Aging, 11,* 621–637.

Payne, J. W. (1976). Task complexity and contingent processing in decision making: An information search and protocol analysis. *Organizational Behavior and Human Performance, 16,* 366–387.

Peters, E., Finucane, M. L., MacGregor, D. G., & Slovic, P. (2000). Appendix C: The bearable lightness of aging: Judgment and decision processes in older adults. In P. C. Stern & L. L. Carstensen (Eds.), *The aging mind: Opportunities in cognitive research.* Washington, DC: National Academy Press.

Petrisek, A. C., Laliberte, L. L., Allen, S. M., & Mor, V. (1997). The treatment decision-making process: Age differences in a sample of women recently diagnosed with nonrecurrent, early-stage breast cancer. *The Gerontologist, 37,* 598–608.

Raz, N. (2000). Aging of the brain and its impact on cognitive performance: Integration of structural and functional findings. In F. I. M. Craik (Ed.), *The handbook of aging and cognition* (2nd ed., pp. 1–90). Mahwah, NJ: Erlbaum.

Reuter-Lorenz, P. A., Stanczak, L., & Miller, A. C. (1999). Neural recruitment and cognitive aging: Two hemispheres are better than one, especially as you age. *Psychological Science, 10,* 494–500.

Salthouse, T. A. (1984). Effects of age and skill in typing. *Journal of Experimental Psychology: General, 113,* 345–371.

Salthouse, T. A. (1987). Age, experience, and compensation. In C. Schooler (Ed.), *Cognitive functioning and social structure over the life course* (pp. 142–157). Stamford, CT: Ablex.

Salthouse, T. A. (1996). The processing-speed theory of adult age differences in cognition. *Psychological Review, 103,* 403–428.

Salthouse, T. A., & Babcock, R. L. (1991). Decomposing adult age differences in working memory. *Developmental Psychology, 27,* 763–776.

Salthouse, T. A., & Somberg, B. L. (1982). Skilled performance: The effects of adult age and experience on elementary processes. *Journal of Experimental Psychology: General, 111,* 176–207.

Sanfey, A. G., & Hastie, R. (2000). Judgment and decision making across the adult life span: A tutorial review of psychological research. In D. C. Park & N. Schwarz (Eds.), *Cognitive aging: A primer* (pp. 253–273). Philadelphia: Psychology Press.

Scheibel, A. B. (1996). Structural and functional changes in the aging brain. In J. E. Birren (Ed.), *Handbook of the psychology of aging* (4th ed., pp. 105–128). San Diego, CA: Academic Press.

Schwarz, N., & Clore, G. L. (1996). Feelings and phenomenal experiences. In E. T. Higgins & A. Kruglanski (Eds.), *Social psychology: Handbook of basic principles* (pp. 433–465). New York: Guilford Press.

Schwarz, N., & Knäuper, B. (2000). Cognition, aging, and self-reports. In D. Park & N. Schwarz (Eds.), *Cognitive aging: A primer* (pp. 233–252). Philadelphia: Psychology Press.

Sen, A. K. (1971). *Behaviour and the concept of preference.* London: London School of Economics and Political Science.

Simonson, I., & Tversky, A. (1992). Choice in context: Tradeoff contrast and extremeness aversion. *Journal of Marketing Research, 29,* 281–287.

Sinnott, J. D. (1989). *Everyday problem solving: Theory and applications*. New York: Praeger Publishers.

Skurnik, I., Yoon, C., Park, D. C., & Schwarz, N. (2005). How warnings about false claims become recommendations. *Journal of Consumer Research, 31*, 713–724.

Taylor, R. N. (1975). Age and experience as determinants of managerial information processing and decision making performance. *Academy of Management Journal, 18*, 74–81.

Tentori, K., Osherson, D., Hasher, L., & May, C. (2001). Wisdom and aging: Irrational preferences in college students but not older adults. *Cognition, 81*, B87–B96.

Tversky, A., & Kahneman, D. (1974, September 27). Judgment under uncertainty: Heuristics and biases. *Science, 185*, 1124–1131.

Tversky, A., & Kahneman, D. (1983). Extensional versus intuitive reasoning: The conjunction fallacy in probability judgment. *Psychological Review, 90*, 293–315.

Tymchuk, A. J., Ouslander, J. G., Rahbar, B., & Fitten, J. (1988). Medical decision-making among elderly people in long term care. *The Gerontologist, 28*(Suppl.), 59–63.

Verplanken, B., & Faes, S. (1999). Good intentions, bad habits, and effects of forming implementation intentions on healthy eating. *European Journal of Social Psychology, 29*, 591–604.

Von Neumann, J., & Morgenstern, O. (1947). *Theory of games and economic behavior* (2nd ed.). Princeton, NJ: Princeton University Press.

Webster, D. M., Richter, L., & Kruglanski, A. W. (1996). On leaping to conclusions when feeling tired: Mental fatigue effects on impressional primacy. *Journal of Experimental Social Psychology, 32*, 181–195.

Wilson, T. D., & Schooler, J. W. (1991). Thinking too much: Introspection can reduce the quality of preferences and decisions. *Journal of Personality and Social Psychology, 60*, 181–192.

Yates, J. F., & Patalano, A. L. (1999). Decision making and aging. In D. C. Park, R. W. Morrell, & K. Shifren (Eds.), *Processing of medical information in aging patients: Cognitive and human factors perspectives* (pp. 31–54). Mahwah, NJ: Erlbaum.

Ybarra, O., Chan, E., & Park, D. C. (2001). Young and old adults' concerns about morality and competence. *Motivation and Emotion, 25*, 85–100.

Ybarra, O., & Park, D. C. (2002). Disconfirmation of person expectations by older and younger adults: Implications for social vigilance. *Journals of Gerontology Series B: Psychological Sciences and Social Sciences, 57*, P435–P443.

Zwahr, M. D., Park, D. C., & Shifren, K. (1999). Judgments about estrogen replacement therapy: The role of age, cognitive abilities, and beliefs. *Psychology and Aging, 14*, 179–191.

IV

TECHNOLOGY AND TREATMENT

10

CUSTOMIZED COMMUNICATION IN PATIENT EDUCATION

MATTHEW W. KREUTER, RICARDO WRAY,
AND CHARLENE CABURNAY

Innovative technology-based approaches to patient education are now being used to enhance adherence to health-related behaviors, medical regimens, and provider instructions. In this chapter, we describe this development, define customized communication and describe the dominant approaches to achieving it, illustrate its applications in health care settings, discuss its roots in theories of information processing and persuasion, and provide recommendations for patient education using this approach.

ENHANCING INFORMATION RELEVANCE TO IMPROVE PATIENT EDUCATION

A major objective in developing or delivering health information to patients is to maximize its relevance to each recipient. Lasswell's (1948) well-known description of communication as *who* says *what* through *which* channel to *whom* and with *what* effect (Lasswell, 1948) provides a useful, if simple, framework for considering how relevance can be achieved in patient education. When planning educational efforts or developing informational materials, every decision made about the source, message, channel, and receiver can influence the extent to which the communication is perceived by the patient as personally relevant and, in turn, whether the information is attended to and effective in achieving its intended objectives. For example, a message source should be perceived as credible by a certain audience for delivering certain kinds of information (Simons, Berkowitz, & Moyer, 1970; Sternthal, Phillips, & Dholakia, 1978), and a message channel should be familiar, comfortable, and accessible to that audience (O'Keefe, Hartwig Boyd, & Brown, 1998; Schooler, Chaffee, Flora, & Roser, 1998). The message content itself can also enhance the relevance of a communication by addressing certain issues in a certain context that reflects awareness of receivers' situation or circumstance. Most recent innovations in patient education have involved either new message delivery channels (e.g., the Internet) or customized content (e.g., tailored messages; Kreuter, Farrell, Olevitch, & Brennan, 1999).

This chapter focuses on the latter of these innovations—new approaches to enhancing information relevance by customizing message content. As in most population subgroups, there is great individual variation among older adults. Because the sources of this variation, which include individual differences in demographic characteristics, acculturation, concerns and fears, health practices, lifestyles, risk factors and disease status, and sources of information, can directly affect adherence to medical regimens, patient education efforts that customize information to match each individual's unique profile should be more effective (Bartlett, 2002; Jamieson et al., 2002; King, Martin, Morrell, Arena, & Boland, 1986; Schnare, 2001; Sennott-Miller, May, & Miller, 1998; Sheikh & Salzman, 1995).

APPROACHES TO CUSTOMIZING HEALTH INFORMATION

Health information ranges from generic (i.e., not customized) to targeted (i.e., designed in response to group characteristics or risk factors) to tailored (i.e., designed in response to individual characteristics or risk factors). Generic materials are typically designed for a general audience and at their best reflect best-practice approaches to design. A best-practice approach utilizes appropriate application of textual and graphic design principles, using plain language and aiming to maximize comprehension and appeal (National Cancer Institute, 1994). We distinguish between two conceptually similar but operationally different approaches to customization: targeted and tailored communication. Both seek to enhance information relevance by presenting messages that address the unique needs of a defined audience, and both base this customization on audience analysis. Whereas targeted communication is directed toward homogeneous groups within the general population, tailored communication is directed toward specific individuals (Kreuter & Skinner, 2000). Traditional approaches to health information, education, and communication, including print materials and mass-mediated campaigns, have typically followed the principles of audience segmentation and have been consistent with a targeted approach. Advances in computer technology during the 1990s made it not only possible but also practical to gather individual-level data from large populations and to use that information to tailor educational and behavior change materials to individuals' unique needs (Kreuter, Strecher, & Glassman, 1999). Operating at the individual level, tailored materials gain the persuasive power of interpersonal communication in that they can respond to a far greater number of constructs and risk factors.

Targeted Communication

Targeted communication is guided by principles of market segmentation, which aim to find a specific group of consumers for a particular product or service (Weinstein, 1994). As applied to the development of patient education materials or other health information, this means the content and presentation of targeted information are based on an understanding of the needs and concerns of a given group of patients or audience segment (Slater, 1996). Similarly, materials are designed according to individual risk factors or theoretically based characteristics, such as self-efficacy. Once an audience segment has been defined, a communication approach can be developed on the basis of a descriptive profile of that segment. With targeted communication, the resulting messages are typically the same for all members of the audience segment.

Strictly generic materials are increasingly rare, because thoughtful patient education planners typically have some audience segment in mind when producing even generic materials. There can be wide variation in the way a segment is defined, and thus the extent and precision of the message targeting varies as well. At the simplest level, segments are defined on the basis of demographic characteristics such as age, race, or sex. This approach might, for example, lead to creating a self-help smoking cessation manual especially for African Americans (Fox Chase Cancer Center, 1992) or breast and cervical cancer screening materials for middle-aged and older women (National Cancer Institute, 1996). Although an improvement over generic information, some targeted communications are based only on simplistic segmentation strategies and, as a result, run the risk of mistaking external attributes (e.g., race) for more complicated and meaningful characteristics (e.g., culture; Kreuter, Lukwago, Bucholtz, Clark, & Sanders-Thompson, 2003). In contrast, some segmentation strategies can be quite detailed, defining population subgroups not just by demographics but also by behavioral, psychosocial, and geographic characteristics or risk factors (Slater, 1996; Weinstein, 1994). Audience segmentation is a well-accepted best practice in health communication based on decades of experience and research (Slater, 1995). Evaluation of targeted materials have generally reported positive results (Davis, Cummings, Rimer, Sciandra, & Stone, 1992; Drossaert, Boer, & Seydel, 1996; Morgan et al., 1996; Rimer & Orleans, 1994; Rimer et al., 1994), including some studies in which the target audience was defined as older adults. Although these studies mistakenly used the terms *tailored* and *targeted* interchangeably (Kreuter & Skinner, 2000), they reported that smoking cessation materials created specifically for smokers ages 50 to 74 were rated more favorably, read more often, and led to higher quit rates than materials that were not targeted to this group (Rimer & Orleans, 1994; Rimer et al., 1994).

Tailored Communication

In contrast to targeted messages that address specific groups of people, tailored messages are intended to reach one specific person. Where targeted communications are based on the profile of a given audience segment, tailored communications are based on the unique characteristics of that one person. To generate such messages, tailored communication requires gathering information about each individual recipient, processing it to determine which messages will best address the person's needs, and generating a communication that conveys that information. In the past 2 decades, computer technologies have made it possible to automate this process using a combination of database and design software (Kreuter, Farrell, et al., 1999). Such computer tailoring programs can easily process large amounts of information in very short periods of time, thus allowing individualized health information to be delivered on a mass scale. Typically, individuals provide personal data that are related to a given health outcome of interest, and those data are examined by algorithms or decision rules in the computer database that determine the most appropriate information or strategies from a library of messages to meet each person's unique needs.

To date, tailored patient education programs have relied heavily on constructs from well-established theories of health behavior as the basis for tailoring messages to promote behavioral change (Kreuter & Holt, 2001). A typical tailoring program might assess individuals' stage of readiness to change (Prochaska & DiClemente, 1983), perceived barriers (Becker, 1974), or self-efficacy (Bandura, 1977) for changing a given behavior and then provide messages to each program participant that address his or her specific stage, barriers, and level of self efficacy. Kreuter, Skinner, et al. (2004) have termed this approach *behavioral construct tailoring* and noted that the evidence base that supports the use of tailored health communication has been built almost solely on intervention studies in which such an approach to tailoring was used (Brug, 1999; Skinner, Campbell, Rimer, Curry, & Prochaska, 1999; Strecher, 1999).

APPLICATIONS OF TAILORED PATIENT EDUCATION PROGRAMS IN HEALTH CARE SETTINGS

To date, few studies have examined the effects of tailored patient education programs among older adult populations. In one exception, Hussey (1994) examined medication compliance among 80 low-income, low-literate, predominantly indigent older adults who received verbal teaching and a medication regimen that either was or was not tailored to the individual's daily schedule. Compliance increased most among those whose scores were low at baseline and who received the tailored regimen (Hussey, 1994). Other studies have also reported positive effects of tailored patient education on screening behaviors (e.g., mammography; Skinner, Strecher, & Hospers, 1994) and management of chronic conditions (e.g., asthma; Thoonen et al., 2002) that certainly apply to older adult populations. We fully expect that tailored patient education will be effective among older adult populations and encourage studies that will help fill this gap.

In the absence of such studies, this section describes other applications of customized communication within clinic-based patient education programs. These programs are conducted either by organizations outside the health care setting or by existing health care staff. The section also discusses the role of health care providers in enhancing the effects of customized communication.

Applications of Clinic-Based Programs

The ABC Immunization Calendar® (Health Communication Research Laboratory & DSA Inc., 1997) program creates computer-tailored monthly calendars for babies ages birth to 2 years. It was designed to promote childhood immunization among new parents by recognizing the value of parents' efforts to follow immunization schedules and providing incentives to encourage them to return. The monthly calendars are full color, tabloid sized (11 inches × 17 inches), and include the following: (a) information about home safety, injury prevention, clinical preventive services, parenting skills, and child development; (b) baby's height and weight; (c) a digital picture of the baby; and (d) a reminder of the baby's next immunization appointment. The content of each monthly calendar is age targeted as well as individually tailored to each specific baby on the basis of information obtained from parents in a brief enrollment interview conducted at the clinic. Calendars are printed immediately; the entire process takes less than 5 minutes. Parents receive calendars for only the months leading up to their baby's next scheduled immunization. When parents return for the baby's next immunization, the baby's picture and other information are updated, and new calendars are printed for the months leading up to the next visit. In a yearlong trial to test the effectiveness of the calendar program, parents of babies ages birth to 1 year ($N = 321$) from 2 urban public health centers in St. Louis, Missouri, received the calendar program. For each baby, an age- and sex-matched control was selected from the same center. Immunization status was tracked through age 24 months. Results found that a significantly higher proportion of intervention than control babies were up to date at the end of a 9-month enrollment period (82% vs. 65%) and at age 24 months (66% vs. 47%; Kreuter, Caburnay, Chen, & Donlin, 2004). Since completion of the study, 6 public health centers in St. Louis, Missouri, and East St. Louis, Illinois, and 12 centers in New York City have adopted the program and are running it with existing health center staff members.

In some clinic-based patient education programs, the patient receives tailored health information by directly interacting with the tailoring program through a computer kiosk. In one such program, Baby, Be Safe!, a computer kiosk located in the waiting room assesses home injury risks among parents of young children and provides them with tailored feedback to reduce these risks. When parents have completed the assessment on the computer, the kiosk immediately prints tailored feedback for the parent to read before being called in to see the doctor. In a Washington, DC, clinic, 213 parents of children ages 6 through 20 months used the kiosk and by random assignment received tailored or generic feedback on home and car safety. At a 3-week follow-up, those receiving tailored feedback were more likely than those receiving generic feedback to have decided to adopt new safety practices (81% vs. 64%), to have actually adopted some practices (65% vs. 41%), and to have had a greater reduction in overall injury risk score (−4.7 vs. −1.5; Nansel et al., 2002).

When it is not possible for the patient to interact directly with the tailoring computer programs, the initial clinical encounter is often used as an opportunity to gather patient information needed to generate tailored materials for delivery at another time. Programs are typically structured in this way when patient information is being processed and tailored materials are being created by a central source located outside the clinic that may be serving multiple provider groups with no relation to one another. In such programs, patient information can be gathered though self-administered paper-and-pencil surveys or medical records data, which are passed along to the central source. When these data have been processed, and tailored materials have been generated, they are sent to patients by mail or e-mail, accessed through Web sites, or delivered by phone counselors. Such approaches have been used to increase healthful dietary habits (Campbell et al., 1994), mammography use (Skinner et al., 1994), smoking cessation (Strecher et al., 1994), and physical activity (Bull, Kreuter, & Scharff, 1999).

As an example, Campbell et al. (1994) assessed the effects of providing tailored nutrition education materials to patients in primary care settings. From four family practices, 558 adult patients completed a self-administered survey while in the family practice office and were then randomly assigned to one of three study groups: a group that received tailored nutrition messages, a group that received nontailored nutrition messages based on the *Dietary Guidelines for Americans* (U.S. Department of Agriculture & U.S. Department of Health and Human Services, 1990), and a control group that did not receive any nutrition messages. The tailored intervention consisted of nutrition education newsletters that were tailored to a participant's dietary intake, stage of change, and psychosocial information. All newsletters were mailed to participants within 3 weeks of completing the baseline survey. At a 3-month follow-up survey, participants who were sent the tailored newsletters were more likely than the nontailored group to remember receiving the newsletter and to have read all of it. Participants in the tailored group also significantly reduced their total fat and saturated fat intakes compared with the control group (percentage reduction in total fat: 23% vs. 3%; in saturated fat: 26% vs. 3%).

Role of Health Care Providers in Enhancing Effects of Customized Communication

The strong association between receiving physician advice and subsequent patient behavior change is well documented. What is less well known is whether advice from a health care provider might also enhance the effects of other patient education efforts. To help answer this question, we undertook a study to examine how physician advice to quit smoking, eat less fat, and exercise more often influenced patients who did and did not receive patient education materials on these same topics. In the study, we assessed smoking, dietary, and exercise behaviors among 493 adult primary care patients and provided patient education materials that matched each patient's needs according to his or her risk factors (i.e., a cigarette smoker would receive smoking cessation materials). We also assessed whether each patient had been told by his or her doctor to quit smoking, eat less fat, or exercise more often prior to receiving the patient education materials.

Analyses compared patients who received physician advice that was concordant with the materials they received with a second group of patients who either received (a) educational materials but not physician advice or (b) educational materials and physician advice that were not concordant. At a 3-month follow-up, patients who had received physician advice prior to receiving concordant educational materials were significantly more likely to report that the materials "applied to me" (44% vs. 31%) and to show the materials to others (51% vs. 34%). They were also significantly more likely to report trying to quit smoking (49% vs. 24%), quitting smoking for at least 24 hours (35% vs. 13%), increasing leisure time physical activity (64% vs. 48%), and reducing fat intake from dairy sources (47% vs. 33%; see Kreuter, Chheda, & Bull, 2000).

Evidence from the aforementioned Baby, Be Safe! program also suggests that physician advice may have a priming effect on patients' use of educational materials. Among all parents in the study, those who received tailored injury prevention materials from the computer kiosk in the waiting room had significantly greater reductions in an injury risk score than did parents who received nontailored materials (−4.7 vs. −1.5). Among those parents who reported that their doctor also talked to them about injury risks during their visit, the magnitude of this reduction doubled (−10 vs. −3), regardless of which type of materials they received (Nansel et al., 2002). These findings have stimulated a replication and extension study, Safe 'n' Sound, in which one group received tailored patient materials, a second group received nontailored materials, and a third group received tailored materials for both the patient and provider. Findings showed that tailored materials were again more effective than nontailored materials, but adding tailored provider prompts did not enhance these effects (Nansel, Weaver, Jacobsen, Glasheen, & Kreuter, in press).

HOW DOES CUSTOMIZED COMMUNICATION WORK?

The elaboration likelihood model (ELM) from Petty and Cacioppo (1981) is a theory of information processing that has received increasing attention in the health promotion literature and provides a theoretical rationale for understanding effects of customized communication like targeting and tailoring. According to ELM, individuals are more likely to process information actively and thoughtfully (i.e., central route processing) if they are motivated and able to process it thoroughly. A principal determinant of motivation is the individual's perception of the relevance of the information. The model proposes that with central route processing, people consider messages carefully, relating them to other information they have encountered and comparing them with their own past experiences. Messages elaborated in this way have been shown to be retained for a longer period of time and are more likely to lead to permanent behavior change (Petty, Cacioppo, Strathman, & Priester, 1994). A rationale for using customized communication follows from this theory and has been summarized in a five-part logic sequence (Kreuter & Holt, 2001): (a) By customizing materials to specific audiences or individuals, superfluous information will be eliminated; (b) the information that remains will be more personally relevant to the recipient; (c) individuals will pay more attention to information they perceive to be personally relevant; (d) information that is attended to is more likely to have an effect than that which is not; and (e) when attended to, information that addresses the unique needs of individuals will help them to become and stay motivated, acquire new skills, and enact and sustain desired lifestyle changes. We would expect, therefore, that patient education programs and materials using customized approaches to health communication will be more likely to lead to behavior change. Following the persuasive steps to behavior change introduced by McGuire (1989), customized communication might elicit greater attention, comprehension, discussion with others, change in cognitive–behavioral mediating constructs (i.e., behavioral intention), and actual behavior change. Findings from tailored patient education interventions in health care settings have generally been consistent with these expectations (Brug, 1999; Kreuter & Holt, 2001; Strecher, 1999).

In a search of the literature, no studies were found that compared the fit of the ELM in different age groups. One study of information processing about drug advertisements in an older adult population compared the relative effects of common ELM variables: credibility of the source, involvement in the topic, and information content of the ads. This experimental study found that in high-involvement conditions, the information content of the ads affected attitudes regardless of credibility. Consistent with research in other age groups, this result suggests that involvement in the topic is also important in an elderly population (Brug, 1999).

To determine whether, as would be predicted by ELM, tailored patient education materials indeed stimulate greater cognitive activity, we conducted a laboratory-based experiment. A community-based sample of overweight adult men and women ($N = 198$) was randomly assigned to receive either tailored or nontailored printed materials on weight loss. Each participant completed a brief survey about his or her weight-related goals, beliefs, and behaviors and then received one of three types of weight loss materials. The first was tailored specifically to his or her responses on the survey. The second was a generic preprinted brochure on weight loss from the American Heart Association (AHA). The third had the same content as the second but was formatted to look like the tailored materials. Inclusion of this third study group provided a mechanism for determining the extent to which content or some other attribute (e.g., design) of the tailored messages was driving any differences in outcomes. If the first and third groups were similar in their information processing and both surpassed the second, we would conclude that effects of tailoring were due more to peripheral route processing (i.e., relying on simple cues such as formatting of the material or attractiveness) than central route processing.

Information processing was measured immediately after participants had received and read their weight loss materials using a thought-listing task. Participants self-rated each idea or thought on their list as positive, neutral, or negative (i.e., polarity). These thoughts were then coded by the project team on four criteria: personal connections to the materials (the extent to which the participants related the material to their lives or to themselves), self-assessment thoughts (the extent to which the participants evaluated themselves in some way), self-efficacy thoughts (the extent to which the thought reflected efficacy beliefs or confidence), and thoughts indicating behavioral intention (the extent to which the thought reflected intention to engage in weight loss behaviors). Findings showed that those who received tailored materials, compared with those who received AHA or AHA formatted materials, listed more positive thoughts about the materials (5.73 vs. 3.96 vs. 4.38), made more positive personal connections to the materials (3.08 vs. 1.79 vs. 1.78), and had more positive self-assessment thoughts (3.25 vs. 1.60 vs. 1.62) and thoughts indicating behavior intention (1.88 vs. 0.74 vs. 0.79), respectively (Kreuter, Bull, Clark, & Oswald, 1999). These thoughts were also associated with attempts to modify weight-related behaviors 1 month later.

These findings suggest that customizing health information to address an individual's unique needs can significantly improve the chances that the information will be thoughtfully considered by the recipient and may even stimulate prebehavioral changes such as self-assessment and intention. However, if ELM is correct that central route processing is stimulated by personally relevant materials, we would also expect to see greater processing not just for tailored materials but also for nontailored materials that were— purely by chance—well suited to a particular individual. To explore this possibility, we classified participants into good-fit, moderate-fit, and poor-fit groups based on the extent to which their weight loss needs matched the goals stated in the generic AHA materials. The goodness of fit was calculated as the proportion of matches (out of 17 possible) between their self-reported weight loss needs and the needs addressed in the AHA materials (17 needs were identified through a content analysis of the text; Kreuter, Oswald, Bull, & Clark, 2000). Findings showed that good-fitting nontailored materials performed as well as or better than tailored materials for a variety of cognitive, affective, and behavioral outcomes, but moderate- and poor-fitting nontailored materials were inferior to both approaches. Thus, we find tailoring-like effects on information processing among nontailored communication that fits an individual well purely by happenstance.

As health care systems increasingly reflect a patient-centered or consumer-driven approach, patient education materials also take on an increasingly important role in clinical care. One example of this is the recommendation that decision aids be used to enhance shared decision making between providers and patients, especially for clinical decisions involving uncertainty (Chan, 2001; Charles, Gafni, & Whelan, 1997; Llewellyn-Thomas, 1995; Rimer et al., 2001). Although materials may provide generic information related to a specific decision (e.g., prostate cancer screening), the concept of shared decision making by definition invokes a customized interpersonal interaction in which the provider and patient share information, preferences, and values to reach a negotiated, mutually agreeable decision (Chan, 2001).

CONCLUSIONS

Patient education programs and materials that are customized to the unique needs of individuals appear to be more effective than generic approaches, perhaps because they stimulate greater cognitive processing of health information. The addition of physician advice that is concordant with the focus of patient education materials seems to further enhance the effects of patient education materials, though tailored physician prompts may not stimulate change in provider behavior. Taken together, these findings suggest a need for coordinated systems of patient education in which information is routinely gathered from patients and used to generate not only customized communication for that patient but also information for use by the providers who will interact with the patient. By providing their patients with strong, clear, and simple advice to make specific changes and pay attention to the educational materials they will receive for help in doing so, providers can become more effective catalysts for change.

REFERENCES

Bandura, A. (1977). Self-efficacy: Toward a unifying theory of behavior change. *Psychology Review, 84,* 191–215.

Bartlett, J. (2002). Addressing the challenges of adherence. *Journal of Acquired Immune Deficiency Syndromes, 29*(Suppl. 1), S2–S10.

Becker, M. (1974). The health belief model and personal health behavior. *Health Education Monographs, 2,* 324–473.

Brug, J. (1999). Dutch research into development and impact of computer-tailored nutrition education. *European Journal of Clinical Nutrition, 53*(Suppl. 2), S78–S82.

Bull, F., Kreuter, M., & Scharff, D. (1999). Effects of tailored, personalized, and general materials on physical activity. *Patient Education and Counseling, 36,* 181–192.

Campbell, M., DeVellis, B., Strecher, V., Ammerman, A., DeVellis, R., & Sandler, R. (1994). Improving dietary behavior: The effectiveness of tailored messages in primary care settings. *American Journal of Public Health, 84,* 783–787.

Chan, E. (2001). Promoting informed decision making about prostate cancer screening. *Comprehensive Therapy, 27,* 195–201.

Charles, C., Gafni, A., & Whelan, T. (1997). Shared decision-making in the medical encounter: What does it mean? (Or it takes at least two to tango). *Social Science and Medicine, 44,* 681–692.

Davis, S., Cummings, K., Rimer, B., Sciandra, R., & Stone, J. (1992). The impact of tailored self-help smoking cessation guides on young mothers. *Health Education Quarterly, 19,* 495–504.

Drossaert, C., Boer, H., & Seydel, E. (1996). Health education to improve repeat participation in the Dutch breast cancer screening programme: Evaluation of a leaflet tailored to previous participants. *Patient Education and Counseling, 28,* 121–131.

Fox Chase Cancer Center. (1992). *Pathways to freedom: Winning the fight against tobacco.* Philadelphia: Author.

Health Communication Research Laboratory, & DSA Inc. (1997). ABC Immunization Calendar (Version 1.0) [computer program]. St Louis, MO: Health Communication Research Laboratory.

Hussey, L. (1994). Minimizing effects of low literacy on medication knowledge and compliance among the elderly. *Clinical Nursing Research, 3,* 132–145.

Jamieson, M., Wilcox, S., Webster, W., Blackhurst, D., Valois, R., & Durstine, J. (2002). Factors influencing health-related quality of life in cardiac rehabilitation patients. *Progress in Cardiovascular Nursing, 17,* 124–131.

King, A., Martin, J., Morrell, E., Arena, J., & Boland, M. (1986). Highlighting specific patient education needs in an aging cardiac population. *Health Education Quarterly, 13,* 29–38.

Kreuter, M., Bull, F., Clark, E., & Oswald, D. (1999). Understanding how people process health information: A comparison of tailored and untailored weight loss materials. *Health Psychology, 18,* 487–494.

Kreuter, M., Caburnay, C., Chen, J., & Donlin, M. (2004). Effectiveness of individually tailored calendars in promoting childhood immunization in urban public health centers. *American Journal of Public Health, 94,* 122–127.

Kreuter, M., Chheda, S., & Bull, F. (2000). How does physician advice influence patient behavior? Evidence for a priming effect. *Archives of Family Medicine, 9,* 426–433.

Kreuter, M., Farrell, D., Olevitch, L., & Brennan, L. (1999). *Tailoring health messages: Customizing communication with computer technology.* Mahwah, NJ: Erlbaum.

Kreuter, M., & Holt, C. (2001). How do people process health information? Applications in an age of individualized communication. *Current Directions in Psychological Science, 10,* 206–209.

Kreuter, M., Lukwago, S., Bucholtz, D., Clark, E., & Sanders-Thompson, V. (2003). Achieving cultural appropriateness in health promotion programs: Targeted and tailored approaches. *Health Education and Behavior, 30*, 133–146.

Kreuter, M., Oswald, D., Bull, F., & Clark, E. (2000). Are tailored health education materials always more effective than non-tailored materials? *Health Education Research, 15*, 305–315.

Kreuter, M., & Skinner, C. (2000). Tailoring: What's in a name? [Editorial]. *Health Education Research, 15*, 1–4.

Kreuter, M., Skinner, C., Steger-May, K., Clark, E., Holt, C., Bucholtz, D., & Haire-Joshu, D. (2004). Reactions to behaviorally vs. culturally tailored cancer communication among African American women. *American Journal of Health Behavior, 28*, 195–207.

Kreuter, M., Strecher, V., & Glassman, B. (1999). One size does not fit all: The case for tailoring print materials. *Annals of Behavioral Medicine, 21*, 276–283.

Lasswell, H. (1948). The structure and function of communication in society. In L. Bryson (Ed.), *The communication of ideas* (pp. 32–51). New York: Harper.

Llewellyn-Thomas, H. (1995). Patients' health-care decision making: A framework for descriptive and experimental investigations. *Medical Decision Making, 15*, 101–106.

McGuire, W. (1989). Theoretical foundations of campaigns. In R. Rice & C. Atkin (Eds.), *Public communication campaigns* (2nd ed., pp. 43–65). Newbury Park, CA: Sage.

Morgan, G., Noll, E., Orleans, C., Rimer, B., Amfoh, K., Phil, M., & Bonney, G. (1996). Reaching mid-life and older smokers: Tailored interventions for routine medical care. *Preventive Medicine, 25*, 346–354.

Nansel, T., Weaver, N., Donlin, M., Jacobsen, H., Kreuter, M., & Simons-Morton, B. (2002). Baby, Be Safe: The effect of pediatric injury prevention tailored communications provided in a primary care setting. *Patient Education and Counseling, 46*, 175–190.

Nansel, T., Weaver, N., Jacobsen, H. A., Glasheen, C., & Kreuter, M. W. (in press). Preventing unintentional pediatric injuries: A tailored intervention for parents and providers. *Patient Education and Counseling.*

National Cancer Institute. (1994). *Clear and simple: Developing effective print materials for low-literate readers* (NIH Publication No. 95-3594). Bethesda, MD: National Institute of Health.

National Cancer Institute. (1996). *Chances are . . . you need a mammogram: A guide for midlife and older women.* Bethesda, MD: National Institutes of Health.

O'Keefe, G., Hartwig Boyd, H., & Brown, M. (1998). Who learns preventive health care information from where: Cross-channel and repertoire comparisons. *Health Communication, 10*, 25–36.

Petty, R., & Cacioppo, J. (1981). *Attitudes and persuasion: Classic and contemporary approaches.* Dubuque, IA: W. C. Brown.

Petty, R., Cacioppo, J., Strathman, A., & Priester, J. (1994). To think or not to think: Exploring two routes to persuasion. In S. Shavitt & T. Brock (Eds.), *Persuasion: Psychological insights and perspectives* (pp. 113–147). Boston: Allyn & Bacon.

Prochaska, J., & DiClemente, C. (1983). Stages and processes of self-change for smoking: Toward an integrative model of change. *Journal of Consulting and Clinical Psychology, 51*, 390–395.

Rimer, B., Halabi, S., Skinner, C., Kaplan, E., Crawford, Y., Samsa, G., et al. (2001). The short-term impact of tailored mammography decision-making interventions. *Patient Education and Counseling, 43*, 269–285.

Rimer, B., & Orleans, C. (1994). Tailoring smoking cessation for older adults. *CANCER Supplement, 74*, 2051–2054.

Rimer, B., Orleans, C., Fleisher, L., Cristinzio, S., Resch, N., Telepchak, J., & Keintz, M. (1994). Does tailoring matter? The impact of a tailored guide on ratings and short-term smoking-related outcomes for older smokers. *Health Education Quarterly, 9*, 69–84.

Schnare, S. (2001). Patient communication in hormone therapy. *International Journal of Fertility and Women's Medicine, 46*, 24–30.

Schooler, C., Chaffee, S., Flora, J., & Roser, C. (1998). Health campaign channels: Tradeoffs among reach, specificity, and impact. *Human Communication Research, 24*, 410–432.

Sennott-Miller, L., May, K., & Miller, J. (1998). Demographic and health status indicators to guide health promotion for Hispanic and Anglo rural elderly. *Patient Education and Counseling, 33*, 13–23.

Sheikh, J., & Salzman, C. (1995). Anxiety in the elderly. Course and treatment. *Psychiatric Clinics of North America, 18*, 874–883.

Simons, H., Berkowitz, N., & Moyer, R. (1970). Similarity, credibility, and attitude change: A review and a theory. *Psychological Bulletin, 73*, 1–16.

Skinner, C., Campbell, M., Rimer, B., Curry, J., & Prochaska, J. (1999). How effective is tailored print communication? *Annals of Behavioral Medicine, 21*, 290–298.

Skinner, C., Strecher, V., & Hospers, H. (1994). Physicians' recommendations for mammography: Do tailored messages make a difference? *American Journal of Public Health, 84*, 43–49.

Slater, M. D. (1995). Choosing audience segmentation strategies and methods for health communication. In E. Maibach & R. Parrott (Eds.), *Designing health messages: Approaches from communication theory and public health practice* (pp. 186–198). Thousand Oaks, CA: Sage.

Slater, M. D. (1996). Theory and method in health audience segmentation. *Journal of Health Communication, 1*, 267–283.

Sternthal, B., Phillips, L., & Dholakia, R. (1978). The persuasive effect of source credibility: A situational analysis. *Public Opinion Quarterly, 42*, 285–314.

Strecher, V. (1999). Computer-tailored smoking cessation materials: A review and discussion. *Patient Education and Counseling, 36*, 107–117.

Strecher, V., Kreuter, M., Den Boer, D., Kobrin, S., Hospers, H., & Skinner, C. (1994). The effects of computer-tailored smoking cessation messages in family practice settings. *Journal of Family Practice, 39*, 262–270.

Thoonen, B., Schermer, T., Jansen, M., Smeele, I., Jacobs, A., Grol, R., & van Schayck, O. (2002). Asthma education tailored to individual patient needs can optimize partnerships in asthma self-management. *Patient Education and Counseling, 47*, 355–360.

U.S. Department of Agriculture & U.S. Department of Health and Human Services. (1990). *Nutrition and your health: Dietary guidelines for Americans* (Home and Garden Bulletin 232, 3rd ed.). Washington, DC: U.S. Department of Agriculture.

Weinstein, A. (1994). *Market segmentation: Using demographics, psychographics and other niche marketing techniques to predict and model customer behavior*. Chicago: Probus.

11

HELPING PATIENTS FOLLOW THEIR DOCTOR'S INSTRUCTIONS: MATCHING INSTRUCTIONAL MEDIA TO TASK DEMANDS

ANNE COLLINS McLAUGHLIN, WENDY A. ROGERS,
AND ARTHUR D. FISK

Bill is a 70-year-old man who has epilepsy. To treat this condition, he has to take a particular medication four times a day. Bill finds it difficult to remember when he should take the medicine or how to adjust the schedule if he sleeps later or gets up earlier. Fortunately, Bill's doctor has given him a phone number that when called delivers personalized audio instructions for Bill so he can organize his medications once in the morning and be set for the day.

Mary was recently diagnosed with diabetes, and at her doctor's office she was shown how to calibrate and use a blood glucose meter. She was

This chapter is based on a presentation given at the conference on "Following Your Doctor's Instructions: Cognitive and Social Psychological Perspectives" in St. Petersburg, Florida (Fisk, Rogers, Sierra, & McLaughlin, 2002). We were supported in part by a grant from the National Institutes of Health (National Institute on Aging) Grant P50 AG11715 under the auspices of the Center for Applied Cognition: Health, Education and Technology (one of the Edward R. Roybal Centers for Research on Applied Gerontology). We thank Edmundo Sierra for his contributions to this research.

able to calibrate it in front of the nurse after some instruction but forgot many of the steps by the time she got home. The next day, when she had to calibrate the meter for a new set of test strips, she accessed the Internet to watch a videotape specially developed to lead her through the steps as well as to educate her about when to calibrate the machine. She is able to watch this video as many times as necessary to calibrate the meter until she is comfortable with the process.

Bob's and Mary's situations are examples of successful telehealth. *Telehealth* is a broad field that includes many types of instruction and aid, from videoconferences that connect doctor and patient at the same point in time to the training videos that often accompany home medical equipment. The field has been defined as "any technology using telecommunication technologies to deliver health services" (Whitten, 2001, p. 127). These examples provide an idea of the potential of telehealth; however, currently telehealth is nowhere near maximum efficiency. The intent of this chapter is to explore the potential of telehealth for the delivery of instruction and to offer guidelines for research and system design that will help to reach that potential.

THE POTENTIAL OF TELEHEALTH

Increasingly, doctors' instructions to their patients are being carried out through telehealth. It is anticipated that the burgeoning area of telehealth will improve the health care of rural communities and other groups that have historically missed out on cutting-edge technology. The federal government currently funds an initiative called the E-Government Directive, which seeks to increase the role of technology in the lives of Americans. Secretary of Agriculture Jill Long Thompson (1999) stated,

> As a result of the E-Government Directive, the Federal government will be making even more benefits and services available over the internet. Classrooms are being connected to the world, and *advanced medical technology is reaching some of the most remote clinics* [italics added]. (¶2)

Effective telehealth can allow groups of people who previously had little or no access to new medical discoveries to be treated or to treat themselves. With the support of the government, hospitals and doctors may realize the potential of telehealth and implement it on a large scale.

Teaching patients to treat themselves is an ambitious task, because 5.5% (roughly 1.94 million) of all hospital admissions result from medication noncompliance (Kohn, Corrigan, & Donaldson, 1999), and it is doubtful that an increase in technology alone will solve this problem. If implemented poorly, technology may even increase patient errors. As recently as 1993, outpatients were 6.5 times more likely to die from medication mistakes than inpatients (Phillips, Christenfeld, & Glynn, 1998). This indicates that not only is technology important for people and patients not directly under a doctor's care, but it is extremely important that the patients understand what they need to do to take care of their own health even if they have already seen a doctor directly. Medication mistakes do not occur because patients do not want to follow their doctor's instructions; it is more likely that training or instructional materials do not provide sufficient support. The need to support health care delivery through human factors interventions was alluded to in the *New England Journal of Medicine*: "Many of these errors are probably due to man's limitations as a data processor rather than to correctable human deficiencies" (McDonald, 1976, p. 1351). The problems do not lie with the motivation of the patient as much as with the limitations of human abilities, the lack of user-centered system design, and the inadequacy of instructions and training.

One advantage of telehealth is that it can provide support to human "data processing." For example, training or instruction can occur on the patient's schedule, whenever the home health product is used, rather than only during normal operating hours for offices and hospitals. Potentially, use of audiotapes, videotapes, animations, and written instructions can augment or take the place of training by doctors or nurses. Such training is referred to as *asynchronous training* because the patient and the instructor are not in the same place or the same time. Also, asynchronous training can be designed to allow the person to repeat the training at will, which can prevent errors due to forgetfulness and can strengthen the associations within the human data processor. An additional benefit of asynchronous training is that it can be individually tailored to the patient, making the training materials more effective than generic materials (see chap 10., this volume).

Another issue in home health care, particularly for older adults, is a feeling of intimidation. Medical equipment is often complex to set up and to operate. As the responsibility of its maintenance and operation falls on the patient, so do the anxiety and emotional stress (Bogner, 1999). The following excerpt is taken from a statement by a 45-year-old woman who was the primary caretaker for her husband, who had to rely on a machine to deliver infusions more than 8 hours per day:

> Obtaining and using home medical equipment carries a great deal of emotional stress, and that affects how we learn about the equipment and how we use and maintain it. Before Leonard was discharged from the hospital, we had a training session. I tried to listen carefully, but it was overwhelming—so many procedures to remember, so much terminology . . . when I got home, I realized I hadn't absorbed half of what

I'd been told. . . . Twice we have gone to the hospital emergency room only to discover that we could have taken care of the problem at home. But we're not doctors or nurses, and we can't always tell whether a problem is urgent. (Smith, Mintz, & Caplan, 1996, p. 6)

This situation consisted of two adults, both of them middle-aged. They felt unable to use the medical device once at home despite in-person training at the hospital and the traditional instructions that accompanied the devices. This example illustrates the difficulties designers encounter when developing training programs; simply providing information is not sufficient. Effective training programs must be tailored to the needs and capabilities of the learner. Moreover, instructions and training materials must be designed to ensure that learning is maintained across time (i.e., that training provided in the hospital will be remembered later in the home). The challenge of developing effective training programs may be exacerbated when the training will be administered asynchronously, where the patient and the instructor are separated in time and space. Further, age-related differences in cognitive and perceptual abilities influence the success of training programs and must be considered during the design process (Rogers, Campbell, & Pak, 2001).

The importance of designing instructions that are tailored to the user group and the task demands is evident in the following example of training younger and older adults to use a glucometer. The effectiveness of the company-designed instructional video can be compared with a video designed by psychologists based on fundamental training principles. Rogers, Mykityshyn, Campbell, and Fisk (2001) assessed the usability of the glucometer following exposure to the manufacturer's video. Younger adults' performance accuracy was approximately 70%, whereas older adults' accuracy was only 25%. In comparison, Mykityshyn, Fisk, and Rogers (2002) found that using a video developed according to known cognitive training principles resulted in both younger and older adults performing the glucometer calibration correctly over 90% of the time. The well-designed training video led to more than 260% improvement in accuracy for the older adults, enabling them to perform at the same level as the younger adults. This example illustrates the potential efficacy of telehealth when its delivery is coupled with design based on principles derived from human factors research.

DEVELOPING TELEHEALTH TRAINING SYSTEMS

How can telehealth training systems be developed to maximally benefit patients and capitalize on the potential of technology? Developing a properly designed training system requires effort (Rogers, Mykityshyn, et al., 2001); developing training to be delivered via telehealth may add to the complexity of the process. One primary issue to be addressed is the medium of delivery, that is, whether the training should be presented via video, audio, text, or some combination of these media. It is important that the medium chosen for the instruction match the demands of the task. For example, an audiotape of how to put together a wheelchair may not match the demands of that task; instructions delivered via an audiotape may not be a good support for an assembly task because of the spatial nature of the task.

Selecting the appropriate medium is not a trivial task. Contrary to intuition, video does not always result in the best performance. Table 11.1 contains a summary of studies that have compared different types of instructional media. This summary shows that there have been mixed findings as to whether video is a better medium for instruction than audio. Some have found audio to be superior, others have found video to produce better performance, some have found that added text enhanced performance, and others have found no differences between media. These findings raise the question of why studies have found such mixed results.

We believe that the success of a particular medium depends on the match between the specific demands of the task and the characteristics of the medium. Tasks may be simple, complex, spatial, sequential, decision making, procedural, memory, discrete, continuous, novel, and so on. Certain media may be better suited to the demands of particular task types. Although many studies have investigated types of media for instruction (see Table 11.1), these studies did not classify the nature of the task to be performed or relate the task demands to the medium. The solution may be to explore what task demands match which media, so that predictions of performance with a medium can be made a priori.

SELECTING THE APPROPRIATE INSTRUCTIONAL MEDIUM FOR A TASK

The selection of an instructional medium depends on understanding the demands of the task, the characteristics of the medium, and the overlap between the two. The first step in matching task demands to instructional media is to perform a task analysis to specify the task demands of the task to be learned. The second step is to conduct a medium analysis to understand the benefits and drawbacks of particular media. The third step is to maximize the match between the demands of the task and the benefits of the medium.

Conducting a Task Analysis

A task analysis is a "science-based and purpose-oriented method or procedure to determine what kind of elements the respective task is composed of, [and] how these elements are arranged and structured" (Luczak,

TABLE 11.1

Previous Research Comparing Instructional and Presentation Media

Author	Media studied	Task	Question	Results	Finding
Anderson et al. (1996)	Audio Audio + video	Travel collaboration	Does video improve audio communication with regard to performance or the ability to solve problems?	No significant differences between audio and video conditions for task performance or the ability to solve problems.	No differences
Boyle, Anderson, and Newlands (1994)	Audio Audio + video	Cooperative problem-solving task	What are the effects of visibility on dialogue performance?	Video can help to disambiguate difficult-to-understand audio.	Video better
Doherty-Sneddon et al. (1997)	Audio Audio + video	Follow directions to draw a path on a map	Does video improve audio-only instruction?	No significant differences in task accuracy or speed were found between audio and video conditions.	No differences
Krauss and Bricker (1967)	Audio Audio + video	Verbal communication	What are the effects of transmission delays on the efficiency of verbal communication?	Words were understood better when the speaker could be seen.	Video better
Meline (1976)	Text Audio Video	Creative problem solving	Which media presentation is better for 6th and 7th grader problem solving?	Audio was better than video. Text was not different from audio or video.	Audio better
Raphael and Wagner (1974)	Text Audio Video	Identification assembly (wires on pegboard) deductive reasoning	Are there any differences among media?	No differences for training using any of the three media for identification or deductive reasoning. Benefit of video for assembly.	No differences

Study	Formats	Task	Question	Result
Toth (1998)	Text Video Text + video + audio Text + video + audio + strategy	Assembly (wooden puzzle)	Which presentation method results in better performance after instruction?	Participants who received the text, video, and audio combination of instructions performed better than other groups.	Combination better
Veinott, Olson, Olson, and Fu (1999)	Audio Audio + video	Reconciling two slightly different maps	Can people who do not speak the language proficiently use video to support a moderately ambiguous task?	The task is performed significantly better with video.	Video better
Hale (1999)	Audio Audio + video	Watching a tennis video, then answering questions	Do people perform better on multiple-choice questions for video or audio information?	Participants performed better when asked questions concerning audio messages.	Audio better

TABLE 11.2
Advantages, Disadvantages, and Task Matches for Instructional Media

Medium	Advantages	Disadvantages	Task matches
Audio	Practical Flexible Cheap Allows task to be practiced while listening Easily stopped Easily restarted No visual display needed	Poor quality produces even worse performance Increases perceived mental workload Difficult to fast-forward or reverse to a specific point Must be at a minimal level to be audible	Some problem-solving tasks Word recall
Video	Decreased quality does not affect performance Produces similar mental workload with both easy and difficult tasks Supports spatial task demands	Expensive to produce Requires visual channel Requires video equipment	Complex tasks Spatial tasks Sequential tasks Assembly tasks
Text	Easily navigated, allowing reviewing or skipping ahead Easily produced and reproduced	May not convey conditional requirements adequately Requires reading ability Requires minimum lighting May not be appropriate for a range of reading abilities	Lengthy tasks that require rereferencing of instruction

1997, p. 341). For an example of a task analysis, see Rogers, Mykityshyn, et al. (2001). Their analysis of a glucometer specified each step to be performed by the user along with potential errors at that step and the cognitive demands imposed on the user. These components should be included in every task analysis (for instruction in task analysis, see Luczak, 1997). After a task analysis has been performed, it will then be possible to categorize the task according to its specific physical (e.g., button presses, component manipulation) and psychological demands (e.g., spatial, verbal, memory).

Conducting a Medium Analysis

Describing the characteristics of a medium is similar to describing the characteristics of a task through a task analysis. The goal is to discover the costs and benefits of a medium through an outline of the demands and allowances of that medium. Table 11.2 provides a summary of various media and their demands and allowances. For example, an analysis of an audio medium such as an instructional cassette tape would suggest that the following criteria be met: (a) The tape must be audible, (b) the listener must possess a minimum level of hearing ability, (c) the audibility must be increased if the tape includes spoken words in addition to alarms, and (d) there must be speakers available to deliver the audio message.

The next step is to outline the allowances of the medium. Using audio as an example again, audio allows performance of a task while listening to the instructions. Audio may be easily stopped and restarted, although it may not be easy to fast-forward or reverse to a specific point. Audio allows information to be presented without a visual display, although one may be used to aid in moving forward or backward in the audio medium.

Matching Tasks to Media

Once a task analysis has been performed and the medium analysis has been conducted for the media available, then the demands of the task should be matched with the demands and allowances of the media. The goal is to find as much overlap as possible between the task demands and the benefits of a medium. For example, a task that requires constant attention and hand motion once the task has begun would overlap best with audio instruction, because the task may be performed while the audio instructions are played, and there is no need to change visual focus from the task to the instructional medium. Finding a medium whose strengths accommodate the demands of the instructional task completely is unlikely. Most task demands and media benefits will overlap only to a certain degree; then it is necessary to decide (a) which has the most overlap, (b) which has overlap for the most crucial task demands, and (c) whether any of the media have drawbacks or costs that supersede the overlapping benefits they have for the instruction. For example, although audio instructions may be best for a particular task, if the task is performed in a noisy environment, the ambient noise may not allow the user to hear the instructions, in which case a visual display may be better.

RESEARCH EXAMPLES

To illustrate the benefit of matching task demands to medium characteristics, we discuss briefly several research studies from our laboratory. In the first such study, on training older and younger adults to load a medication organizer, we examined the benefits of audio versus video instructions for that task (Campbell, Rogers, & Fisk, 2000).

Loading a medication organizer is a common task that patients perform at home without the assistance of a nurse or doctor. Most older adults take medications, and it is up to the patient to remember when to take them and what to take. It has been reported that 75% of older adults use prescription drugs (Kart, Dunkle, & Lockery, 1994), and there is evidence that a considerable number of older adults are not taking their medications properly. Kart et al. (1994) found that 15% of all individuals over the age of 70 who were admitted to hospitals for acute care were there because of adverse drug reactions. Older adults have difficulty loading over-the-counter medication organizers correctly (Park, Morrell, Frieske, Blackburn, & Birchmore, 1991), which may account for a number of adverse drug reactions.

A typical medication organizer is a plastic case divided into compartments, with each compartment labeled with a day of the week or hour of the day. The idea of the organizer is to reduce prospective memory demands when taking medications. If the organizer is used properly, the patient can easily tell whether a certain medication was already taken or still needs to be taken in a day (for a more detailed discussion of prospective memory issues in medication adherence, see chap. 3, this volume). Once the medications are properly loaded in the organizer, the patient will benefit from the memory support provided by the organizer, as demonstrated by Park, Morrell, Frieske, and Kincaid (1992). However, loading the organizer correctly can be difficult for the patient, who must coordinate the schedules of each medicine along with differences in medication-specific requirements. Examples of conditional requirements would be medications that must be taken with food or without food, medications that require alcohol avoidance, medications that cannot be taken with other medications, and medications that must be taken at a certain time or not at all. A doctor may instruct a patient on his or her medication schedule and conditions, but once the patient is at home it is up to him or her to remember the doctor's orders. The only memory aids are the instructions on the side of the medicine bottle, which rarely include conditional requirements such as other medications to avoid.

A task analysis of loading an organizer would show that the task demands of loading a regimen into a medication organizer include long-term memory, working memory, and some spatial and motor skills for physically loading the pills into the organizer. These demands may even be slightly different among patients, depending on their prescribed regimen. Once the task analysis has been completed, an instructional medium may be chosen. Two ways to provide instructions for loading a medication organizer are via audiotape or videotape. Both of these methods allow the patients to learn to load their organizer at any time and provide personalized instructions, and they can provide meta-information to the patient, such as medications that should not be combined or other conditional requirements.

Campbell et al. (2000) focused on determining the optimal instructional medium for tasks that place demands on long-term and working memory, using the medication-loading task as an example. Using the research design method of testing different media with task demands, we compared video instruction with audio instruction wherein the audio and video instructions contained the same information. Because loading a medication organizer is a task defined by substantial memory demands, a prediction could be made that there would be no difference between audio and video instruction for this task.

The measures for the study were the speed at which participants loaded the organizer, the accuracy with which they loaded it, the subjective mental workload (self-rated) they experienced, and their performance on a test of their memory for the medication schedules at the end of the study. As predicted, there were no differences between the audio and video groups on any of the measures. Therefore, it seems true that video adds little support for the performance of memorization tasks. There is nothing magical about the medium of video that makes it superior to audio instruction.

Studies by Campbell et al. (2000) and others (see Table 11.1) have demonstrated that video does not show a benefit for all types of tasks. When does video support performance? In a another study (McLaughlin, Rogers, & Fisk, 2002), we assessed the benefits of video, if any, for the calibration of a glucometer. A task analysis of glucometer calibration showed that the task was complex, with sequential and spatial components with some memory demands (Rogers, Mykityshyn, et al., 2001). We hypothesized that the complex, sequential, and spatial nature of the task would be better trained through video than audio. These demands capitalized on the benefits video provides in that the task as a whole can be shown, including advance organizers (such as an outline or list of concepts). The steps of the task may be shown in order and the components of the glucometer illustrated rather than described.

As predicted, participants in our study (McLaughlin et al., 2002) showed better performance after viewing a video of glucometer calibration than after listening to the same information via audio; these findings illustrate the importance of matching the instructional medium to the task demands. Video supported the demands placed on the user because it was a better match for the task, whereas audio was a poorer match and hence provided less effective support.

However, even participants in the video condition did not perform the task perfectly. Thus although the video was the better match for these task demands, the training system was not optimal. Calibration of a glucometer is a complex task, and there may have been other demands that were not supported by the video, such as remembering the code on the meter after it disappears from the screen and then comparing that number held

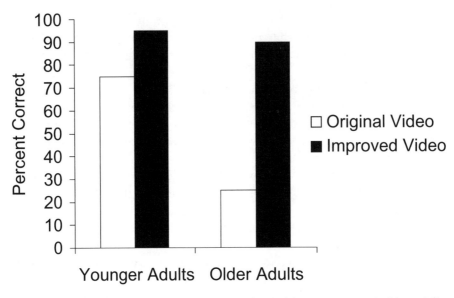

Figure 11.1. Percentage of correct steps performed by younger and older adults receiving instruction on how to calibrate a glucometer either with the company-provided video (original video) or a video based on psychological training principles (improved video). Data from Rogers, Mykityshyn, et al. (2001) and Mykityshyn et al. (2002).

in memory with the number on the side of the test strip bottle. There are two possibilities: (a) Video is the best match of all media types, even if it does not produce perfect performance, or (b) video may support most of the task demands for glucometer calibration, but the best instruction may require a combination of different types of media to fill in any gaps left by the video. Hybrid instructions also would be acceptable; however, it then becomes important to make sure the instructions themselves are not increasing the demands placed on the user. For example, trying to read additional information while watching a video would likely result in poorer performance, not improved performance.

TASK AND MEDIA DEMAND INTERACTIONS

Figure 11.1 illustrates how poor instruction can harm performance. Because instructions typically vary in quality, it is important to know how instruction quality might interact with the medium of instruction, in this case video, to influence task performance in younger and older adults. When instruction quality is high (in the improved video condition), the type of medium may not have a large effect on performance in either younger or older adults; however, when instructional supports are poor, the effect of the optimal medium may be magnified in older adults.

Sierra, Fisk, and Rogers (2002) assessed the benefits of video for different levels of instruction quality and task difficulty. The hypothesis was that video might support performance far better than audio when the instructional quality was poor and the task was complex. We investigated whether the support of video for the task demands remained strong as the quality of instruction declined.

For this study, the task itself was changed, but the type of task demands remained the same: complex, sequential, and spatial. This was to further support that the demands of the task drive the effect, not the task itself. The task was an assembly task wherein participants assembled figures from step-by-step instructions. The design of the study was Medium (audio vs. video) × Instruction Quality (simple vs. complex) × Task Difficulty (easy vs. difficult). Participants received either audio or video instructions. Within the audio and video instructional group, participants received either simple or complex instructions and built either easy or difficult objects.

There was an interaction between complexity of instructions and the instructional medium when subjective mental workload was measured. When instructions were simple, there was little difference in the subjective mental workload between the mode of presentation and younger and older adults. However, when the instructions were complex, participants in the audio condition experienced a high degree of mental workload, whereas participants in the video condition did not report changes in mental workload. Thus, participants perceived their mental workload to be higher when given complex audio instructions than when given complex video instructions. Therefore, if the task analysis mandates complex instructions, such instructions will be easier to follow if presented via video for a sequential and spatial task.

Subjective mental workload was not the only variable affected by instructional medium. There was also an interaction between presentation medium and difficulty for the accuracy of assembly. As difficulty increased, accuracy for the participants in the audio condition decreased significantly, whereas performance stayed nearly constant for the participants in the video condition. When learning conditions were less than optimal (as with complex instructions for a difficult task), having audio instructions was particularly detrimental to accuracy. This is further support for video instruction being used for a complex, sequential, spatial task, especially for difficult tasks. It is up to the practitioner to use this information when choosing an instructional medium.

Advice for Practitioners

Knowing the demands of the task for which instructions are being developed is the first step in matching instructional media to task demands.

The decision to use audio, video, animation, or written documentation should not be made arbitrarily but only after careful consideration. Conducting a task analysis will allow an examination of the cognitive demands each task places on the user and will result in instructions that are easier to use for the patient. Considering the advantages and disadvantages of each medium and how they match the demands of the task will improve the final desired result. Table 11.2 shows the advantages and disadvantages of different media. Although the media in Table 11.2 are not the only avenues for instruction, they represent ones that are more commonly used. It is important for practitioners to perform a task analysis of what they expect their patients to do and then perform a comparison of the task demands with the benefits provided by different instructional media to determine the best match.

Advice for Researchers

Thus far, experiments that have predicted that a match between instruction and media can come from task analysis have shown that for complex, sequential, and spatial tasks, video is the preferred instructional method. However, there is no benefit of video for tasks that require retrieval from long-term memory or rehearsal in working memory (Campbell et al., 2000). Although there appears to be an unlimited number of tasks that can be presented to patients, these can be categorized into a finite number of groups according to the type of task they represent. The goal for researchers should be to define matches between task types and media types. This can be done through experiments such as those discussed herein: Define a priori the demands of the task and use them to make predictions. Then use the experimental results to fill in the medium and task type matches to enable practitioners in the future to choose the correct medium, or combinations of media, for their instructions. Thus far, the media of audio and video have received the most focus; however, all potential instructional media need to be explored.

CONCLUSION

For instructions to be designed and delivered appropriately, practitioners and researchers must work together to discover matches for task types and instructional methods. As more tasks are adapted for telemedicine, practitioners should use the tools provided by researchers to develop optimal instructions. Researchers need to continue their exploration of the costs and benefits of different media, enabling them to provide a finer grained outline of different media and combinations to practitioners. Both practitioners and researchers need to keep in mind that improvements in technology alone do not lead to improvements in telehealth. Because a new technology is available does not mean it is desirable. However, by matching task requirements to instructional medium characteristics, telehealth will move toward its potential.

REFERENCES

Anderson, A. H., Newlands, A., Mullin, J., Fleming, A., Doherty-Sneddon, G., & Van der Velden, J. (1996). Impact of videomediated communication on simulated service encounters. *Interacting With Computers, 8,* 193–206.

Bogner, M. S. (1999). "How do I work this thing?" Cognitive issues in home medical equipment use and maintenance. In D. C. Park, R. W. Morrell, & K. Shifren (Eds.), *Processing of medical information in aging patients: Cognitive and human factors perspectives* (pp. 223–232). Mahwah, NJ: Erlbaum.

Boyle, E. A., Anderson, A. H., & Newlands, A. (1994). The effects of visibility on dialogue and performance in a cooperative problem solving task. *Language and Speech, 37,* 1–20.

Campbell, R. H., Rogers, W. A., & Fisk, A. D. (2000). Providing environmental support through the use of a visual channel. In *Proceedings of the IEA2000/ HFES 2000 Congress* (Vol. 4, pp. 34–37). Santa Monica, CA: Human Factors and Ergonomics Society.

Doherty-Sneddon, G., Anderson, A. H., O'Malley, C., Langton, S., Garrod, S., & Bruce, V. (1997). Face-to-face and video mediated communication: A comparison of dialogue structure and task performance. *Journal of Experimental Psychology: Applied, 3,* 1–21.

Fisk, A. D., Rogers, W. A., Sierra, E., & McLaughlin, A. C. (2002, February). *Facilitating user's cognitive knowledge: Matching instructional media to task demands.* Paper presented at the conference, "Following Your Doctor's Instructions: Cognitive and Social Psychological Perspectives," sponsored by Center on Aging and Cognition: Health Education, and Training, St. Petersburg, FL.

Hale, J. J. (1999). The visual superiority effect: Retention of audio visual messages. *Dissertation Abstracts International: Section B. The Sciences and Engineering, 60,* 0849.

Kart, C. S., Dunkle, R. E., & Lockery, S. A. (1994). Self-health care. In B. R. Bonder & M. B. Wagner (Eds.), *Functional performance in older adults* (pp. 136–147). Philadelphia: Davis.

Kohn, L. T., Corrigan, J. M., & Donaldson, M. S. (Eds.). (1999). *To err is human.* Washington, DC: National Academy Press.

Krauss, R. M., & Bricker, P. D. (1967). Effects of transmission delay and access delay on the efficiency of verbal communication. *Journal of the Acoustical Society of America, 41,* 286–292.

Luczak, H. (1997). Task analysis. In G. Salvendy (Ed.), *Handbook of human factors and ergonomics* (2nd ed., pp. 340–416). New York: Wiley.

McDonald, C. J. (1976). Title protocol-based computer reminders, the quality of care, and the non-perfectibility of man. *New England Journal of Medicine, 295,* 1351–1355.

McLaughlin, A. C., Rogers, W. A., & Fisk, A. D. (2002, October). *Effects of training presentation mode on glucometer calibration.* Paper presented at the annual meeting of the Human Factors and Ergonomics Society/International Ergonomics Association, Baltimore, MD.

Meline, C. W. (1976). Does the medium matter? *Journal of Communication, 26,* 81–89.

Mykityshyn, A. L., Fisk, A. D., & Rogers, W. A. (2002). Learning to use a home medical device: Mediating age-related differences with training. *Human Factors, 44,* 354–364.

Park, D. C., Morrell, R. W., Frieske, D., Blackburn, A. B., & Birchmore D. (1991). Cognitive factors and the use of over-the-counter medication organizers by arthritis patients. *Human Factors, 33,* 57–67.

Park, D. C., Morrell, R. W., Frieske, D., & Kincaid, D. (1992). Medication adherence behaviors in older adults: Effects of external cognitive supports. *Psychology and Aging, 7,* 252–256.

Phillips, D. P., Christenfeld, N., & Glynn, L. M. (1998). Increase in US medication-error deaths between 1983 and 1993. *The Lancet, 351,* 643–644.

Raphael, M. A., & Wagner, E. E. (1974). Training via text, audio tape or TV makes a difference: or does it? *Training and Development Journal, 28,* 3–5.

Rogers, W. A., Campbell, R. H., & Pak, R. (2001). A systems approach for training older adults to use technology. In N. Charness, D. C. Park, & B. A. Sabel (Eds.), *Communication, technology, and aging: Opportunities and challenges for the future* (pp. 187–208). New York: Springer Publishing Company.

Rogers, W. A., Mykityshyn, A. L., Campbell, R. H., & Fisk, A. D. (2001). Analysis of a "simple" medical device. *Ergonomics and Design, 9,* 7–14.

Sierra, E. A., Jr., Fisk, A. D., & Rogers, W. A. (2002, October). Matching instructional media with instructional demands. In *Proceedings of the Human Factors and Ergonomics Society 47th Annual Meeting* (Vol. 4, pp. 2089–2093). Santa Monica, CA: Human Factors and Ergonomics Society.

Smith, C., Mintz, S., & Caplan, A. (1996). Caregivers. In R. L. Klatzky, N. Kober, & A. Mavor (Eds.), *Safe, comfortable, attractive, and easy to use: Improving the usability of home medical devices* (pp. 5–7). Washington, DC: National Academy Press.

Thompson, J. L. (1999). *E-commerce: Bringing new opportunity to rural America.* Retrieved December 1, 2002, from http://www.rurdev.usda.gov/rd/newsroom/1999/ecomm.htm

Toth, L. S. (1998). Comparison of video demonstration vs. written instruction in teaching a psychomotor task. *Dissertation Abstracts International: Section A. Humanities and Social Sciences, 58,* 4189.

Veinott, E. S., Olson, J. S., Olson, G. M., & Fu, X. (1999). Video helps remote work: Speakers who need to negotiate common ground benefit from seeing each other. In *Proceeding of the CHI 99 Conference on Human Factors in Computing Systems* (pp. 302–309). New York: ACM Press.

Whitten, P. (2001). The state of telecommunication technologies to enhance older adults' access to health services. In W. A. Rogers & A. D. Fisk (Eds.), *Human factors interventions for the health care of older adults* (pp. 121–146). Mahwah, NJ: Erlbaum.

12

USING TELECOMMUNICATION
TECHNOLOGIES TO DELIVER
HOME-BASED CARE TO SENIORS

PAMELA WHITTEN

It has been demonstrated that as people age, cognitive, perceptual, and motor abilities decline (Salthouse, 1991). Despite this fact, older adults make up a large number of technology users. For instance, a 2004 investigation by the Pew Internet & American Life Project indicated that approximately 22%, nearly one quarter, of Internet users are older adults. Of the older adults online, 66% had utilized the Internet for finding health-related information. Previous investigations with technology use, particularly computer use, have shown that older adults are fully capable of performing tasks with computers, particularly with the help of conscientious design of interfaces as well as adaptive technologies (Worden, Walker, Bharat, & Hudson, 1997). This has enormous implications for the potential success of telehome care equipment for older populations. In fact, many telehealth investigations have indicated that seniors were pleased with the care received through telehealth interventions as well as comfortable with the technology used, particularly as the intervention proceeded (Demiris, Speedie, & Finkelstein, 2001; Finkelstein et al., 2004; Lamothe, Fortin, Labbe, Gagnon, & Messikh, 2006).

Today is an exciting yet challenging time to be an aging American. The number of older adults in the United States is projected to grow dramatically over the next 50 years. Currently there are more than 35 million Americans over the age of 65, accounting for approximately 12% of the U.S. population. By 2030, it is estimated that this number will climb to more than 71 million (Administration on Aging, 2003). As the largest consumer segment in the health industry, the shifting age demographics in the United States point toward a need to analyze the impact of this shift on health care expenditures and resources.

Health care spending in the United States is projected to reach $4 trillion in 2015, up from an estimated more than $2 trillion in 2005, according to a report by the Centers for Medicare and Medicaid Services, Office of the Actuary (2006). The report stated that health spending is expected to grow at an average annual rate of 7.2% from 2005 to 2015. As a percentage of gross domestic product, health care spending is expected to reach 20% in 2015, up from a projected 16.2% in 2005.

As a result of the dramatically increasing hospital and nursing home costs for older adults, policy analysts are looking for alternatives to help patients remain at home rather than face admission into expensive institutions. Home health care services have emerged as one viable solution. Home health care is provided to individuals and families in their place of residence for the purpose of promoting, maintaining, or restoring health or for maximizing their level of independence while minimizing the effects of disability and illness, including terminal illness (National Center for Health Statistics, 2002).

The recent transition of the home health service infrastructure from a fee-for-service model to prospective payment–managed care and the mandate for outcomes assessment have paved the way for innovative home care models. *Telemedicine*, the use of telecommunication technologies to deliver health services, has garnered significant attention during recent years as a solution to address access and cost concerns. The present chapter examines the potential impact of telemedicine in the delivery of home health services to older adults. I begin by setting the stage with a general overview of the impact of home health care in the United States. Next, I present an overview of telemedicine and telehome health care, followed by lessons learned from telehome health care evaluation. I conclude with a discussion of future issues related to telehome health care.

HOME HEALTH CARE

In 2001, about 20,000 health care providers delivered home care to almost 8 million Americans requiring services because of acute illness, long-term health conditions, permanent disability, or terminal illness. Annual expenditures for home health care exceeded $41 billion in 2001 (National Association for Home Care and Hospice, 2001). Numerous studies have documented the economic and health efficiencies of home health care over hospital or nursing home care. For example, Hughes et al. (1992) found that a home care program for terminally ill veterans reduced hospital per capita costs by $971. In the 6-month study, patients receiving home care demonstrated 5.9 fewer hospital admission days than those in the control group. No differences were found in patient survival, activities of daily living, cognitive functioning, or morale. However, patient and caregiver satisfaction with care was significantly better among the patients receiving home care. The impact of intensive home care monitoring on the morbidity rates of elderly patients with congestive heart failure (CHF) was the focus of another study (Kornowski et al., 1995). The study found that with intensive home care surveillance, the total hospitalization rate dropped from 3.2 admissions per year to 1.2 admissions per year, and the length of stay decreased from 26 days per year to 6 days per year. Cardiovascular admissions declined from 2.9 admissions per year to 0.8 admissions per year, and length of stay decreased from 23 days per year to 4 days per year. This in-home program also resulted in significant functional status improvement in elderly patients with CHF (Kornowski et al., 1995).

Home care is a cost-effective service not only for individuals recuperating from a hospital stay but also for those who, because of a functional or cognitive disability, are unable to take care of themselves. In 2000, the average cost of hospital charges per day was $2,753, the average skilled nursing facility charges per day were $421, and the average home health charge per visit was $100 (National Association for Home Care and Hospice, 2001).

Yet, cost-effectiveness is not the only rationale for home care. Many health care providers argue that home care is a compassionate way to deliver health care. Home care reinforces and supplements the care provided by family members while simultaneously maintaining the recipient's dignity and independence. In addition, home care allows patients to play an active role in their own health. A variety of studies have documented enhanced overall quality of life for patients receiving home health care services. For example, in a study conducted at Duke University, researchers found that patients with heart disease receiving home visits after hospital discharge reported better quality of life than those who received no visits. The researchers believed that the perceived enhanced quality of life translates into better health outcomes for heart disease patients ("Heart Disease," 2003). The home health care patient is not the only beneficiary of improvements in quality of life. Family members serving as caregivers also demonstrate significant benefits when home health care services are delivered to their loved ones. Dufault (2003) found that family caregivers for patients receiving high-quality pain management services at home reported fewer sleep disturbances from the patient's pain, less overall personal financial strain, fewer upsetting symptoms, and fewer changes to personal plans due to the patient's illness.

Just as the savings, efficiencies, and enhanced quality of life resulting from home health services have been documented and accepted, the health industry has faced new challenges placing limitations on the delivery of home health services. The first of these challenges has resulted from policy changes that have forced home health care agencies to seek more efficient ways to deliver services. For example, the Medicare Home Health Prospective Payment plan resulted from the prospective payment system for Medicare home health mandated by the Health Care Financing Administration (HCFA; now known as the Centers for Medicare and Medicaid Services). The rationale for the move from the modified fee-for-service payment system to a prospective payment system was that by setting a national payment rate, providers would provide care more efficiently (Medicare Program; Prospective Payment System, 2000). In addition to mandated efforts to streamline efficiencies, the home health industry is also addressing constraints facing the general health care industry, namely, health care provider shortages. The combination of policy constraints and labor shortages is challenging the home health care industry. The Bureau of Labor Statistics estimated that 671,600 people were employed in home health care agencies in 1998. HCFA recorded 240,136 full-time equivalents employed in Medicare-certified agencies as of December 2000, a decline of 170,972 since December 1997. According to both the Bureau of Labor Statistics and HCFA, the largest numbers of employees were home care aides and registered nurses (National Association for Home Care and Hospice, 2001).

With the potential to provide high-quality, humane care in cost-effective ways, home health care is an important segment of health care for older adults, and with the aging U.S. population, its role will only increase. Yet home health agencies are challenged to provide more services with fewer resources. One potential solution for this challenge is the use of communication-mediated technologies to supplement the delivery of home health care.

Telemedicine is emerging as one viable alternative. Indeed, Wootton et al. (1998) conducted a content analysis of data from almost 1,000 episodes of patient home care that indicated approximately 45% of all home nursing visits could be delivered via telemedicine. The next section provides a brief definition and background of telemedicine, highlighting the field of telehome health care.

TELEMEDICINE AND TELEHOME HEALTH CARE

Telemedicine has been defined in a variety of ways, ranging from very specific to broader in scope. Park (1974) defined *telemedicine* very narrowly, with a focus on the technology, when he described it as the use of interactive or two-way television to provide health care. Others have described telemedicine in terms of diagnosing or treating a patient who is at a different location (Willemain & Mark, 1971). Bennet, Rappaport, and Skinner (1978) coined the term *telehealth*, which includes education, administration, and patient care. The Office for the Advancement of Telehealth (n.d.) has defined *telehealth* as "the use of electronic information and telecommunication technologies to support long-distance clinical care, patient and professional health-related education, public health and health administration" (¶4).

The use of telecommunication technologies for medical diagnosis, care, and education has traditionally involved the use of interactive video for synchronous delivery of care. *Interactive video* refers to real-time videoconferencing that occurs between two or more sites. The quality of the interactions depends on the equipment and transmission speeds used. A handful of specialty applications use asynchronous or store-and-forward solutions, including radiology, pathology, and dermatology. Store-and-forward connections permit audio clips, video clips, still images, or data to be held now and transmitted or received at a later date. The recipient is free to choose the actual time that he or she reviews the contents of the transmission.

Telemedicine techniques have developed over the past 4 decades. Wittson, Affleck, and Johnson (1961) in 1959 were the first to use telemedicine for medical purposes when they set up telepsychiatry consultations via microwave technology between the Nebraska Psychiatric Institute in Omaha and the state mental hospital 112 miles away. In the same year, Montreal, Quebec, Canada, was the site for Jutra's (1959) pioneering teleradiology work. The advent of teleradiology allowed for the asynchronous transmission of radiographic images to experts located at distant sites.

In the 1970s, there was a flurry of telemedicine activity as several major projects developed in North America and Australia, including the Space Technology Applied to Rural Papago Advanced Health Care project of the National Aeronautics and Space Administration in southern Arizona; a project at Logan Airport in Boston, Massachusetts; and programs in northern Canada (Dunn, Conrath, Action, & Bain, 1980). These initial projects provided valuable insight into technological constraints and acceptance issues that paved the way for future telemedicine endeavors such as telehome health care.

Although data are limited, early reviews and evaluations of these programs suggest the equipment was reasonably effective at transmitting the information needed for most clinical applications, and users were mostly satisfied (Conrath, Buckingham, Dunn, & Swanson, 1975; Dongier, Tempier, Lalinec-Michaud, & Meunier, 1986; Fuchs, 1974; Murphy & Bird, 1974). It is interesting that with the exception of one simple program at Memorial University Hospital of Newfoundland in Canada, no telemedicine programs survived past 1986. When external sources of funding were withdrawn, the programs simply folded.

The decades of the 1960s, 1970s, and 1980s exhibited a series of telemedicine pilot and demonstration projects, and the 1990s proved to be a period of rapid growth. In the early 1990s, new, fairly inexpensive, and commonly available digital technologies enabled video, audio, and other imaging information to be digitized and compressed. This facilitated the transmission of information over telephone lines with relatively narrow bandwidths instead of through more expensive satellites or relatively unavailable private cable or fiber-optic lines. In 1990, there were 4 active telemedicine programs. By 1997, there were almost 90 such programs, and by 1998, there were 200 documented telemedicine programs (Federal Telemedicine Update, 2002). Today, so many health systems use some form of telecommunication technology to deliver health services or education that it is no longer possible to quantify the number of telemedicine programs. The fact that the U.S. federal government spent close to $1 billion in 2001 on telemedicine research, grants, and other funding is strong evidence of telemedicine's growing proliferation. Major funding areas include research and development, infrastructure development, information management, and health care delivery.

One of the fastest growing segments of telemedicine has occurred in the home health care field. Telehome services are typically delivered in one of three ways: transmission of data only, transmission of video–audio only, and transmission of data and video–audio simultaneously.

The data-only modality (often called *telemonitoring*) requires patients to attach or place a medical device on their body to capture vital signs that are transmitted and typically stored in a database at the home health care agency. The video/audio-only modality uses some form of videophone technology. A real-time visit is conducted with the patient by a home health care provider such as a nurse. During the visit, the provider and patient are able to hear and see one another on the videophone. Usually no electronic record of the visit is maintained, but it is common for a visit note to be included within the patient's chart. Finally, the combination data and video–audio modality has garnered the most attention to date in telehome health care projects. In this modality, a real-time visit is conducted during which the patient and home health care provider can see and hear each other. At the same time, patient data are gathered through medical peripheral devices attached to the videophone unit (e.g., stethoscope, blood pressure monitor, glucometer, pulse oximeter). The data are typically transmitted to a nurse's base station, where they are stored in the patient's electronic chart. Rarely is an electronic version of the video portion of the visit captured. Table 12.1 provides project examples for each of the three modalities of telehome care. Whether based on the transmission of data only, video–audio only, or a combination of data and video–audio, hundreds of articles have been published regarding telehome health projects. The next section summarizes the lessons from these publications.

LESSONS FROM TELEHOME HEALTH EVALUATION

Most publications in this field have provided project descriptives or utilization activities. However, many publications have reported research rationales in line with two overarching theoretical approaches for understanding telehome health.

The first and most common theoretical underpinning can be linked to Rogers's (1995) classic work on the diffusion of innovations. Rogers's theory stipulates that the diffusion and rate of adoption for any innovation can be understood by studying its evolution through six steps, beginning with recognizing a need and concluding with understanding the consequences that result from the diffusion of a solution for this need. Rogers also stressed that *diffusion* is a communication phenomenon "in which participants create and share information with one another in order to reach a mutual understanding" (pp. 6–7).

Application of diffusion theory in the study of telehome health has been a fairly popular implicit and explicit approach. Frantz (2001) outlined how telehome care should be evaluated using Rogers's (1995) five attributes affecting the rate of innovation adoption:

- *Relative advantage:* the degree to which an innovation is perceived as being better than the current process. A common research theme for telehome health within this attribute is economic advantage or cost benefit.
- *Compatibility:* the degree to which the technology is compatible with professional and patient values and needs. A common research theme for telehome health within this attribute is satisfaction and perceptions.
- *Complexity:* the degree of complexity of operations. A common research theme for telehome health within this attribute revolves around specifications of the technology and ease of use.
- *Trialibility:* the concept of piloting the new technology before making a decision to fully integrate. Many publications in the

TABLE 12.1
Exemplar Telehome Health Projects by Modality

Citation	Project description
	Data only
Artinian, Washington, and Templin (2001)	The purpose of this pilot study was to determine whether people who participated in nurse-managed home telemonitoring (HT) plus usual care or those who participated in nurse-managed community-based monitoring (CBm) plus usual care would have greater improvement in blood pressure from baseline to 3 months' follow-up than would people who receive usual care only. Both the HT group and the CBm group had clinically and statistically significant ($p < .05$) drops in systolic and diastolic blood pressure at 3 months' follow-up, with participants in the HT group demonstrating the greatest improvement.
De Lusignan et al. (2000)	The researchers conducted a trial of a wireless device for continuous cardiopulmonary monitoring. The telehome health system recorded the heart rate and respiratory rate, blood pressure, electrocardiogram (ECG), and body temperature, and the results were transmitted automatically to a central monitoring station. The accuracy of the measurements was checked by a comparison system and also by conventional measurements performed by a nurse. The system was acceptable to patients and functioned satisfactorily in the home.
Yatim (1997)	Shahal, a for-profit company, put telemonitoring on a production basis, providing home cardiac and pulmonary care from central nursing stations, first in Israel and then in Singapore and Italy. Data-based services included the following: (a) a cardiac monitoring and emergency response system, with a transtelephone ECG device transmitting a full 12-lead ECG within 42 seconds; (b) a pulmonary monitoring system for asthmatics and chronic obstructive pulmonary disease sufferers, in which subscribers perform their own pulmonary tests from home by breathing into a handheld measurement device, with results transmitted via phone to the remote monitor center, analyzed, and stored in a database; and (c) a blood pressure monitoring system that uses the "TelePress" device, which automatically measures and transmits heart rate and blood pressure values to the remote monitoring center.
	Video–audio only
Whitten, Doolittle, Mackert, and Rush (2003)	Hospice of Michigan participated in a telehospice project designed to use telemedicine technology to enhance end-of-life care. In each participating rural and urban office, nurses accessed videophone technology that operated over regular analog phone lines. With this technology, hospice nurses were able to connect with and assess patients from their offices through videophones located in patients' homes.

(continued)

TABLE 12.1 *(Continued)*

Citation	Project description
	Video–audio only *(continued)*
Magnusson (1999)	Assisting Carers Using Telematics Interventions to Meet Older Persons' Needs (ACTION) was a 3-year European project aimed at improving the lives of the elderly and their carers. The project was particularly beneficial to carers who were unable to go out or who lived in remote areas. It also helped to give the elderly and carers a more active role in health care.
Whitten, Mair, and Collins (1997)	In a project developed to study provision of home care to elderly residents, nurses provided home health services from "telenursing cockpits" located in three separate sites in Kansas. A cable television–based interactive video system was used to transmit video pictures at 30 frames per second with 288 horizontal lines of resolution. Contrary to expectations, the technology was not an important issue for the participants. They did not express any particular worry or excitement about it. Nor did they describe difficulties in adapting to its use. Use of telemedicine technology did not appear to have any negative effects on communication.
	Video–audio and data
Johnston, Wheeler, Deuser, and Sousa (2000)	A home health department in the Sacramento, California, facility of a large health maintenance organization provided supplemental home health services via a video system that included peripheral medical equipment for assessing cardiopulmonary status. Services were provided for newly referred patients diagnosed as having congestive heart failure, chronic obstructive pulmonary disease, cerebral vascular accident, cancer, diabetes, anxiety, and need for wound care.
Yoo, Huh, Jeon, and Yun (1998)	Project administrators computerized patients' data and offered periodic health reminders to patients for health promotion by using a LifeTime Health Monitoring Program (LHMP). The project connected LHMP to the Internet by Common Gateway Interface as an electronic medical record, enabling reference to patients' medical records anywhere. The study also made possible video teleconsultation and constructed a multimedia database to provide health-related information to the patients.
Dansky, Palmer, Shea, and Bowles (2001)	This Pennsylvania-based telehome care project used personal computers and video equipment to transmit data and video over ordinary telephone lines and allowed home health care providers to monitor patients and provide care at a much lower cost than earlier technologies that required wider bandwidth telephone lines and more complex equipment.

(continued)

TABLE 12.1 *(Continued)*

Citation	Project description
	Video–audio and data *(continued)*
Finkelstein, Speedie, and Potthoff (2006)	In this investigation, two telehome care conditions (video–audio and video–audio plus data) were compared with a control group for patients with CHF, COPD, or chronic wound care. Data indicated that discharge to a higher level of care as well as average cost per visit was greater in the control condition than it was in the telehome care conditions using communication technologies (with the video–audio and data condition having the least percentage of patients discharged to a higher level and the video–audio condition having the lowest average cost per visit).
Paré, Sicotte, St.-Jules, and Gauthier (2006)	This investigation, comparing a video–audio and data telehome care condition to a control group receiving standard home health care, found that fewer home visits and hospitalizations were required in the condition utilizing the telehome care technologies than in the control group. In addition, telemonitoring over a 6-month time period yielded cost savings for patients. Finally, patients in the telehome care condition were accepting of the technologies.

telehome health care field address pilot studies and their outcomes.

- *Observability:* ability of the user to observe the outcomes of the technology's predicted results. Within this attribute, a host of researchers have evaluated clinical efficacy or outcomes.

A second theoretical underpinning of many telehome health care projects is related to the concept of social support. Because of policy and technological constraints, many telehome health care projects are based on the premise that the technology can be used to provide supplementary services in addition to traditional care for patients and their family members or informal caregivers. Numerous studies have documented that social support is linked to psychological and physical health outcomes (Cohen & Wills, 1985).

Two general models of social support have evolved from many years of research: the stress-buffer model and the direct effects model. In the stress-buffer model, social support protects individuals from the effects of stressful situations. However, the success of the buffering effect depends on the level of stress (Cohen & Wills, 1985). In the direct effects model of social support, a tangible outcome is identified from the provision of social support.

Telehome health research has answered a number of preliminary questions regarding this innovative service. In line with the theoretical approaches discussed here, a summary of research results is provided in the following sections.

Satisfaction and Perceptions

Patient satisfaction and perceptions of telehome health care are the most commonly evaluated aspects of this service. The vast majority of studies report extremely high patient satisfaction. For example, Meyer (2002) reported a 90% patient satisfaction rate with a telehome health care project launched through the Veterans Administration Home and Community Care Service Line in Georgia, Florida, and Puerto Rico. In an ongoing study of patient satisfaction with telehome health care services delivered in Michigan's Upper Peninsula, patients continue to provide extremely high means for various aspects of telehome health care services, including very strong agreement with the statements, "I found the telehealth equipment easy to use"; "I think telehealth is a good way to provide home health care for patients with heart/lung disease"; "It was easy to communicate with the other person during the telehome health consult"; and "Overall, I am satisfied with the telehome health service that I received" (Marquette General Health System, 2002, Tables 1 and 2).

A handful of studies have also sought to document provider perceptions of telehome health care. In a study of telehome hospice nurses' preperceptions, nurses were cautiously enthusiastic about the service but were also skeptical about the comparable quality with traditional visits (Whitten & Doolittle, 2002). However, additional research related to telehospice provider perceptions revealed that in many cases, the provider is predisposed to avoid the use of telehome health equipment and ultimately serves as a gatekeeper preventing patients from accessing this service (Whitten, Doolittle, Mackert, & Rush, 2003). Dansky and Bowles (2002) found that nurses' responses to telehome care varied but were positive overall. These researchers noted a significant learning curve among nurses and stated that nurses' comfort and ease with the technology will increase as it becomes more pervasive in the industry. In a telehome health care study conducted in Minnesota, Demiris, Speedie, and Finkelstein (2000) concluded that telehome health care providers felt that for the great majority of visits (92%), the televisit would not have been significantly better if performed in person.

Overall, researchers have concluded that patients are very satisfied with telehome health services. Many patients even have expressed frustration that the telehome health care system is not used more frequently (Whitten

& Doolittle, 2002). Studies also have demonstrated high levels of satisfaction by providers, though often with some initial reservation.

Technologies and Pilot Projects

To date, telehome health services have most often relied on technologies that transmit over regular analog phone lines, better known as POTS (plain old telephone system). However, some studies have toyed with alternative solutions for delivering data and video images to the home. In Nova Scotia, Canada, project managers have launched an Internet protocol–based home telehealth solution that uses high-speed broadband networks to provide high quality and secure remote monitoring and early intervention services to patients in their homes (Lowenstein & Scott, 2002).

Rigau et al. (2002) developed a portable forced oscillation device for respiratory home monitoring that has significant potential to monitor respiratory mechanics in ambulatory and home care applications. Another prototype that has demonstrated some interesting new features is the DIABNET system, developed to assist patients affected by diabetes mellitus in their home monitoring. This system is designed to manage asynchronous data acquisition and management tasks as well as synchronous communications (e.g., telephone or videoconferencing; Bellazzi, Montani, Riva, & Stefanelli, 2001).

Innovative pilot projects are being launched throughout the world for older adults. In one project, developers have created an Internet-based system for providing arm movement therapy for stroke victims. The system operates over the World Wide Web using client-side JAVA applets and can track user movement recovery over time and report it to a remote server computer. Data from home use by individuals with stroke have demonstrated the feasibility of using the system to direct a therapy program and track movement improvement (Reinkensmeyer, 2002). Wireless technologies are generating great enthusiasm in a wide array of interesting pilot applications, many of which are proposing wearable solutions. For example, Wolf (2000) advocated the use of a techno-savvy T-shirt to facilitate accurate and unobtrusive remote health monitoring for all patients, from the oldest to the youngest.

Researchers warn of a potential disadvantage of telehome services that should be considered in the design and implementation of projects. Specifically, there is concern about the possibility that an unauthorized source will be able to more easily steal private health information, or greater risk of a simple misunderstanding between patients and health care providers that could lead to breaches in privacy, particularly for data transmitted via the Internet (Kokdemir & Gorkey, 2002).

Clinical Outcomes

Although only limited clinical outcome trials have been conducted in the field of telehome health, a handful of publications show the potential of this type of care. For example, Levine et al. (2002) developed the MyCare-Team Web site to help people with diabetes to better manage their disease and provide them with access to their health care team in between clinic visits. A feasibility study of this site was conducted at Georgetown University in Washington, DC, with interesting results. Over a 6-month period, patients exhibited a statistically significant reduction in HbA1c (an indicator of glucose control). In a study conducted with 10 patients with CHF over 65 years of age, Chetney, Strickland, and Jordan (2002) concluded that tele-home health patients demonstrated a 31% decrease in hospital admissions and a 36% decrease in emergency room visits as well as a 52% improvement in quality-of-life scores. In the Kaiser Permanente telehome health project, researchers documented no difference in quality indicators (e.g., medication compliance, knowledge of disease, and ability for self-care) between the telemedicine group and the control group (Johnston, Wheeler, Deuser, & Sousa, 2000).

A number of current studies are using more rigorous standards to evaluate clinical outcomes for telehome health. For example, a project being conducted in Michigan's Upper Peninsula is using a randomly controlled trial study to compare chronic obstructive pulmonary disease and CHF telehome patients with a control group receiving no intervention (Whitten & Mickus, in press). In addition, the Centers for Medicare and Medicaid Services (2001) has funded 16 disease management and remote monitoring demonstration projects to evaluate the role of telemonitoring in reducing overall health care costs by targeting patients with chronic health problems (Chin, 2002). Results from such studies will play an important role over the next 5 to 10 years in determining appropriate uses for telehome care.

Social Support

Both patients and caregivers perceive enhanced support from home health care providers through telehome health. For example, patients from a telehome health project conducted by the Visiting Nurses Association in southern Massachusetts credited the telehome health equipment with increasing their sense of security because they felt more closely connected to staff (Cardoza & Glaskell, 2002). In their summary of videotelephony for telehome care, Arnaert and Delesie (2001) explained that this technology addresses several of the special needs and expectations of the elderly in relation to their autonomy, specifically the need to feel a sense of belonging that is often countered by their social isolation. These authors explained that videotelephony allows health care providers to offer health information and advice in a personal and interactive way that can be adapted to the older adult's capacities. Video telephony is also credited with offering an alternative means for dealing with personal matters, such as loss and death, worries, complaints, emotions, and loneliness.

In research looking at the delivery of telehome hospice services, Whitten and Doolittle (2002) shipped videophones to distant family members to serve as a stress buffer. Through this technology, family members and dying patients were able to establish a somewhat intimate form of communication resulting in enhanced social support for both patients and their loved ones. The equipment has also been used for direct support. In the same Michigan telehospice project mentioned earlier, Whitten and colleagues (Whitten, Doolittle, Mackert, & Rush, 2003) used telehealth technology to provide support so that a wife could provide end-of-life care to her husband. In this case, telehospice was put into a home of an actively dying patient, something that was not usually done because of the high levels of anxiety in the home at that time. The caregiver and social worker felt the telemedicine equipment would decrease the caregiver's and patient's level of anxiety. During the patient's last night, the wife called the extended coverage staff stating that her husband was having a hard time breathing and was very congested. A nursing visit was offered but the wife declined, wanting to be alone with her husband but still needing the support. The nurse encouraged her to get on the telehospice unit with her so the nurse could see what was going on and provide support and encouragement to the wife throughout her husband's final night.

Cost-Effectiveness

Numerous telehome health projects make claims regarding the cost benefits of using telemedicine for home care. In their Pennsylvania-based telehome health study, Dansky and Bowles (2002) compared the costs of telehome care intervention with traditional skilled nursing visits. Their analysis of costs showed that telehome care does add additional costs to a home health agency but that these costs may be offset by the potential for fewer home visits. In a study evaluating the cost-effectiveness of telemedicine for home-based hospice services, Doolittle (2000) concluded that for two studied time periods, the average costs per visit for traditional hospice services were $126 and $141, respectively, compared with an average cost of $29 for a telehospice visit. A telehome health study conducted by Kaiser Permanente in northern California also documented the potential for long-term cost savings for telemedicine interventions. In this study, researchers documented that even though the average cost was $1,830 for the telemedicine group and $1,167 for the traditional group, the total mean costs of care for patients (excluding home health care costs) were $1,948 in the telemedicine group and $2,674 for the traditional group (Johnston et al., 2000). Other studies have documented peripheral cost savings to health organizations provided by telehome health. For example, Jerant, Rahman, and Nesbitt (2001) tested the use of telehome health care for patients discharged after hospitalization for CHF. This study concluded that the telemedicine recipients had fewer CHF-related emergency department visits.

Even though many studies have made positive claims regarding the cost-effectiveness of telehome health services, the reader is advised to approach many of these studies with caution. Whitten et al. (2002) published a telemedicine cost-effectiveness meta-analysis in the *British Medical Journal*. This article identified 612 articles specifically addressing costs associated with the telemedicine intervention through an extensive database search. This analysis was not limited solely to telehome health publications but did include these in the overall analysis. Of these 612 articles, 557 did not include any type of cost data. Of the 557 articles that lacked cost data, only 2% made claims of negative economic outcomes. From the remaining 55 articles with cost data, only 24 included criteria qualifying them for a full systematic review. Most studies failed to make clear the perspective and boundaries used in the analysis and used inappropriate economic analytical techniques. In general, Whitten et al. found no uniformity of analysis, and the studies reviewed were plagued by poor design and inadequate technical quality.

In summary, evaluation data indicate that there is potential for significant cost savings with telehome health. However, these studies require close scrutiny. A number of studies looking at both patient and provider satisfaction indicate that both parties are willing to accept this alternative health delivery model, though providers with predisposed negative perceptions can prevent their patients from accessing telehome services. A wide range of new technological solutions and pilot studies continues to be demonstrated. Preliminary evidence of efficacy and positive health outcomes exist, but much more rigorous outcomes research is needed. Finally, the role of telehome health technologies to provide both a stress buffer and direct social support is an important potential contribution of this innovation. Each of these research areas will play an important and often recursive role in the ability of telehome health to positively affect patients' willingness and ability to follow the care plan and instructions provided by their physicians. Demonstrated clinical and cost outcomes will pave the way for more physicians to prescribe telehome health services. Patients will then be able to take advantage of the benefits of the technology to enjoy the results of their medical instructions. These benefits will arise from the immediate feedback offered by telehome health and the enhanced social support and quality of life. Yet, telehome health as an industry is in its infancy and has a long way to go before it is fully integrated into the continuum of home health care.

TOWARD A TELEHOME HEALTH CARE FUTURE

Telehome health care offers a wide range of potential advantages for both patients and health care providers. Increased accessibility is an important trait of this technology. This enhanced access includes linkages to services that previously would have required hospitalization or nursing home admissions. Patients can receive frequent televisits to monitor a wide range of health problems. In addition to preventing utilization of more costly health services, telehome health also increases home health patients' access to additional home health services, particularly for patients living in rural areas. Patients can receive multiple visits during the same day without requiring a nurse to drive to their home for each visit. Patients and family members can call the after hours or extended-coverage nurse on duty and prevent a problem by having an immediate consultation rather than waiting for the next business day. Health care providers can use the technology to check on patients whom they are worried about or offer more frequent social support services. Telehome care provides a consultation resource, a monitoring device, and a means to provide immediate feedback to anxious patients and their families (Jenkins & White, 2001). The potential to provide this increased access at lower costs is another significant advantage of telehome health care.

Perhaps the most important yet least stated advantage of telehome health care concerns the issue of allowing patients to remain at home. Even though this has important economic implications, it also has crucial quality-of-life implications. The longer patients can remain in familiar surroundings with the people and routines that make them happy, the better their final years of life will be. Telehome health will offer seniors more autonomy in decisions regarding their own lifestyle and health care. This is an important consideration for societies concerned with humane and ethical treatment of aging adults.

Even with these obvious advantages, a number of challenges must be overcome for this innovation to reach its full potential. Certainly legal and regulatory issues must be simplified and resolved. The current Medicare prospective payment system must become more reimbursement friendly in the coming years. The Health Insurance Portability and Accountability Act of 1996 guidelines must also be clarified if home health care agencies are to feel more comfortable with adopting new technologies (Center for Telehealth and eLaw, 2006; Center for Telemedicine Law, 2003; Goodwin, 2001; Jacobson & Selvin, 2000; Whitten & Mackert, 2005).

Organizational issues at the home health care agency level must also be addressed. Too many agencies have made the mistake of purchasing telehome health equipment and expecting immediate utilization. Shaul (2000) recommended that home health care agencies address a number of key issues in the development stage of telehome health, including the following:

- Determine the percentage of the agency caseload covered under managed care contracts or other types of insurance that allow for flexibility in deciding service delivery patterns that include telemedicine.
- Identify the types of patients who will benefit from telehome health care.
- Plan how telehome health care will be integrated within the agency's routine services and include providers who are clinically competent and well respected in the planning process.
- Choose equipment that can be used to deliver the predetermined services and is simple to install and operate.
- Plan nursing time to allow nurses to complete the telehome health visit, which is often shorter than a traditional visit, while still allowing them time to perform coordination and follow-up activities.
- Develop clear procedures and protocols and provide ample training and practice time for health providers and patients.

In addition to organizational considerations, home health care agencies need to consider equipment and human factors issues. For example, when implementing telehome health care, an agency should place the equipment in a room that is private, quiet, and secure. Security issues must be addressed. A computer base station, for example, must be password protected. The quality of the actual transmission should be considered. Lighting must be bright but not glaring to maximize video images. Equipment should be placed in the patient's home in a location that is conducive to easy telecommunication linkage yet also meets the needs of bed-bound patients. Although these might seem like obvious issues, too many home health care agencies consider them only as afterthoughts. One bad experience can be enough to dissuade a patient or health care provider from future use.

Health care providers interested in launching telehome health care need to consider initial startup costs, ongoing reimbursement and security requirements, organizational and delivery issues, and technical considerations. To obtain the necessary information, significant research questions still need to be addressed, including consistently rigorous economic evaluations from multiple perspectives. Does telehome health care save money for home health care agencies? Does it save funds for public and private payers? How about individuals? Do they have fewer out-of-pocket overall health expenses?

Health outcomes are another ripe area for research. Specific and quantifiable ways that access is improved via telehome health care should be documented. Data are needed that demonstrate whether health outcomes remain the same or actually improve via this technology. Studies are necessary that increase understanding with regard to which home health care services are enhanced by telehome health care and which should not be delivered in this fashion. What new and unique clinical and support services are available through the advent of telehome health care? What is the real impact on quality of life for both patients and caregivers?

Because health care is such a complex service industry, research needs to provide information regarding the delivery or organizational mechanisms of telehome health. Do telehome health care services need to be tailored to the age of the patient? Are unique forms of training, resources, or protocols required? Documentation is crucial with regard to maintaining the integrity of patient security and confidentiality when an intervening technology is used to deliver health care services.

Finally, researchers need to publish articles that will enhance understanding related to the societal impacts of telemedicine innovations. Do these technologies open new avenues for involvement of family and friends in patient care? Do these technologies possibly create an environment that encourages older adults to remain shut in their homes for all health services or, instead, do they open up new horizons for older adults by expanding the people and services they can access? By addressing this wide scope of questions ranging from economic and health outcomes to societal impacts, advocates for the elderly are better poised to influence legislation and policy that will ensure telehome health care's positive impact on older adults.

REFERENCES

Administration on Aging. (1999). *Table: Older population by age: 1900 to 2050.* Retrieved December 11, 2002, from http://www.aoa.gov/aoa/stats/AgePop 2050.html

Administration on Aging. (2003). *A statistical profile of older Americans aged 65+.* Retrieved August 13, 2006, from http://www.aoa.gov/press/fact/pdf/ss_stat_ profile.pdf

Arnaert, A., & Delesie, L. (2001). Telenursing for the elderly: The case for care via video-telephony. *Journal of Telemedicine and Telecare, 7,* 311–316.

Artinian, N. T., Washington, O. G. M., & Templin, T. N. (2001). Effects of home telemonitoring and community-based monitoring on blood pressure control in urban African Americans: A pilot study. *Heart and Lung, 30,* 191–199.

Bellazzi, R., Montani, S., Riva, A., & Stefanelli, M. (2001). Web-based telemedicine systems for home-care: Technical issues and experiences. *Computer Methods and Programs in Biomedicine, 64,* 175–187.

Bennet, A. M., Rappaport, W. H., & Skinner, E. L. (1978). *Telehealth handbook* (Publication No. PHS 79-3210). Washington, DC: U.S. Department of Health, Education and Welfare.

Cardoza, C. L., & Glaskell, S. M. (2002, September/October). Determining the value of home telemonitoring for CHF patients. *The Remington Report,* 16–20.

Center for Telehealth and eHealth Law. (2006). *Telehealth & emerging technologies.* Retrieved August 15, 2006, from http://www.ctel.org/Telehealth.html

Center for Telemedicine Law. (2003). *Telemedicine reimbursement report.* Retrieved August 15, 2006, from ftp://ftp.hrsa.gov/telehealth/licen.pdf

Centers for Medicare and Medicaid Services. (2006). *National health care expenditures projections: 2005–2015.* Retrieved August 13, 2006, from http://www.cms.hhs.gov/NationalHealthExpendData/downloads/proj2005.pdf

Centers for Medicare and Medicaid Services, Office of the Actuary. (2001). *National health expenditure projections 2001–2011.* Retrieved May 16, 2003, from http://cms.hhs.gov/statistics/nhe/

Chetney, R., Strickland, P., & Jordan, L. (2002). Telemedicine: Making a difference in home care CHF patients. *Telemedicine Journal and e-Health, 8,* 200.

Chin, T. (2002). *Remote control: The growth of home monitoring.* Chicago: American Medical Association. Retrieved November 19, 2002, from http://www.ama-assn.org/sci-pubs/amnews/pick_02/bisa1118.htm

Cohen, S., & Wills, T. A. (1985). Stress, social support, and the buffering hypothesis. *Psychological Bulletin, 98,* 310–357.

Conrath, D. W., Buckingham, P., Dunn, E. V., & Swanson, J. N. (1975). An experimental evaluation of alternative communication systems as used for medical diagnosis. *Behavioral Science, 20,* 296–305.

Dansky, K. H., & Bowles, K. H. (2002, April). Lessons learned from a telehome care project. *Caring,* 18–22.

Dansky, K. H., Palmer, L., Shea, D., & Bowles, K. H. (2001). Cost analysis of telehome care. *Telemedicine Journal and e-Health, 7,* 225–232.

De Lusignan, S., Althaus, A., Wells, S., Johnson, P., Vandenburg, M., & Robinson, J. (2000). A pilot study of radiotelemetry for continuous cardiopulmonary monitoring of patients at home. *Journal of Telemedicine and Telecare, 6*(Suppl. 1), 119–122.

Demiris, G., Speedie, S. M., & Finkelstein, S. (2000). A questionnaire for the assessment of patients' impressions of the risks and benefits of home telecare. *Journal of Telemedicine and Telecare, 6,* 278–284.

Demiris, G., Speedie, S. M., & Finkelstein, S. (2001). Change of patients' perceptions of telehomecare. *Telemedicine and e-Health, 7,* 241–248.

Dongier, M., Tempier, R., Lalinec-Michaud, M., & Meunier, D. (1986). Telepsychiatry: Psychiatry consultation through two-way television: A controlled study. *Canadian Journal of Psychiatry, 31*, 32–34.

Doolittle, G. (2000). A cost measurement study for a home-based telehospice service. *Journal of Telemedicine and Telecare, 6*(Suppl. 1), 193–195.

Dufault, M. (2003, January 6). Study helps agencies ease suffering. *Pain and Central Nervous System Week.* Available at http://www.newsrx.com/newsletters/Pain-and.-Central-Nervous-System-Week

Dunn, E., Conrath, D., Action H., & Bain, H. (1980). Telemedicine links patients in Sioux Lookout with doctors in Toronto. *Canadian Medical Association Journal, 22*, 484–487.

Federal Telemedicine Update. (2002) *Federal telemedicine update.* Retrieved October 30, 2002, from http://www.federaltelemedicine.com/

Finkelstein, S. M., Speedie, S. M., Demiris, G., Veen, M., Lundgren, J. M., & Pothoff, S. (2004). Telehomecare: Quality, perception, satisfaction. *Telemedicine and e-Health, 10*, 122–128.

Finkelstein, S. M., Speedie, S. M., & Potthoff, S. (2006). Home telehealth improves clinical outcomes at lower cost for home healthcare. *Telemedicine and e-Health, 12*, 128–136.

Frantz, A. K. (2001, September). Evaluating technology for success in home care. *Caring, 20*, 10–12.

Fuchs, M. (1974). Provider attitudes toward STARPAHC, a telemedicine project on the Papago Reservation. *Medical Care, 17*, 59–68.

Goodwin, K. (2001). *Payment, licensure are barriers to telemedicine.* Retrieved August 15, 2006, from http://www.ncsl.org/programs/health/barriers.htm

Heart disease: Home health care improves perceived quality of life for patients. (2003, April 20). *Heart Disease Weekly.* Available at http://www.newsrx.com/newsletters/Pain-and.-Central-Nervous-System-Week

Health Insurance and Portability Act of 1996, 29 U.S.C. § 11814 *et seq.* (1996).

Hughes, S. L., Cummings, J., Weaver, F., Manheim, L., Braun, B., & Conrad, K. (1992). A randomized trial of the cost effectiveness of VA hospital-based home care for the terminally ill. *Health Services Research, 6*, 801–817.

Jacobson, P. D., & Selvin, E. (2000). Licensing telemedicine: The need for a national system. *Telemedicine and eHealth, 6*, 429–439.

Jenkins, R. L., & White, P. (2001). Telehealth advancing nursing practice. *Nursing Outlook, 49*, 100–105.

Jerant, A. F., Rahman, A., & Nesbitt, T. S. (2001). Reducing the cost of frequent hospital admissions for congestive heart failure. *Medical Care, 39*, 1234–1245.

Johnston, B., Wheeler, L., Deuser, J., & Sousa, K. H. (2000). Outcomes of the Kaiser Permanente tele-home health research project. *Archives of Family Medicine Journal, 9*, 40–45.

Jutra, A. (1959). Teleroentgen diagnosis by means of videotape recording. *American Journal of Roentgenology, 82*, 1099–1102.

Kokdemir, P., & Gorkey, S. (2002). Are telemedicine/telehealth services ethical? *Sendrom, 14,* 86–92.

Kornowski, R., Zeeli, D., Averbuch, M., Finkelstein, A., Schwartz, D., Moshkovitz, M., et al. (1995). Intensive home-care surveillance prevents hospitalization and improves morbidity rates among elderly patients with severe congestive heart failure. *American Heart Journal, 129,* 762–766.

Lamothe, L., Fortin, J. P., Labbe, F., Gagnon, M. P., & Messikh, D. (2006). Impacts of telehomecare on patients, providers, and organizations. *Telemedicine and eHealth, 12,* 363–369.

Levine, B. A., Smith, K. E., Ming-Jye, T. H., Alaoui, A., Clement, S., & Mun, S. K. (2002). Results of MyCare Team Feasibility Study. *Telemedicine Journal and e-Health, 8,* 196.

Lowenstein, S., & Scott, R. (2002). The virtual homecare visit: Using broadband connectivity to support remote homecare delivery. *Telemedicine Journal and e-Health, 8,* 191.

Magnusson, L. (1999, October 20). Careers tap into the information superhighway: Use of videotelephony for elders and their carers. *Nursing Times, 95,* 48–50.

Marquette General Health System. (2002). *Results/evaluation telehealth network.* Retrieved December 11, 2002, from http://www.mgh.org/telehealth/resultseval.html

Medicare Program: Prospective Payment System for Home Health Agencies. (2000, July 3). 65 Fed. Reg. 41128–41214 (July 3, 2000).

Meyer, M. (2002). "Virtually Healthy" integrating technology and coordination: A two year success story. *Telemedicine Journal and e-Health, 8,* 218.

Murphy, L. H., & Bird, K. T. (1974). Telediagnosis: A new community health resource. *American Journal of Public Health, 64,* 113–119.

National Association for Home Care and Hospice. (2001). *2001 home care statistics.* Retrieved December 11, 2002, from http://www.nahc.org/Consumer/hcstats.html

National Center for Health Statistics. (2002). *National home and hospice care survey.* Retrieved December 11, 2002, from http://www.cdc.gov/nchs/about/major/nhhcsd/nhhcsdes.htm

Office for the Advancement of Telehealth. (n.d.) *Welcome.* Retrieved December 11, 2002, from http://telehealth.hrsa.gov/welcome.htm

Paré, G., Sicotte, C., St.-Jules, D., & Gauthier, R. (2006). Cost-minimization analysis of a telehomecare program for patients with chronic obstructive pulmonary disease. *Telemedicine and e-Health, 12,* 114–121.

Park, B. (1974). *An introduction to telemedicine: Interactive television for delivery of health services.* New York: New York University, Alternative Media Center.

Reinkensmeyer, D. J. (2002). JAVA therapy: Web-based movement rehabilitation after stroke. *Telemedicine Journal and e-Health, 8,* 216.

Rigau, J., Farre, R., Roca, J., Marco, S., Herms, A., & Navajas, D. (2002). A portable forced oscillation device for respiratory home monitoring. *European Respiratory Journal, 19,* 146–150.

Rogers, E. (1995). *Diffusion of innovations* (4th ed.). New York: Free Press.

Salthouse, T. A. (1991). *Theoretical perspectives on cognitive aging*. Hillsdale, NJ: Erlbaum.

Shaul, M. P. (2000). What you should know before embarking on telehome health: Lessons learned from a pilot study. *Home Healthcare Nurse, 18*, 470–475.

Skurnik, I., Yoon, C., Park, D. C., & Schwarz, N. (2005). How warnings about false claims become recommendations. *Journal of Consumer Research, 31*, 713–724.

Whitten, P., & Doolittle, G. C. (2002). Telehospice in Michigan and Kansas: Year two study results. *Telemedicine Journal and e-Health, 8*, 199–200.

Whitten, P., Doolittle, G. C., Mackert, M., & Rush, T. (2003). Telehospice: End-of-life care over the lines. *Nursing Management, 34*, 36–39.

Whitten, P., & Mackert, M. (2005). Addressing telehealth's foremost barrier: Provider as initial gatekeeper. *International Journal of Technology Assessment in Health Care, 21*, 517–521.

Whitten, P., Mair, F., & Collins, B. (1997). Home telenursing in Kansas: Patients' perceptions of uses and benefits. *Journal of Telemedicine and Telecare, 3*(Suppl. 1), 67–69.

Whitten, P., Mair., F., Haycox, A., May, C. R., Williams, T. L., & Hellmich, S. (2002). Systematic review of cost-effectiveness studies of telemedicine interventions: Economic benefits of new technology are assumed, rather than known. *British Medical Journal, 324*, 1434–1437.

Whitten, P., & Mickus, M. (in press). Telehome care for COPD/CHF patients: A measurement of outcomes and perceptions. *Journal of Telemedicine and Telecare*.

Willemain, T. R., & Mark, R. G. (1971). Models of health care systems. *Biomedical Science Instrument, 8*, 9–17.

Wittson, C. L., Affleck, D. C, & Johnson, V. (1961). Two-way television group therapy. *Mental Hospital, 12*, 2–23.

Wolf, J. (2000, December). Wearable wireless wonder: Remote monitoring transmits data for patient assessment in the field. *Health Management Technology, 21*, 30–31.

Wootton, R., Loane, M., Mair, F., Allen, A., Doolittle, G., Begley, M., et al. (1998). A joint US–UK study of home telenursing. *Journal of Telemedicine and Telecare, 4*(Suppl. 1), 83–85.

Worden, A., Walker, N., Bharat, K., & Hudson, S. (1997). Making computers easier for older adults to use: Area cursors and sticky icons. *Proceedings of the SIGCHI Conference on Human Factors in Computing Systems*. Available at http://acm.org/sigchi/chi97/proceedings/paper/nw.htm

Yatim, L. (1997, December). Israeli telenursing call center: Home cardiac telemonitoring: Revisiting Israel's Shahal. *Telemedicine Today, 5*, 26–27, 33.

Yoo, T., Huh, B. Y., Jeon, H., & Yun, Y. H. (1998). Home telecare system integrated with periodic health reminder and medical record and multimedia health information. *Medinfo '98: Proceedings of the Ninth World Congress on Medical Informatics, 9*, 265–268.

AUTHOR INDEX

Numbers in italics refer to listings in reference sections.

Engle, R. W., 62, 69, *74*
Erkinjuntti, T., *121*
Eslinger, P. J., 152, *163, 164*
Espley, A., 171, *196*
Estes, C. L., 124, *142*

Faes, S., 70, *75*, 185, *199*, 220, *232*
Farah, M. J., 62, *74*
Farinacci, S., 105, *116*
Farre, R., *289*
Farrell, D., 236, 238, *246*
Farrow, T. F. D., 152, *163*
Faulkner, A., 123, *142*
Federal Telemedicine Update, *288*
Feigelman, S., *199*
Fiedler, F. E., 149, *163*
Fiedler, K., 37, *44*
Figueredo, A., 72, *74*
Finkelstein, A., *289*
Finkelstein, S. M., 269, 278, 279, *287,*
        288
Finucane, M. L., 205, 207, *228, 231*
Fishbein, M., 24, 29, *44*, 169, 172, 174,
        175, 181, *192, 193*
Fisk, A. D., 97, 99, *117, 119, 120*, 251,
        254, 259, 261, 263, *265, 266*
Fiske, S. T., 149, *163*
Fitten, J., 214, *232*
Fleisher, L., *248*
Fleming, A., *265*
Flora, J., 236, *248*
Flynn, M. F., 172, *193*
Folkman, S., 125, 126, 132, *143*
Forsthoff, C. A., 133, *142*
Fortin, J. P., 269, *289*
Fox Chase Cancer Center, 237, *246*
Fozard, J. L., 94, *117*
Frankel, R., 111, 115, *120*
Frantz, A. K., 275, *288*
Freund, A. M., 137, *144*
Friedmann, E., 111, *117*
Fries, J. F., 104, *117*
Frieske, D. A., 8, 9, *20*, 95, 98, *117, 120,*
        153, *163, 164, 230*, 260, *266*
Fu, X., 257, *267*
Fuchs, M., 274, *288*
Fuhrmann, A., 190, *195*

Gafni, A., 245, *246*
Gagnon, M. P., 269, *289*

Gaines, C. L., 4, *21, 120, 164, 230*
Galajda, J., 111, *121*
Galbraith, J., *199*
Gallois, C., 179, *193*
Gandek, B., 110, *118*
Garrity, T. F., 148, *163*
Garrod, S., *265*
Gauthier, R., 278, *289*
Gigerenzer, G., 210, *228*
Gispen, W. H., 108, *116*
Glasgow, R. E., 171, *194*
Glasheen, C., 242, *247*
Glaskell, S. M., 281, *287*
Glass, J. M., 107, 108, *116, 117, 119*
Glasser, M., 113, *120*
Glassman, B., 237, *247*
Gleicher, F., 175, *199*
Glick, P., 149, *163*
Glynn, L. M., 253, *266*
Godin, G., 173, 176, *193*
Goff, L. M., 57, 58, *74*
Goldberg, L. R., 140, *142*
Goldstein, D., 11, *19*
Gollwitzer, P. M., 16, 18, 24–26, 29–41,
        43, 44–47, 70, 74, 182, 184–189,
        192–194, 199, 220, 228
Gonder-Frederick, L. A., 131, *142*
Goodwin, K., 285, *288*
Gordon-Salant, S., 94, *117*
Gorkey, S., 280, *289*
Gottschaldt, K., 31, *46*
Gould, O. N., 161, *163*
Graesser, A. C., 103, *117*
Greene, M. G., 109, 111, 113, *115, 117*
Greenfield, S., 110, 111, *118*
Gregory, S. S., 147, *164*
Greve, W., 130, *141*, 181, *194*
Griffiths, K., 108, *116*
Grisso, T., 202, *227*
Grol, R., *249*
Guinote, A., 182, *196*
Gutmann, M., 104, *119*, 133, *143*, 171,
        195
Guynn, M. J., 51, 52, *73*, 183, *194*

Hagenah, M., 27, 28, *46*
Hagger, M. S., 170, 171, 173, 175, 176,
        194, 196
Haire-Joshu, D., *247*
Halabi, S., *248*

SUBJECT INDEX

Internet, 12–13
    e-government via, 252
    health information available on, 226
    medical information on, 202
    older adults as users of, 269
Interruptions
    effects of, on prospective memory
        tasks, 60–69
    overcoming effects of, 69–71
Intimidation, 253–254
Intrusions, control of, 35–40
    with blocking adverse situational in-
        fluences, 38–40
    with blocking detrimental self-states,
        36–38
    with suppression, 35–36
Isolation, 282

Judgments, 203, 205

Labeling, 79–80
Learning (of health information), 93–115
    age differences in, 96–100
    and cognitive aging, 95–96
    and cognitive effects of medical
        conditions/treatments, 106–110
    and prior knowledge, 100–106
    and psychosocial issues, 110–113
    and sensory aging, 94
Lifestyle, 125
Life-threatening diseases
    and non-life-threatening with com-
        mon symptoms, 83–85
    vigilance-inducing, 87–88
List format, 14, 98
Logs, 59
Long-term memory, 95

Meaningfulness, 130
Media
    analysis of, 258–259
    instructional. *See* Instructional
        media
    mass, 12–13
Medical adherence, 3–18
    cognitive influences, 4
    comprehension/memory in, 6–14
    contextual influences, 4–5

    definition of, 3
    and diminished cognition, 5–6
    future directions for, 18
    and implementing medical instruc-
        tions, 14–17
    importance of, 123–124
    psychosocial influences, 4
Medical conditions, cognitive effects of,
    106–108
Medical decision, 202
Medical devices, learning to use, 99
Medical equipment, 253–254
Medical judgment, 202
Medical model, 80–81
Medical treatments, cognitive effects of,
    108–109
Medicare, 284
Medicare Home Health Prospective Pay-
    ment plan, 272
Medication Event Monitoring System
    (MEMS), 15
Medication labels, 7, 8
Medication mistakes, 253
Medication organizers
    as external aids, 59, 98
    learning to use, 259–261
    types of, 7–9
Medium analysis, 258–259
Memory
    and acquiring new information,
        10–11
    and dyad collaboration, 13
    of familiar false statements, 11–12
    media influences on, 13
    medication organizers to aid, 7–9
    picture-recognition, 7, 8
    of regime/instructions, 6–14
Memory decline, 10
MEMS (Medication Event Monitoring
    System), 15
Mental availability, 211
Mental contrasting, 25–29
    and efficiency in health service man-
        agers, 28
    health behavior changed by, 26–27
    patient–provider communication
        changed by, 27–28
Mental fatigue, 213
Metacognitive failures, 7
Microchips, 15
Modifiable diseases, 125

Primary appraisal, 132
Prior knowledge, 100–106
    inaccurate, 104–105
    and learning medical information,
        101–104
    and older adults as "medical ex-
        perts," 100–101
    and repeated warnings, 105–106
Privacy, 280
Problem solvers, 125
Prospective memory, 49–73, 206, 221
    definition of, 49
    and delays/interruptions, 60–71
    event- vs. time-based, 50–53
    habitual, 53–57
    and imagined actions, 57–60
Prospective memory tasks, 14–17
Prospective payment system, 272
Protection-motivation theory, 170–172
Provider perceptions, 279–280
Psychosocial influences, 4
Psychosocial issues, 110–113
    older patients' behaviors in medical
        encounters, 110–111
    physicians' behaviors toward older
        patients, 111–113
    third-person impact on medical en-
        counter, 113

Quality of life, 284

Reading ability, 207
Reading materials, 106, 112
Reasoned action, theory of, 172–173
Rebound, 41
Recall tasks, 95
Recency effect, 157, 158, 212
Recognition tasks, 50
Recollection, 96
Regularity axiom, 218
Rehearsal, 62–66, 220, 225–226
Relative advantage (of telehealth), 275
Relevance, 235–236
Repetition, 14, 105–106, 224
Repetition errors, 55–56
Representativeness, 213
Resistance to acquiring information,
    10–11
Restating illness beliefs, 104–105

Retrieval processes, 50
Rigidity, 40
Risk aversion, 81
Routinization, 15–16
Ruling-out strategy, 216–217

Safe 'n' Sound, 242
"Schema-copy plus tag" model of text
    comprehension, 103
Search behavior, 217
Secondary appraisal, 132
Self-assessment thoughts, 244
Self-complexity, 138
Self-concept differentiation, 138, 139
Self-control, 190
Self-efficacy thoughts, 244
Self-maintenance, 189
Self-regulation
    effective, 37–38
    of goal setting, 25–27
    and pursuit of complex goals,
        188–191
Self-report habit index (SRHI), 188
Self-representations
    age effects on, 137–138
    definition of, 127–128
    linking illness representations with,
        131–132
    in patient–doctor relationship,
        128–130
    physician assessment of patients',
        138–140
    role of, 134–136
Sensitive soma, 88
Sensory changes, age-related, 94
Sensory experiences, 60
7-day without times organizers, 8–9
7-day with times organizers, 8–10
Severity heuristic, 80
Severity of disease, 131
Silent but life-threatening diseases, 85–86
Similarity, 213–214
Skepticism, 208
Social loafing phenomenon, 39
Social self, 129
Social support, 281–282
Social support models, 278
Social vigilance, 208
Speed of processing, 152–155, 205
SRHI (self-report habit index), 188

ABOUT THE EDITORS

Denise C. Park, PhD, is professor of psychology at the University of Illinois at Urbana–Champaign, where she is codirector of the Center for Healthy Minds at the Beckman Institute. She is past chair of the Board of Scientific Affairs of the American Psychological Association and a former member of the American Psychological Society's board of directors. She has published extensively on cognitive aging and medical issues and has focused much of her recent work on the cognitive neuroscience of aging.

Linda L. Liu, PhD, focuses her research on aging and cognition, with a special emphasis on medical adherence and judgment and decision-making processes. She holds a PhD in cognitive psychology from Northwestern University, Evanston, Illinois, and a BS in biology and psychology from Duke University, Durham, North Carolina. She conducted postdoctoral work at the University of Michigan, Ann Arbor, and is now a research assistant professor in the Department of Psychology at Northwestern University.